# Childhood Brain & Spinal Cord Tumors

## A Guide for Families, Friends & Caregivers

Tania Shiminski-Maher
Patsy Cullen
Maria Sansalone

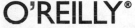

# O'REILLY®

Beijing • Cambridge • Farnham • Köln • Paris • Sebastopol • Taipei • Tokyo

*Childhood Brain & Spinal Cord Tumors: A Guide for Families, Friends & Caregivers*
by Tania Shiminski-Maher, Patsy Cullen, Maria Sansalone

Copyright © 2002 O'Reilly & Associates, Inc. All rights reserved.
Printed in the United States of America.

Published by O'Reilly & Associates, Inc., 1005 Gravenstein Hwy N., Sebastopol, CA 95472.

*Editor:* Nancy Keene

*Production Editor:* Tom Dorsaneo

*Cover Designer:* Kristen Throop

*Printing History: January 2002, First Edition*

Many of the designations used by manufacturers and sellers to distinguish their products are claimed as trademarks. Where those designations appear in this book, and O'Reilly & Associates, Inc. was aware of a trademark claim, the designations have been printed in caps or initial caps.

This book is meant to educate and should not be used as an alternative for professional medical care. Although we have exerted every effort to ensure that the information presented is accurate at the time of publication, there is no guarantee that this information will remain current over time. Appropriate medical professionals should be consulted before adopting any procedures or treatments discussed in this book.

**Library of Congress Cataloging-in-Publication Data:**

Shiminski-Maher, Tania,
    Childhood brain & spinal cord tumors: a guide for families, friends & caregivers /
Tania Shiminski-Maher, Patsy Cullen, Maria Sansalone
        p. cm.—(Patient-centered guides)
    Includes bibliographical references and index.
    ISBN 0-596-50009-2
    1. Brain—Tumors—Popular works. 2. Spinal cord—Tumors—Popular works. 3. Tumors in children—Popular works. I. Title: Childhood brain and spinal cord tumors. II. Cullen, Patsy, 1955– III. Sansalone, Maria, 1960– IV. Title. V. Series.

RC280.B7 S48 2001
618.92'99481--dc21                                                    2001052057

[M]

# Table of Contents

# Foreword

The diagnosis of a brain or spinal cord tumor in a child generates an extraordinary degree of pain, suffering, and turmoil in a family. The pain is compounded by the almost universal belief in the lay community that a brain or spinal cord tumor is invariably a lethal process with no hope of cure. Accordingly, it becomes virtually impossible for a family to respond to this news in an objective, sophisticated, and intellectual fashion. Instead, the family is thrust into an almost paralyzing torrent of emotion that makes it almost inconceivable for things to proceed in a calm and calculated fashion. Furthermore, a family that has never faced a child with cancer does not have the knowledge base that is required to address all of the different issues: how to cope with procedures and hospitalization, how to work in a positive fashion with the healthcare team, and how to deal with the intricacies of each of the different treatment options.

This book fills an extraordinary void for families in whom a child has been diagnosed with a brain or spinal cord tumor. Written in comprehensive and straightforward prose, it will give a family virtually everything they need to know in order to deal with this most frightening diagnosis. Although reading this book will not, of course, ensure a successful outcome for their child, it will provide a framework for them to understand all of the issues they are dealing with on the path from diagnosis to treatment and to either a successful outcome or the loss of their child.

A review of the table of contents in this book shows the remarkable breadth of information available to the reader. A family is introduced to the kind of tumor that their child might have and offered help with painful procedures that can prove frightening to child and family alike. They are taught how to work creatively with the healthcare team and, when necessary, make a change, and are introduced to the major modalities used to treat a child with a brain or spinal cord tumor. Additionally, equally critical issues that are rarely discussed with a family and poorly detailed in the literature include how to deal with school, how to find additional support for the family, how to deal with either the joy and fear of end of successful therapy or, for those children who relapse and die, how to deal with those issues and how the family can continue to survive.

This book is a gifted and welcome addition to the field of pediatric neuro-oncology. It will help countless families and healthcare providers alike learn all the ramifications of diagnosing a brain or spinal cord tumor in a child and the incredible turmoil that is subsequently produced in a family. This book should be on the shelf of every healthcare professional who deals with children with brain and spinal cord tumors and should be made available to every family in whom a tumor is diagnosed.

—Henry S. Friedman, MD
James B. Powell, Jr., Professor of Neuro-Oncology
The Brain Tumor Center at Duke
Durham, North Carolina

# Preface

*We are all in the same boat, in a stormy sea,*
*and we owe each other a terrible loyalty.*

—G.K. Chesterton

*Maria's story:* I'm a mom of a 6-year-old bundle of energy, who happens to have a low-grade astrocytoma.

Our family has two stories, actually. The first begins in 1970. Albert, my husband's brother, an honor student and just 15, was having increasingly intense bouts of headaches, dizziness, and problems with balance. His parents turned to their doctor, who chalked it up to growing pains. A year went by. The symptoms were no better, they were worsening, and no one was helping to point the family to better resources. Albert was spending more time at home, mostly in bed. The doctor eventually sent him for a brain scan, but nothing was found. Finally, they were referred to a neurosurgeon. He immediately performed surgery, searched for the tumor, but could only find and remove a small portion. They planned to do whole brain radiation, standard treatment at the time, but there wasn't an opportunity. Albert passed away shortly after surgery. The course pointed toward a malignant brain tumor possibly on or near the brainstem.

Our 2-year-old son was diagnosed in 1997 with a low-grade astrocytoma. Because of the location and the size of the tumor, we were referred to an experienced pediatric neurosurgeon at a children's hospital two hours from home. Surgery removed part of the tumor. We then had a period of observation, followed by a year-plus course of chemotherapy. It has been two years since we finished treatment, and we're happy to say that we still have no change in the residual. And, truly, I do mean "we." My family survives this diagnosis only through the combined efforts of medical specialists, family members and friends, our son's school team, and especially coworkers and employers.

My husband and I are very proud of our son, who is entering first grade, loves his school, and is doing well with academic modifications.

Thirty years have gone by between Albert's experience and ours. Many wonderful advances have been made. But there needs to be greater public awareness, more pediatric clinical trials for both high-grade and low-grade tumors, and a faster track to cure.

*Tania's story:* It seems logical that I would write this book for parents of children with brain and spinal cord tumors. Each phase of my life has evolved into choices or decisions that have guided the path to the next phase. I became a nurse because I chose at age 15 to live with my grandmother, a diabetic who needed a companion. Upon graduation from nursing school, the only position that I could get in pediatrics was on a pediatric oncology floor. After spending five years there and completing a nurse practitioner masters program, I became aware of how important it is for chronically ill children to have a healthcare provider who integrates normal childhood growth and development into their care. The only available position with this approach was in pediatric neuro-oncology, and from there I moved a few years later to pediatric neurosurgery.

I have spent most of my career working with children and families of children who have brain and spinal cord tumors. My job has been to translate the medical terminology into an understandable language, do innumerable blood pokes, listen to crying and screaming children and adults, laugh, cry, and hold hands. I have learned how parents long for information—any information—to read that will help them through this long and arduous road of life with a brain and spinal cord tumor. When I was approached to write this book, it seemed appropriate that I translate my everyday interactions into a resource for patients and families. After all, it was the next fork in the road.

*Patsy's story:* As a nursing student at the University of California Medical Center in San Francisco in the late 1960s, I determined very early that pediatrics was my area of interest and that pediatric oncology was my chosen area of practice. In those days, the survival rate for all children with cancer was very poor, with the vast majority of children dying within one year of diagnosis. After graduation, I worked for a number of years at the medical center on the pediatric unit and had the good fortune to work with Gail Perin, an advanced practice nurse in pediatric oncology. Gail generously shared her knowledge and expertise with me and was a role model in every sense of the word.

In 1974, I moved to Kansas City, Missouri, taught nursing at St. Luke's School of Nursing, and joined the staff at Children's Mercy Hospital. The oncology program at Children's was just starting in those days, but I let it be known early on that I was interested. Five years later, Dr. John Cullen returned from his pediatric oncology fellowship at M.D. Anderson to join Dr. Donald Forgue in the department. They decided they needed a nurse, and I interviewed for the job. I got the job and, as they say, "the rest is history." These two physicians mentored me from my first day in the department. I was encouraged and funded to attend Children's Cancer Group meetings, and I was able to reestablish my professional relationship with Gail Perin, the first chair of the Nursing Discipline Committee.

Dr. Denman Hammond, the Group Chair of CCG, agreed to assign a few nurses to select clinical trial protocol committees in the mid-1980s. I was one of the fortunate few and elected to become involved in the CNS tumor group. I was appointed to the high-grade glioma study, chaired by Dr. Jonathan Finlay, and the high-risk medulloblastoma study, chaired by Dr. Paul Zeltzer. Both of these physicians welcomed me to their committees, listened to my ideas, and gave me meaningful tasks to perform. Eventually, I was appointed to represent nursing on the CNS Tumor Strategy Group, a position I have held to this day.

Tania and I first met by phone in mid-1986. We agreed to get together at the fall CCG meeting that year and begin her involvement with the group. Unfortunately, my personal and professional train got "derailed" in October, 1986, when I discovered a breast lump, underwent surgery, and learned that I had breast cancer. I was 38 years old, and I was scared to death. Needless to say, I didn't attend the meeting that fall!

Tania called me after the meeting. She made me laugh by saying in an accusatory way: "I waited and you never showed up!" I liked her immediately. That started a professional and personal friendship that has continued to this day. For the next six months I was both a cancer patient and a cancer nurse. The support I received from patients, families, friends, and colleagues was a sustaining factor and a motivating force.

I moved to Denver, Colorado, in 1987 and continued my work as a pediatric oncology nurse practitioner, first at The Children's Hospital and then at Childhood Hematology-Oncology Associates and Presbyterian-St. Luke's Medical Center, where I am on staff today. I continued to work with CNS tumor patients as much as possible and worked closely for many years with Dr. Ed Arenson, a neuro-oncologist who now cares primarily for adults. John Cullen and I eventually married, and Tania and I worked closely on many projects related to the care of children with CNS tumors. We knew that someday we needed to write "the book." Eventually, Nancy Keene approached us about undertaking this project and we agreed to take up the challenge. It is my sincere hope that this book will provide a framework for patients and families embarking down this long, winding road of treatment and, hopefully, survival.

# Why we wrote this book

While living with and working with children with cancer, we amassed not only a library of medical information, but scores of first-person accounts of how individual parents coped. It saddened us to think that most parents of children with brain and spinal cord tumors have to expend precious time and energy to collect, assess, and prioritize information vital to their child's well-being. After all, parents are busy providing much of the treatment that their child receives. They make all appointments, prepare their child for procedures, buy and dispense medicines, deal with all of the physical and emotional side effects, and make daily decisions on when the child needs medical attention. In a sense, this book grew out of our wish to collect in one volume the basic information that newly diagnosed families need to begin to cope.

# What this book offers

This book is not intended to be autobiographical. Instead, we wanted to blend basic technical information in easy-to-understand language with stories and advice from many parents and survivors. We wanted to provide the insight and experiences of veteran parents, who have all felt the hope, helplessness, anger, humor, longing, panic, ignorance, warmth, and anguish of their children's treatment for cancer. We wanted parents know how other children react to treatment, what to expect, and provide tips to make the experience easier.

Obtaining a basic understanding of such topics as medical terminology, common side effects of chemotherapy, and how to interpret blood counts can only improve the quality of life for the whole family suffering along with their child. Learning how to develop a partnership with your child's physician can vastly increase your family's comfort and peace of mind. Hearing parents describe their own emotional ups and downs, how they coped, and how they molded their family life around hospitalizations is a tremendous comfort. Just knowing that there are other kids on chemotherapy who refuse to eat anything but tacos or who have frequent rages makes one feel less alone. Our hope is that parents who read this book will encounter medical facts simply explained, will find advice that eases their daily life, and will feel empowered to be a strong advocate for their child.

The parent stories and suggestions in this book are true, although some names have been changed to protect children's privacy. Every word has been spoken by the parent of a child with a brain or spinal cord tumor, a sibling, or a survivor. They wanted to share with others what they have learned.

# How this book is organized

We have organized the book sequentially in an attempt to parallel most families' journey through treatment. We all start with diagnosis, learn about brain and spinal cord tumors, try to cope with procedures, adjust to medical personnel, and deal with family and friends. We all seek out various methods of support, and struggle with the strong feelings of our child with cancer and our other children. We try to work with our child's school to provide the richest and most appropriate education for our child. And, unfortunately, we must grieve, either for our child or for the child of a close friend we have made in our new community of cancer.

Because it is tremendously hard to focus on learning new things when you are emotionally battered and extremely tired, we have tried to keep each chapter short.

Because half of the children diagnosed with brain tumors are boys and half are girls, we did not adopt the common convention of using only masculine personal pronouns. Because we do not like using he/she, we have alternated personal pronouns within chapters. This may seem awkward as you read, but it prevents half of the parents from feeling that the text does not apply to their child.

All of the medical information contained in this book is current for 2001. As treatment is constantly evolving and improving, there will inevitably be changes. You will learn in this book how to discover the newest and most appropriate treatment for your child.

To give you more places to find help for your cancer journey, we have included four appendices for reference: blood counts and what they mean, resource organizations, books and online sites, and a list of pediatric neurosurgeons. Finally, we have included an indispensable health record to be filled out at the end of treatment and copied and given to each subsequent caregiver for the rest of your child's life. This personal long-term follow-up guide educates your healthcare providers about the types of treatment given and the follow-up schedule necessary to maintain optimum health.

# How to use this book

While researching this book, we were repeatedly told by parents to "write the truth." Because the "truth" varies for each person, over one hundred parents, children with brain and spinal cord tumors, and siblings share portions of their experiences. This book is full of such snapshots in time, some of which may be hard to read, especially by those families of children newly diagnosed. Here are our suggestions for a positive way to use the information contained in this book:

- Consider reading only sections that apply to the present or immediate future. Even if your child's prognosis indicates a high probability of cure, reading about relapse or death can be emotionally difficult.

- Realize that only a fraction of the problems that parents describe will affect your child. Every child is different; every child sails smoothly through some portions of treatment, but encounters difficulties in others. The more you understand about the variability of cancer experiences, the better you will be able to cope with your own situation as well as be a good listener and helpful friend to other families you meet with differing diagnoses and circumstances.

- Take any concerns or questions that arise to your pediatric oncologist and/or pediatric neurosurgeon for answers (or more questions). The more you learn, the better you can advocate for your family and others.

- We have struggled to keep each chapter short and the technical information easy to read. If you want to delve into any topic in greater depth, Appendix C, *Books and Online Sites,* is a good place to start. It contains a list of books and web sites for parents as well as children of all ages. Reading tastes are a very individual matter, so if something suggested in the appendix is not helpful or upsets you, put it down. You will probably find something else on the list that is more appropriate for you.

- Share the book with family and friends. Usually they desperately want to help and just don't know how. This book not only explains the disease and treatment, but also offers dozens of concrete suggestions for family and friends.

Best wishes for a smooth journey through treatment and a bright future for the entire family.

# Acknowledgments

This book is truly a collaborative effort: without the help of many, it would simply not exist. Our heartfelt thanks to our family and friends who supported us along the way.

Tania gives special thanks to her husband, Spencer, for his love, patience, tolerance, and support and to her daughter, Emily, whose "spirit" never dwindles. To her parents, James and Barbara Shiminski, and to Spencer's mother, Gertude Maher, thank you for all of your advice and wisdom. All of her coworkers, especially Kathleen,

Eileen, Linda, Fred, Rick, George, Karl, Jeff, and Joao, deserve thanks for continual positive reinforcement. And, lastly, thanks to the hundreds of children and families who have touched her life over the years.

Patsy would like to thank her husband and colleague, John, for his support, encouragement, humor, and mentoring over the last twenty years. To her mom and dad for allowing her to grow up always believing that she could achieve her goals. To the physicians, nurses, and support staff with whom she works at Childhood Hematology-Oncology Associates, sincere thanks for allowing her the time to bring this idea to fruition. Finally, special thanks to her Children's Oncology Group nursing colleagues for providing twenty years of inspiration, support, encouragement, and, most of all, friendship.

Maria wishes to thank Tania, Patsy, and Nancy Keene for asking her to represent the families for this project. She'd like to give thanks for her husband, Jim, for being the best partner anyone could ask for, for sharing in the joys and lightening the worries, and especially for his love and enthusiasm. Together, they'd like to say: We love you William! She would also like to express her family's gratitude to each doctor, nurse practitioner, vision specialist, teacher, rehab therapist, and insurance coordinator they've ever come to rely upon. And special thanks to family, friends, and coworkers at Merriam-Webster and American International College, who time and again extend their support.

Special thanks to our editor, Nancy Keene, for having the drive to keep three busy authors "on track" and writing per the schedule; for having humor, patience, tact, and honesty when needed; and for having a love of the subject and a desire to help patients and their families. Special thanks to Shawnde Paull, Director of Operations, for handling the avalanche of details with competence, aplomb, and good cheer. Thanks to Kristin Throop for making the interior design and cover gorgeous, and to Tom Dorsaneo for producing superb books in just a few short months. And special thanks to Tim O'Reilly, for believing in and supporting the Patient-Centered Guides.

This book is a true collaboration between families of children with brain and spinal cord tumors and medical professionals. Many well-known and respected members of the pediatric community, members of national organizations, and parents carved time out of their busy schedules to make invaluable suggestions and catch errors. We especially appreciate the patient and thoughtful responses to our many emails and phone calls. Thank you: Jeffrey C. Allen, MD; Diane Barounis, MSW, LCSW; Roberta Calhoun, ACSW; Debbie Civello, RN, MA, CPON; Cass Cooney, MSN, PNP; Jillann Demes, MSW, LSW; Geri Jo Duda, RN; Fred Epstein, MD; Henry Friedman, MD;

Russ Geyer, MD; Sharon Grandinette, MS Ed; Deneen Hesser, RN, BS, OCN; George Jallo, MD; Larry Kun, MD; Mary Lovely, PhD, RN; Maureen McCarthy, BSCCLS, Child Life Specialist; Tobey J. MacDonald, MD; Paul McKay; Gigi McMillan; Al Musella, DPM; Elizabeth A. Seay; Yvonne Soghomonian, RN; Nancy Tarbell, MD; Kathy Warren, MD; Sheri and Greg White; Catherine Woodman, MD; Jeanne Young, BA.

Special thanks to George Jallo, MD, for his help with the scans used for illustrations.

More than words can express, we are deeply grateful to the parents, children with brain and spinal cord tumors, their siblings, and others who generously opened their hearts and relived their pain while sharing their experiences with us. To all of you whose words form the heart and soul of the book, thank you: Kathleen A. Barry; Cynthia Baumann-Retalic, mom of Kevin; Kathleen Bell; Kathy Bucher; Nancy Bullard, mother of three incredible young women; Tonya M. Burwell; Angie M. Cheeks; Patricia V. Christiansen, mom to John V. Christiansen; Debbie Civello, RN, CPON; Lisa M. Clark, Christopher's mom; Grace Coville-McKenna; Maureen Colvin; Cheryl Coutts; Karen Covell, mother of two wonder boys, Christopher and Cameron; Aimee Dion Crisanti; Melissa and Andrew Croom; Renee Curkendall; Evan Darlington; Carol Dean, Mandy's mom; Lucindy M. DeLuca PTA; Wade Demmert, proud dad of Mandy; Laura Duty, mother of Benjamin Duty; Sharon Eaton, Super "T's" Mom; Mark, loving husband of Janet; Fred Epstein; Wes and Vicki Fleming; Tracy Flinders; Drew Head, father of Alissa; Cindy Herb and son Michael; Kellie Hicks; Shawn Honohan; Linda Horvat; Debbie Hoskin; Mary L. Hubbell; Margie Huhner, mom to Anna; George Hunter; Janie, Megan's Mom; Marcia Jacobs, angel Anjuli's mommy; Jenny Jardine; Darlene Behrend Jones; Larry Junck, MD; Susan Junghans, mother of angel David; Carolyn, mother of Paul Kazakos; Jan Klooster, mother of Dan Steven; Kathy Knight; C.J. Korenek, mom to Emily; Louise and John Lamp, parents of Victoria; Missy Layfield; Debbie Lentini; Aidan Leslie; Melanie Logan and son, Darren Klawinski; Rachel Lourie; Christina McCarter; Maureen A. McCarthy; Mrs. Danielle McCauley; Gillian McGovern; Alannah, Susan, and Paul McKay; Gigi McMillan; Susan Milliken; Katy Moffitt, proud mom of angel Jessica Ann Moffitt; Berendina Norton; Sandra M. Norton; Lauren Ott, RN; Josie and Kylie Pace; MaryJo Palermo-Kirsch, Kevin's momma; Stephanie Paul, proud mother of Derick Corey; Jane Peppler, mother of Ezra Farber; Diane Robinson Phillips; Robin and Emily Pierce; David Rank; Jim and Sally Reeves, parents of Jordan; Kris Riley, mom of Matt; Alison C. Roberto; Dona M. Ross; Ruth Sansalone; Carole-Lynn Saros; Kelly Saunders, mom to Hunter Goodon; Mindy Schwartz, Mikey's mom;  Elizabeth A. Seay; Lee D. Smolen; Carol J. Sorsdahl; Loice Swisher, mother of Victoria Middleton; Trish Telcik; Bob Thomas and Megan Thomas; Terra Trevor; Denise Turek, mom to Jen; Greg and Sheri White; Catherine Woodman;

Marcey, mom to Madison; Mark, father of Deli; Carolyn; and those who wish to remain anonymous.

Thank you also to Nancy Keene and Honna Janes-Hodder for sharing their words. Some of the text for this book comes from their previous books for families of children with cancer: *Childhood Leukemia: A Guide for Family, Friends, and Caregivers,* by Nancy Keene, and *Childhood Cancer: A Parent's Guide to Solid Tumor Cancers,* by Honna Janes-Hodder and Nancy Keene.

Despite the inspiration and contributions of so many, any errors, omissions, misstatements, or flaws in the book are entirely our own.

# CHAPTER 1

# Diagnosis

THE DIAGNOSIS OF A BRAIN or spinal cord tumor in a child is the beginning of a parent's worst nightmare. To hear the word "brain tumor" or "spinal cord tumor" used in the same sentence as your child's name is terrifying. From that point forward, life is never the same. Families are forced into a strange new world that feels like an emotional roller coaster ride in the dark. Once the initial shock of diagnosis has passed, however, the reality that some children are cured provides strength and hope.

## Signs and symptoms

The brain and spinal cord make up the central nervous system (CNS). These organs coordinate all of the functions necessary for life, including breathing, heart rate, thinking, and moving. Tumors of the CNS begin with the transformation of a single cell. This renegade cell reproduces, creating more abnormal cells. Eventually, this collection of abnormal cells forms a tumor in the brain or spinal cord. The location of the tumor (also called a mass), its rate of growth, and associated swelling determine the signs and symptoms that develop in a child. Chapter 3, *Types of Tumors,* provides an in-depth explanation about the various types of brain and spinal cord tumors.

Parents are usually the first to notice that something is wrong with their child. Occasionally, a pediatrician notices a problem during a well-baby visit, or the tumor is discovered by chance on a scan or other test. Unfortunately, some of the signs and symptoms of CNS tumors mimic common childhood illnesses, sometimes making diagnosis difficult.

The following are some of the signs and symptoms that may indicate the presence of a childhood brain tumor:

* Headaches (often with early morning vomiting)
* Dizziness
* Seizures (convulsions)
* Staring spells

- Loss of peripheral vision

- Double vision

- Nystagmus (jiggling of eyeball)

- Inability to look up

- Eye turns inward or outward

- Weakness in hands on one or both sides of the body

- Unsteady walk

- Change in speech

- Trouble swallowing

- Drowsiness

- Facial drooping or asymmetry

- Nausea relieved by vomiting

- Hormonal or growth problems

- Hearing loss

- Changes in appetite or thirst

- Behavior changes

- Change in school performance

These symptoms can be present for a long or short period of time, depending upon the location and rate of growth of the tumor. A child with a brain or spinal cord tumor usually has a combination of the above symptoms, not just one.

The following are signs and symptoms that may indicate the presence of a spinal cord tumor in a child:

- Back or neck pain, which may awaken child from sleep

- Scoliosis (curvature of the spine resulting in leaning of shoulders to one side or a hump noticeable in the back)

- Torticollis (tilting of the head and upper spine to one side)

- Weakness or sensory changes in arms or legs

- Changes in bowel and bladder control

Most parents react to their concerns by taking their child to a doctor. Often the symptoms are attributed to a normal childhood illness and parents bring their child in for one or more visits before a brain tumor is suspected. This is easier to understand when you consider that, in their entire careers, most pediatricians see only one or two children with brain or spinal cord tumors. Ultimately, the doctor orders a scan (MRI or CT) or refers the child to a specialist, such as a pediatric neurologist, for further tests (see Chapter 4, *Coping with Procedures*).

*Alannah was 4 years old when she was diagnosed with a brainstem glioblastoma. On December 23, 1999, my daughter's school called my wife to have her pick up Alannah because she had vomited, although she appeared fine afterward.*

*On Christmas Eve, Alannah woke up, and after playing for awhile, began complaining of a headache. We assumed she had picked up some sort of virus at her school.*

*Later that day, we went to my parent's house for a traditional Christmas Eve gathering. Alannah began displaying difficulty in walking, and appeared to be looking at everything with her eyes shifted to the left. We laid her down in the guest room and a few minutes later, she threw up again. We still figured that we were dealing with a "bug", so we cleaned her up and went home. The following morning, she seemed fine except that her eyes were still fixed to the left. Later in the day, she started to have trouble with her balance and walking again. We took her to our local urgent care, still expecting to be told that she had a virus.*

*First, she was examined by a nurse practitioner. After checking Alannah's eyes, she quickly called in the doctor on duty. After a brief examination, he told me that he wanted to send her to the hospital by ambulance for a CT scan. He said that while it might be a virus affecting her brain, he wanted the scan done to be sure that nothing else was wrong. Once we arrived at the hospital, several doctors examined Alannah. After waiting for about two hours, the CT scan was performed. Shortly thereafter, the physician called my wife and I out of the room and showed us the scan. She showed us what she called a "mass" on Alannah's brainstem, and told us that she would admit Alannah to the hospital and order an MRI. After another couple of hours in the ER we were transferred to a room on the fifth floor, in shock and disbelief, waiting for them to discover their mistake, and send us home.*

The diagnosis of a CNS tumor is often not as quick as Alannah's:

> The first signs were so subtle: the slight but constant inward turn of our son's left eye became apparent to us within the first few months of life. By the time he was seven months old, we were concerned enough to bring it to our pediatrician's attention. He felt it was just normal uncoordinated eye movement. Every well-baby visit we brought the same problem to his attention. When our son was a year old, we were finally referred to an eye specialist—a pediatric ophthalmologist. Another year of visits began: the specialist insisted his eye was fine. We were just as certain the eye wasn't right, and we thought we could now see the eyeball jiggling. Then the ophthalmologist referred us to a pediatric orthoptist at a local Lions' Club clinic. She listened to our concerns, examined our son's eyes, and wrote a letter for our pediatrician verifying the abnormalities. Based on her report, our pediatrician agreed to schedule an MRI. Our son was two years and two months old by the time he was diagnosed with a moderately large optic glioma.

# Where should your child receive treatment?

After tentatively diagnosing a CNS tumor, most physicians refer the child to the closest major medical center with expertise in treating children with tumors. Every child with a brain or spinal cord tumor should be treated at a facility that uses a multidisciplinary team approach. A multidisciplinary team often includes pediatric specialists in the areas of neurosurgery, neuro-oncology, neurology, neuropathology, radiation oncology, neuroradiology, rehabilitation, neuro-opthalmology, and endocrinology. Nurse practitioners, child life specialists, social workers, educational specialists, and pastoral ministers are also part of the team. These institutions provide state-of-the-art treatment, offering your child the best chance for cure, remission (disappearance of disease in response to treatment), or disease control.

> Just after surgery, a number of doctors came by and introduced themselves as members of our team. At first, I was startled to learn that a radiation oncologist had been assigned to us, because radiation was not part of our son's current treatment plan. But then she explained that each member of the team would see us whenever we came to the children's hospital pediatric brain tumor clinic. I feel better knowing our child isn't an unknown quantity to these specialists, in case we ever do need them.

# Physical responses

Many parents become physically ill in the weeks following diagnosis. This is not surprising, given that most parents stop eating or grab only fast food, normal sleep patterns are a thing of the past, and staying in the hospital exposes them to all sorts of illnesses. Every waking moment is filled with excruciating emotional stress, which makes the physical stress so much more potent.

> Our daughter had many strong seizures while in the hospital, and my stomach would churn. I'd have to leave the bedside when the nurse would come to help. I had almost uncontrollable diarrhea. Every new stressful event just dissolved my gut; I could feel it happening.

Parental illness is a very common event. To attempt to prevent its occurrence, it is helpful to try to eat nutritious meals, get a break from your child's bedside to take a walk outdoors, and find time to sleep. Care needs to be taken not to overuse drugs or alcohol in an attempt to control anxiety or cope with grief. Whereas physical illnesses usually end or improve after a period of adjustment, emotional effects continue throughout treatment.

# Emotional responses

The shock of diagnosis results in an overwhelming number of intense emotions for the child and the parents. The length of time people experience each of these feelings differs greatly, depending on pre-existing emotional issues and coping strategies. Many of these emotions reappear at different times during the child's treatment. Some of the feelings that parents experience are described below. Children and teens' emotional responses to diagnosis are discussed in Chapter 15, *Feelings, Communication, and Behavior.*

## Confusion and numbness

In their anguish, most parents remember only bits and pieces of the doctor's early explanations about their child's disease. This dreamlike state is an almost universal response to shock. The brain provides protective layers of numbness and confusion to prevent emotional overload. This allows parents to examine information in smaller, less threatening pieces. Pediatric neurosurgeons and oncologists understand this phenomenon and are usually quite willing to repeat information as often as necessary.

Many centers have nurse practitioners who translate medical information into understandable language and answer questions. It is sometimes helpful to write down instructions, record them on a small tape recorder, or ask a friend or family member to help keep track of all the new and complex information.

> When I left the doctor's office, I was a mass of hysteria. I couldn't breathe and felt as if I was suffocating. Tears were flowing nonstop. I had lost total control of myself and had no idea of how to stop my world from turning upside down.

· · · · ·

> For a brief moment I stared at the doctor's face and felt totally confused by what he was explaining to me. In an instant that internal chaos was joined with a scream of terror that came from some place inside me that, up until that point, I never knew existed.

## Denial

In the first few days after diagnosis, many parents use denial to shield themselves from the reality of the situation. They simply cannot believe that their child has a life-threatening illness. Denial may serve as a useful method to survive the first few days after diagnosis, but a gradual acceptance must occur so that the family can begin to make the necessary adjustments to treatment. Life has dramatically changed. Once parents accept the doctor's prognosis, push their fears into the background, and begin to believe that their child can survive, they are better able to advocate for their child and their family.

> I walked into the empty hospital playroom and saw my wife clutching Matthew's teddy bear. Her eyes were red and swollen from crying. I had no idea what had happened. A minute later the doctor came into the room with several residents (doctors who are receiving specialized training). He told me that Matthew had a tumor and that he was very sick. I remember thinking that there had to have been a mistake. Maybe he was reading the wrong chart? My initial reaction was that it was physically impossible for one of my children to have a tumor. Tumors only grow in the elderly. Kids don't get tumors!

## Guilt

Guilt is a common and normal reaction after a diagnosis of a brain or spinal cord tumor. Parents sometimes feel that they have failed to protect their child, and they blame themselves. It is especially difficult because the cause of their child's tumor, in most instances, cannot be explained. There are questions: How could we have prevented this? What did we do wrong? How did we miss the signs? Why didn't we bring her to the doctor sooner? Why didn't we insist that the doctor do a scan? Did he inherit this from me? Why didn't we live in a safer place? Maybe I shouldn't have let her drink the well water. Was it because of the fumes from painting the house? Why? Why? Why? It may be difficult to accept, but parents need to remember that nothing they did caused their child's illness.

Nancy Roach describes some of these feelings in her booklet *The Last Day of April:*

> *Almost as soon as Erin's illness was diagnosed, our self-recrimination began. What had we done to cause this illness? Was I careful enough during pregnancy? We knew radiation was a possible contributor; where had we taken Erin that she might have been exposed? I wondered about the toxic glue used in my advertising work or the silk screen ink used in my artwork. Bob questioned the fumes from some wood preservatives used in a project. We analyzed everything—food, fumes, and TV. Fortunately, most of the guilt feelings were relieved by knowledge and by meeting other parents whose children had been exposed to an entirely different environment.*

## Fear and helplessness

A diagnosis of brain or spinal cord tumor strips parents of control over their child's daily life. Previously, parents established routines and rules that defined family life. Children woke up, washed and dressed, ate breakfast, perhaps attended daycare or school, played with friends, and performed chores. Life was predictable. Suddenly, the family is thrust into a new world populated by an ever-changing cast of characters (neurosurgeons, oncologists, radiologists, radiation oncologists, ophthalmologists, rehabilitative specialists, endocrinologists, interns, residents, fellows, IV teams, nurses, nurse practitioners, social workers) and containing a new language (medical terminology): a new world full of hospitalizations, procedures, and drugs.

Until adjustment begins, parents sometimes feel utterly helpless. Physicians whom they have never met are presenting treatment options for their child. Even if parents are comfortable in a hospital environment, feelings of helplessness may develop because there is simply not enough time in the day to care for a very sick child, deal with their own emotions, begin to educate themselves about the disease, notify friends and family, make job decisions, and restructure the family to deal with the crisis.

*I stood at the elevator bank in the basement of Children's Hospital waiting for the elevator, saying to all those around me: "I can't even say those words out loud! Come on everybody say it with me: My daughter has a brain tumor! A brain tumor! A b-r-a-i-n t-u-m-o-r! Now that we know how to spell it, let's say it over and over ... braintumorbraintumor braintumorbraintumorbraintumor!" Needless to say, I'm sure all the docs, nurses, and patients who were standing there with me just chalked it up to my temporary insanity, shock, denial, and complete flip-out that I was going through.*

· · · · ·

*My daughter Alexandra (age 3½) was diagnosed with an hemangioma in her brainstem. It is a non-cancerous type of "tumor" which does not require radiation. It is benign except for its location, location, location. She required two surgeries and we are hoping, praying, and pleading with the powers that BE, that it shrinks and stops causing a problem. Hemangiomas are those purplish-red birthmark things you see on children's faces sometimes. They serve no purpose except to traumatize families until they go away ... if they go away.*

Parents also experience different levels of anxiety, including fear and panic. Many parents have trouble sleeping and feel overwhelmed by fears of what the future holds. Their world has turned inside out—they have gone from adults in control of their lives to helpless people who cannot protect their child.

Many parents state that helplessness begins to disappear when a sense of reality and control returns. They begin to make decisions, study their options, learn about the disease, and grow comfortable with the hospital and staff. However, feelings of fear, panic, and anxiety periodically erupt for many parents at varying times throughout their child's treatment.

*It's not a nice way to have to live. What's waiting around the next corner? That's a scary question. One of my biggest fears is the uncertainty of the future. All that we can do is the best we can and hope that it's enough.*

· · · · ·

*Sometimes I would feel incredible waves of absolute terror wash over me. The kind of fear that causes your breathing to become difficult and your heart to beat faster. While I would be consciously aware of what was happening, there was nothing I could do to stop it. It's happened sometimes very late at night, when I'm lying in bed, staring off into the darkness. It's so intense that for a brief moment, I try to comfort myself by thinking that it can't be real, because it's just too horrible. During those moments, these thoughts only offer a second or two of comfort. Then I become aware of just how wide my eyes are opened in the darkness.*

## Anger

Anger is a common response to the diagnosis of life-threatening illness. However, spouses often have very different ways of responding to stress. One may talk non-stop while the other clams up. When the inescapable anger is directed at each other, it can be very destructive.

> *Life isn't fair, but yet the sun still comes up each morning. To be angry because your child has a brain tumor is normal. The question is where to direct that anger. Sometimes I feel as if I'm angry at the entire world. In my heart, though, my outrage is directed solely at each and every tumor cell feeding on my child.*

Expressing anger is normal and can be cathartic. Attempting to suppress this powerful emotion is usually not helpful. It is nobody's fault that children are stricken with a CNS tumor. Since parents cannot direct their anger at the disease—they target doctors, nurses, spouses, siblings, and sometimes even the ill child. Because anger directed at other people can be very destructive, it is necessary to devise ways to express the anger. Some suggestions from parents for managing anger follow.

Anger at healthcare team:

- Try to improve communication with doctors
- Discuss feelings with one of the nurses or nurse practitioners
- Discuss feelings with social workers
- Talk with parents of other ill children, either locally or by joining an on-line support group

Anger at family:

- Exercise a little every day
- Do yoga or relaxation exercises
- Keep a journal or tape-record feelings
- Cry in the shower or pound a pillow
- Listen to music

- Read other people's stories about CNS tumors
- Talk with friends
- Talk with parents of other ill children
- Join or start a support group
- Improve communication within family
- Try individual or family counseling
- Live one day (or sometimes one hour) at a time

Anger at God:

- Share your feelings with spouse or close friends
- Discuss feelings with clergy or church members
- Re-examine your faith
- Know that anger at God is normal
- Pray
- Give yourself time to heal

It is important to remember that angry feelings are normal and expected. Discovering healthy ways to cope with anger is a vital tool for all parents.

## Loss of control

Parents sometimes feel overwhelmed by the sudden loss of control after their child is diagnosed with a tumor. This is especially true for parents who are used to having a measure of power and authority in the workplace or the home.

> My husband had a difficult time after our son was diagnosed. We have a traditional marriage, and he was used to his role as provider and protector for the family. It was hard for him to deal with the fact that he couldn't fix everything.

Parents can regain some control over the situation by learning about their child's disease and its treatments. This knowledge can be used to advocate for their child. They can also gain some control by becoming active participants in their child's treatment. They can ask the doctor what tests and appointments are negotiable. They can have a say in what time clinic appointments are, which days to have tests done, what times to give medications, and more. Molding treatment around family life increases a sense of control. For more information, see Chapter 7, *Forming a Partnership with the Medical Team.*

## Sadness and grief

Parents feel an acute sense of loss when their child is diagnosed with a CNS tumor. They feel unprepared to cope with the possibility of death, and they fear that they may simply not be able to deal with the enormity of the problems facing the family. Parents describe themselves as feeling engulfed by sadness. Parents grieve the loss of normalcy: the realization that life will never be the same. They grieve the loss of their dreams and aspirations for their child. Some parents also feel shame and embarrassment. Cultural background, individual coping styles, basic temperament, and family dynamics all affect the type of emotions experienced.

> I have an overwhelming sadness and, unfortunately for me, that means feelings of helplessness. I wish I could muster up a fighting spirit, but I just can't right now.

· · · · ·

> While I have moments of deep sadness and despair, I try not to let them turn into hours and certainly not days. I am too aware of the fact that I may have the rest of my life to grieve.

Parents also grieve the loss of the child they knew. Children who achieve remission or cure from a CNS tumor often have permanent late effects from treatment. The loss of the child as he once was can be very difficult for all members of the family.

Parents travel a tumultuous emotional path where overwhelming emotions subside, only to resurface later. All of these are normal, common responses to a catastrophic event. For the majority of parents, some of the strong emotions begin to fade as hope grows.

## Hope

After being buffeted by illness, anger, fear, sadness, grief, and guilt, most parents welcome the growth of hope. Hope is the belief in a better tomorrow. Hope sustains the will to live and gives the strength to endure each trial. Hope is not a way around, it is a way through. There is reason for hope.

Twenty-five years ago, very few children with CNS tumors were cured. Technological advances, including computer-assisted surgical planning, advanced imaging techniques, newer chemotherapy drugs, and focused radiation therapies, have changed that. Over the last two decades, because of these advances as well as research and participation in clinical trials (see Chapter 9, *Clinical Trials*), many children are now long-term survivors.

Families often discover a renewed sense of both the fragility and beauty of life after the diagnosis. Outpourings of love and support from family and friends provide comfort and sustenance. Many parents speak of a renewed appreciation for life and consider each day with their child as a precious gift.

> *When we were given the diagnosis of glioblastoma multiforme (GBM) in June, 1999, it took time and layers of understanding before we could come to grips with everything. This whole concept of brain disease is so frightening and so surreal, it can't possibly be grasped in a few weeks. We realized that the adjustment wouldn't be made in a single step, but that we'd reach plateaus of "new normal" along the way. In other words, don't be surprised if you feel like you have a pretty good grip on things and then suddenly lose it one day. As with life as usual, some days will be better than others. If you feel deeply sad or completely overwhelmed one day, remind yourself that it's a mood like all the others in your repertoire, there is an excellent reason for it, but in time you will feel better able to cope.*

# The immediate future

It is important for you to know that you are not alone. Many have traveled this path before you. Although it is sad to know that others are forced into this terrifying journey, you can take some small solace from knowing that you are not the only parents to experience these feelings. You can call upon these parents as resources and fountains of support.

The next several chapters provide specific disease-related information: how to get the best doctors and treatment plan, what type of catheter to choose, whether your child should be enrolled in a clinical study, and various forms of treatment for children with CNS tumors. Veteran parents explain what choices they made, how they adjusted, learned, and became active participants in their children's treatment. Sharing experiences with parents and survivors of childhood central nervous system tumors may help your family develop its own unique strategy for coping with the challenges ahead.

*A Mother's View*

> *Memory is a funny thing. I'd be hard pressed to remember what I had for dinner last night, but like many people, the day of the Challenger explosion and, even further back, the day of John Kennedy's death are etched in my mind to the smallest detail.*

And like a smaller group of people, the day of my child's diagnosis is a strong and vivid memory, even seven years later. Most of the time, I don't dwell on that series of images. It was, after all, a chapter in our lives, and one that is now blessedly behind us. But early each autumn, when I get a whiff of the crisp smell of leaves in the air, it brings back that dark day when our lives changed forever.

Many of the memories are painful and, like my daughter's scars, they fade a little more each year, but will never completely disappear. While dealing with the medical and physical aspects of the disease, my husband and I also made many emotional discoveries. We sometimes encountered ignorance and narrow-mindedness, which made me more sad than angry. Mistakes were made, tempers were short, and family relations were strained. But we saw the other side, too. Somehow, our sense of humor held on throughout the ordeal, and when that kicked in, we had some of the best laughs of our lives. There was compassion and understanding when we needed it most. And people were there for us like never before.

I remember two young fathers on our street, torn by the news, who wanted to help but felt helpless. My husband came home from the hospital late one night to find that our lawn had been mowed and our leaves had been raked by them. They had found a way to make a small difference that day.

Another time, a neighbor came to our house bearing a bakery box full of pastries and the message that his family was praying for our daughter nightly around their supper table. The image of this man, his wife, and his eight children joining in prayer for us will never leave me.

A close friend entered the hospital during that first terrible week we were there, to give birth to her son. I held her baby, she held me, and we laughed and cried together.

Sometimes, when I look back at that time, I feel as though everything that is wrong with the world and everything that is right are somehow distilled in one small child's battle to live. We learned so very much about people and about life.

Surely people who haven't experienced a crisis of this magnitude would believe that we would want to put that time behind us and forget as much of it as possible. But the fact is, we grew a little through our pain, like it or not. We see through new eyes. Not all of it is good or happy, but it is profound.

*I treasure good friends like never before. I view life as much more fragile and precious than I used to. I think of myself as a tougher person than I was, but I cry more easily now. And sure, I still yell at my kids and eagerly await each September when they will be out of my hair for a few hours each day. But I hold them with more tenderness when they hop off the school bus into my arms. And I like to think that some of the people around us, who saw how suddenly and drastically a family's life can change, hold their children a little dearer as well.*

*Do I want to forget those terrible days and nights seven years ago? Not on your life. And I hope the smell of autumn leaves will still bring the memories back when I'm a grandmother, even if I can't remember what I had for dinner last night.*

—Kathy Tucker
CURE Childhood Cancer Newsletter

# CHAPTER 2

# The Brain and Spinal Cord

IF SOMEONE YOU LOVE has a brain or spinal cord tumor, it's helpful to understand the basics of brain and spinal cord anatomy. Learning about the structure and function of the brain and spinal cord makes it easier to understand your doctor's explanations about types of tumors and treatment plans.

This chapter provides an overview of brain and spinal cord anatomy, with several figures to help you visualize the different parts of the brain. It then discusses symptoms associated with tumors in various locations in the brain and spinal cord. The chapter also includes a summary table describing location of tumor and associated symptoms.

## The brain

The brain, cushioned by watery fluid on all sides, resides inside the skull. It resembles a fleshy, shelled walnut in shape. Like a walnut, it has two distinct but tightly connected halves. These are called the left and right cerebral hemispheres—and although they appear to be mirror images of each other, similar-looking parts of each hemisphere do different things.

Like a walnut's exterior, the brain's surface folds in and out. These wrinkles increase the surface area of the brain. Its surface is divided by especially deep grooves, called fissures or sulci. The brain contains several major nerves—such as the optic nerves, which connect it to the eyes. The brain has no pain receptors of its own. Blood vessels carry oxygen and nutrients to all parts of the brain, and channels called aqueducts allow fluid to move through some areas.

## Cerebrum

The largest region in the brain is called the cerebrum (also called the supratentorial region). It is made up of two cerebral hemispheres (left and right). The two hemispheres are separated by a large groove, called the cerebral fissure. Deep within the cerebral fissure is a bundle of nerve fibers called the corpus callosum, which transmits information between the two sides.

The cerebrum interprets sensory input from all parts of the body and also controls body movements. It is the part of the brain responsible for thinking, emotions, memory, reasoning, learning, and movement. Symptoms of tumors in this area include:

- Seizures
- Memory difficulties
- Headaches
- Weakness or paralysis of arms and legs
- Speech abnormalities
- Changes in personality
- Visual loss

Symptoms can be generalized (from changes in pressure regulation) or focal (from tissue destruction or compression from the tumor). Generalized symptoms include irritability, lethargy, early morning vomiting, headache, loss of appetite, and behavior changes.

The cerebrum is divided into four areas (called lobes) on each side of the brain: the frontal, temporal, parietal, and occipital lobes. The corpus callosum connects the two parts of each lobe. Any movement of the arms and legs on the right side of the body is controlled by the left cerebral hemisphere.

Your child's physicians will attempt to determine which side of your child's brain is dominant. Dominance is important for tumors that are near the motor or speech (parietal/temporal) areas. It may be difficult for the surgeon to remove all of the tumor on the dominant side in these areas without injuring speech or limb function. Pre-operative testing and intraoperative monitoring (mapping) are vital in dealing with tumors in the dominant hemisphere. These are discussed in Chapter 8, *Surgery*. These tools assist the surgeon in removing as much tumor as possible while preserving function. The parts of the cerebrum are shown in Figure 2-1, *Basic brain anatomy*.

## Frontal lobes

The frontal lobes, located directly behind your forehead, are your mind's main planning and personality centers. They process and store information that helps you think ahead, use strategy, and respond to events based on past experiences and other knowledge. A small part of the frontal lobe is involved in articulating speech. Another small strip of the frontal lobe helps control movement. Malfunctions in the frontal lobe may lead to poor planning, impulsiveness, and certain types of speech

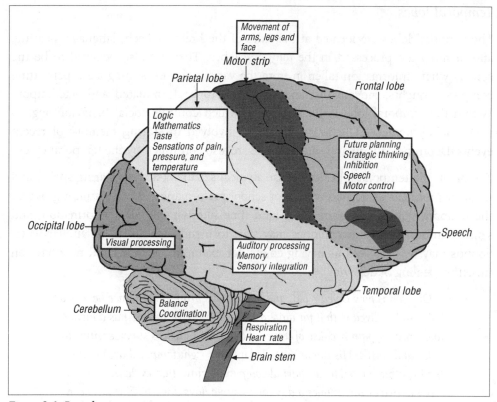

Figure 2-1. Basic brain anatomy

problems. Symptoms are most pronounced if the tumor crosses the corpus callosum and affects both frontal lobes. Symptoms of tumors of the frontal lobe are:

- Seizures

- Changes in ability to concentrate

- Poor school performance

- Changes in social behaviors and personality

Toward the back section of the frontal lobe is the motor area, a strip of the brain that controls movement of the head and body parts on the opposite side of the body. Because the location of motor nerves varies a little in each person, mapping of the motor area either prior to or during surgery helps doctors know the exact location of these functions so they are not injured during tumor removal. For more information, see the intraoperative monitoring section of Chapter 8.

## Temporal lobes

The temporal lobes are located at the sides of the brain. Speech, language, hearing, and memory are processed in the temporal lobes. They are also believed to be the centers where information taken in from the various senses is integrated, permitting complex thoughts, movements, and sensations to be formulated and acted upon. Within the temporal lobe is the amygdala, which controls social behavior, aggression, and excitement. The hippocampus is involved in storing memory of recent events. Depth perception and sense of time are also controlled by the temporal lobes.

Tumors in the temporal lobes can cause atypical seizures (such as staring spells) and memory problems associated with poor school performance. When a tumor grows in the temporal lobes, the brain has a hard time filtering out extra information, and sensory information and memories may start to blend together in unfamiliar ways. Sounds may be perceived as having colors, for example, or your child may have an unsettling feeling of déjà vu.

> Our son is now 6 years old, and he's had his brain tumor since he was a baby, so he's lived with it for quite a while. I'm pretty sure he has a higher tolerance for pain because of it, yet at the same time he's supersensitive to noise and smells. His tumor extended into the right temporal area and to the hypothalamus. He has partial complex seizures that cycle from one a week to two or three times a day for a couple days a week. This has been going on regardless of what medication we've used, so far.
>
> They start with a blank stare, then he says, "Um, um" or "Mom, Dad" a few times, or sometimes, if it's at night, he may be more disoriented and cry out. Then he flushes pink, sometimes he smacks his lips or picks at his clothes with his fingers. At one point, you can tell he can't hear or even see, but then he becomes more aware, and he'll take a breath when we ask. Then he usually spits up and wants to nap.
>
> And the medications can cause their own side effects, like dull affect, behavior changes, and light sensitivity. Our neurologist's office had a poster up about an epilepsy support group in the area, so I've been going to those.

## Parietal lobes

Directly behind the frontal lobes and above the temporal lobes are the parietal lobes. The parietal lobes process all sorts of sensory information coming in from the body, including data about temperature, pain, and taste. The parietal lobes also control

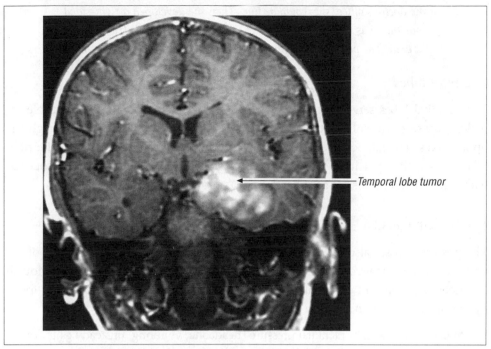

Temporal lobe tumor

*Figure 2-2 . MRI showing temporal lobe tumor responsible for seizures in a child*

language and the ability to do arithmetic. Numbers may be read, but calculations may be a challenge because of difficulty in knowing left from right. When the parietal lobes are not functioning properly, sensory information is not processed correctly, and your child may have a hard time making sense of her environment.

The rear of the parietal lobe, next to the temporal lobe, has an area important in processing auditory and visual information needed for language. When children have tumors in this area, they do not understand when someone speaks to them, but they are able to make sounds themselves.

Abnormal movements or weakness in the arms and legs, memory problems, and seizures are associated with tumors in these areas. During a seizure affecting the parietal lobe, strange physical sensations may be felt, such as a crushing pressure or a tingle in part of the body.

> Megan was 20 months old when we found out that she had an anaplastic
> ependymoma occupying the entire left occipital-parietal region of her brain
> (about half the size of her little head). For six to eight weeks, she had
> sporadic vomiting and crabbiness in the morning. By the time we'd arrive

*at the doctor's office, she would be fine. Then she developed a right-sided*
*tremor that was so strong it shook her whole body when she tried to use her*
*right arm. The pediatrician ordered an MRI and found the brain tumor.*

## Occipital lobes

The occipital lobes serve as the visual centers of the brain. They are responsible for
making sense of the information that comes to the brain from the eyes through the
optic nerves. The left occipital lobe deals with input from the right eye, and the right
lobe deals with input from the left eye. Tumors in the occipital lobe are associated
with visual field cut (loss of peripheral vision) on one side or the other.

# Posterior fossa

The posterior fossa (also called the infratentorium) is located at the very back of the
brain, atop the spinal cord. It includes the cerebellum, the brainstem, and the fourth
ventricle. Sixty percent of all childhood brain tumors originate in the posterior fossa.
Symptoms of tumors in this area of the brain include:

- Signs of increased intracranial pressure (headache, vomiting, unsteady gait, double
  vision, sleepiness, or lethargy)
- Weakness of cranial nerves (visual or hearing problems, weakness or drooping
  on one side of the face, eye movement problems, difficulty swallowing, difficulty
  breathing)
- Unsteady gait (ataxia)

## Cerebellum

The cerebellum is about one-eighth the size of the cerebrum. Tumors growing in the
cerebellum can cause coordination and balance problems. The child may have an
uneven walking pattern or may continually fall to one side. Difficulty judging distances or reaching for and grabbing an object are symptoms of a tumor in this area. If
the tumor grows towards or puts pressure on the fourth ventricle, normal flow of
cerebrospinal fluid (CSF) is blocked, causing a condition called hydrocephalus.

> *Red-headed, 2-year-old Matthew had vomiting almost every day. After*
> *three months of running back and forth to the doctor, the babysitter and I*
> *noticed some "tipsy walking" as we called Matt's ever-so-subtle dizziness.*
> *A call to the doctor with this report led us to the office of a neurologist. A*
> *neurological exam and a little observation found us with an order to have*

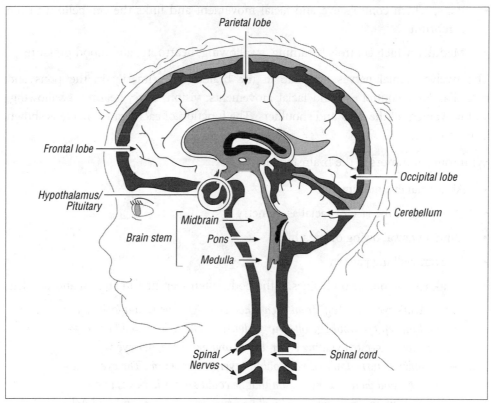

Figure 2-3 . Side view of the brain

*an MRI to rule out a brainstem tumor. The neurologist was sure the diagnosis was going to be benign vertigo of infancy, something usually outgrown by the age of three. Whew, one more year of the vomiting and we'd be done. Wrong again. On February 6, 1996 the neurologist told us our son had a brain tumor (medulloblastoma, on the floor of the 4th ventricle), that it was malignant, and he would need surgery as soon as possible. His tumor was located in the cerebellum, at the base of the brainstem, right where the circuits for all vital functions are connected.*

## Brainstem

The brainstem is the relay center for transmitting messages between the brain and other parts of the body. The three parts of the brainstem are:

- Midbrain, which processes vision and hearing and coordinates sleep and wake cycles

- Pons, which controls eye and facial movement and links the cerebellum to the cerebrum

- Medulla, which controls breathing, swallowing, heart rate, and blood pressure

The twelve cranial nerves originate in the brainstem, primarily in the pons and medulla. They control eye and facial movements, vision, taste, hearing, swallowing, and movement of the neck and shoulders. The function of each cranial nerve is shown in Figure 2-4.

Symptoms of tumors in the brainstem are:

- Abnormal eye movements

- Drooping of the face or facial asymmetry

- Difficulty swallowing or breathing

- Uneven walking pattern

- Weakness on one or both sides of the body, often seen first in an arm and/or a leg

> Ayla's eyes were "off" from each other. Her right eye would look at you and the left eye would go off. Our pediatrician thought it could be cross-eye, and suggested waiting it out, but in another week, her eye was completely turned in and you couldn't even see the pupil. The eye doctor we saw said there was no reason that he could see for her eyes to cross, so we went to a neurologist, who did a neurological exam, and said Ayla showed no neuro problems. But, he ordered a scan just in case, not expecting to find anything. He thought it could possibly be a virus. The scan found a 5×5 cm tumor in the posterior fossa, cerebellopontine angle, fourth ventricle, and arising from the brainstem.

## Fourth ventricle

The fourth ventricle is the fluid compartment that sits between the brainstem and the cerebellum. CSF flows from the ventricles above through the fourth ventricle and down into the spinal cord or to the outside of the brain. Tumors can grow inside the fourth ventricle or into the fourth ventricle from the brainstem or cerebellum. The tumor can block the normal flow of CSF, causing hydrocephalus. For more information on hydrocephalus, refer to Chapter 8.

> My son Paul had multiple admissions for pneumonia and a collapsed lung as a baby. The doctors were sure he had cystic fibrosis. After many tests, they decided maybe they were wrong. Summer started and everything was going well. In August he again started getting sick. Over

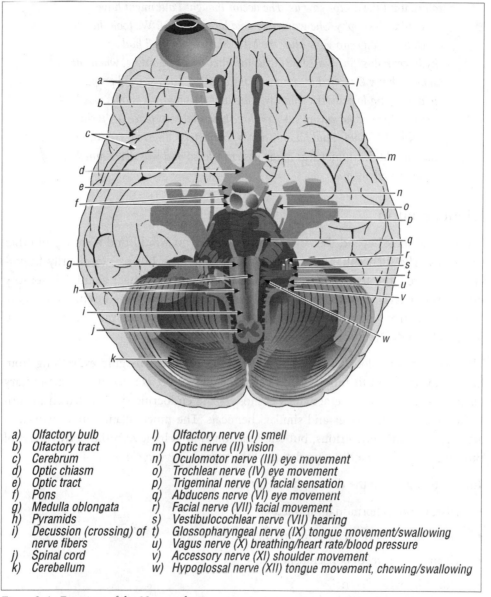

a) Olfactory bulb
b) Olfactory tract
c) Cerebrum
d) Optic chiasm
e) Optic tract
f) Pons
g) Medulla oblongata
h) Pyramids
i) Decussion (crossing) of
   nerve fibers
j) Spinal cord
k) Cerebellum

l) Olfactory nerve (I) smell
m) Optic nerve (II) vision
n) Oculomotor nerve (III) eye movement
o) Trochlear nerve (IV) eye movement
p) Trigeminal nerve (V) facial sensation
q) Abducens nerve (VI) eye movement
r) Facial nerve (VII) facial movement
s) Vestibulocochlear nerve (VII) hearing
t) Glossopharyngeal nerve (IX) tongue movement/swallowing
u) Vagus nerve (X) breathing/heart rate/blood pressure
v) Accessory nerve (XI) shoulder movement
w) Hypoglossal nerve (XII) tongue movement, chewing/swallowing

*Figure 2-4 . Functions of the 12 cranial nerves*

the next two months, Paul's balance deteriorated. By October he could no longer walk. Our family doctor sent us to see a neurologist. On the day of our appointment, we went to the neurologist and were told we didn't have an appointment, that we would have to reschedule. The nurse had forgotten to write us in the book. I insisted we be seen and we sat in the *office until the doctor saw us. The doctor thought Paul might have muscular dystrophy. She wanted to do a baseline MRI. We took the films back to her office to view after the MRI. She told us Paul had hydrocephalus. She was showing us the films and explaining, when she said, "Oh my God, he has a tumor. I'm so sorry." They started preparing to admit him to pediatric intensive care unit. His hydrocephalus was life-threatening and he was in surgery three hours later to place a VP shunt. On Nov. 14, 1994, Paul had his tumor completely removed. He was 21 months old. His tumor was in the posterior fossa and was determined to be an ependymoma.*

## Diencephalon

If you could look beyond the surface of the brain, you would find a variety of other structures. The diencephalon is made up of several tiny but extraordinarily important structures: the thalamus, the hypothalamus, and the pineal gland. All sensory information passes through the thalamus before being sent to the forebrain for more advanced interpretation—except for information gathered via the sense of smell, which takes a different route.

The hypothalamus looks small, but it has a big role in managing everything from hunger to digestion to muscle contractions. It has direct control over the pituitary gland, which manages the activities of most of the endocrine system, which in turn makes and uses hormones and similar chemicals. The pineal gland's inner workings are still somewhat mysterious, but one function is to help govern the body's sense of time and rhythm, including regulation of the reproductive cycle.

Tumors that grow in the diencephalon cause:

- Disruption in hormonal production
- Abnormal growth (usually delayed growth)
- Changes in level of consciousness
- Difficulty with vision
- Memory problems
- Weakness of one or both sides of the body

> *Florence has recovered from a germinoma, a malignant tumour of the pituitary gland. She was ill from age eleven to fifteen and the diagnosis took two years. This tumour seems to be very rare. Prior to diagnosis,*

there was a long period of weight loss, incessant thirst, and teachers and doctors who kept saying this was all psychological. Florence would get up in the morning, go to the kitchen, and start the awful drinking, glass after glass. One time I really lost it. I shouted at her, "Why are you doing this? Do you know what you are doing? You are going to make yourself very ill. Do you know what manipulative behaviour is?" I shouted and shouted, she didn't argue or cry. She just stood there and smiled at me sadly. She said, "I just can't help it." I thought, "That is it. This is a real illness." By then she was thin and she hadn't grown for months.

A young doctor gave her an injection of vasopressin. The effect was miraculous, she ran along the corridor, skipped up and down, she felt marvelous. The young doctor came back, very excited. He said, "We have a very good result." I stared at him. He said, "Well, perhaps a bad result from your point of view. Florence has diabetes insipidus. This is a permanent condition, the hormone which governs her kidneys is not being produced, she has been drinking to stop herself from dying of dehydration." After more searching, I finally found a consultant, and when he heard the symptoms, he said he knew what the cause could be. It was a germinoma—a rare tumour whose symptoms often begin with diabetes insipidus.

## Optic pathway

The optic nerves carry information from the eyes to the occipital lobe via the optic pathways. The nerve from the right eye goes to the left occipital lobe, and the nerve from the left eye goes to the right occipital lobe. These two nerves cross at a place called the optic chiasm, near the hypothalamus. Tumors that affect the optic pathway or the optic chiasm cause changes in vision. Visual acuity (the ability to see) or visual fields (peripheral vision) are disrupted.

After they discovered the optic tract tumor on the MRI, they sent us to vision specialists at the eye clinic. There Jamie saw an ophthalmologist who checked for optic nerve swelling, an orthoptist who checked acuity, and a visual function specialist, who found a complete loss of left-sided peripheral vision. The field cut is especially noticeable when he's in new environments, and he bumps into things on the left, although mostly he remembers to make the extra effort to turn his head to check out things on that side.

The following table summarizes the symptoms associated with tumors in various parts of the brain.

| Part of the brain | Symptoms of tumors |
|---|---|
| Frontal lobes (cerebral hemisphere) | Problems with learning and concentration, changes in behavior, personality changes, seizures, weakness of arm or leg on side opposite of tumor |
| Parietal lobes (cerebral hemisphere) | Seizures, difficulty processing information, language disorders |
| Temporal lobes (cerebral hemisphere) | Atypical seizures (partial complex), behavior problems (aggressive, impulsive) |
| Occipital lobes (cerebral hemisphere) | Loss of peripheral vision |
| Cerebellum | Problems with balance, uncoordinated gait |
| Brainstem | Abnormal eye movements, decreased hearing, asymmetry of the face, problems with breathing and swallowing, problems with balance and strength |
| Midbrain/thalamus | Sleepiness, weakness of arms or legs |
| Diencephalon | Disruption of hormonal secretion (decreased growth, diabetes insipidus, underactive thyroid), memory/academic problems, puberty problems |
| Optic pathway | Visual changes: loss of visual field, decrease in visual acuity |

A good starting point for understanding the workings of the brain is *Neuroscience for Kids,* a comprehensive web site for children and adults, which can be found at: *http://faculty.washington.edu/chudler/neurok.html.* Another great resource for understanding brain structure is a coloring book published in 1985 by Marian C. Diamond, called *The Human Brain Coloring Book.*

# Ventricular system

The CNS has several protective coverings that prevent injury to the brain and spinal cord. The outermost protection is the bones of the skull and the spine. Inside the skull are three thin membranes called the meninges, which surround the brain and spinal cord. The CNS is also protected by cerebrospinal fluid, which flows between the layers of meninges (called the subarachnoid space).

The ventricular system, shown in Figure 2-5, is made up of four chambers in the brain, called ventricles. At the base of the brain CSF exits from the fourth ventricle into the subarachnoid spaces that surround the brain and the spinal cord. Under normal conditions, the brain produces approximately one pint of CSF a day. This equals the amount absorbed by the body.

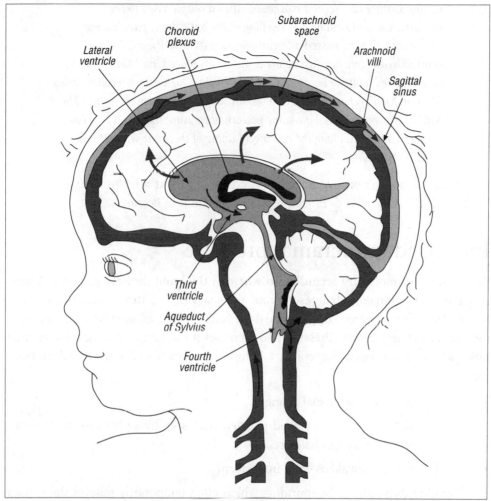

Figure 2-5. The ventricular system

Disruptions in the balance between the amount of CSF produced and reabsorbed can result in an increase in cerebrospinal fluid and pressure. Fluid buildup, called hydrocephalus, occurs in two ways:

- A tumor grows in or pushes into a ventricle, blocking the normal flow of CSF.
- Blood, tumor cells, a scar, or dead tissue obstructs the subarachnoid space and prevents the absorption of CSF.

> *Danny (age 8) began having infrequent bouts of headaches and vomiting at odd times, not always in the morning. He also told me that he was*

*having strange half-second blackouts. After a couple visits to the
pediatrician, we found he had swelling of the optic discs, papilledema.
Other than that, he passed all neurological tests. Finally, a CT scan
showed hydrocephalus. Just before a shunt was placed, an MRI of the
head showed multiple lesions all over the brain. Our doctors recommended
a spinal MRI to check if the brain lesions were spread from the spine. The
MRI of the spine showed the same pattern of unusual lesions. It was like
a sugar coating all along the meningeal lining of the spine without any
hard central mass.*

For more information on hydrocephalus and its treatment refer to *Hydrocephalus: A
Guide for Patients, Families & Friends* listed in Appendix B, *Resources*.

# Increased intracranial pressure

Symptoms of tumors vary according to where in the brain they are growing. A general term for symptoms that result from the mass of the tumor occupying space within the brain is "increased intracranial pressure." As the mass grows it compresses the brain causing pressure. Pressure also increases if the tumor obstructs the normal fluid pathways causing hydrocephalus. Symptoms of increased intracranial pressure include:

- Double vision or other visual changes
- Pressure on the optic discs (called papilledema), seen by a physician when looking into eyes with an ophthalmoscope
- Headache (which awakens child from sleep)
- Vomiting (typically in the morning, which often temporarily relieves the nausea and headache)
- Unsteady gait
- Sleepiness or lethargy
- Memory problems

*On July 3, 1999, Jennifer (age 20) had her second appointment with
a doctor in one week's time because her headaches were so severe. The
primary physician sent Jennifer to the hospital for a CT scan. I figured it
would be in a couple of weeks due to the holiday weekend. He said within
two hours. The nurse was drawing Jennifer's blood, when another nurse
came in and said that the hospital wants Jennifer down there as soon as*

*possible. They were holding the radiologist there, waiting on Jennifer. We left the primary physician's office around 11:00, and at noon, I was informed that Jennifer had an abnormality found on the brain. We were told to go to lunch and then report to the MRI department around 1:00. We reported to the MRI department and were told that Jennifer would be admitted to the hospital as soon as the MRI was done. I asked, "Would someone like to tell me what is going on?" I saw a telephone and called Jennifer's primary physician. This was the first time that I did not have to speak to a nurse; he got right on the phone. He said, "I am so sorry, I was waiting on the results of the MRI and was going to talk to you and Jennifer. The CT scan revealed a huge mass on the left side of the brain."*

# Spinal cord

At the base of the hindbrain, the brain becomes the spinal cord—a long, tough bundle of nerve fibers that runs down the back and is protected from harm by the vertebrae. The spinal cord is the pathway for nerve impulses that travel to and from the brain to all parts of the body. Tumors can grow inside or outside the spinal cord or, in some cases, twine around the cord. Symptoms of tumors in the spinal cord include:

* Back or leg pain that awakens child from sleep

* Curvature of the spine

* Weakness in arms or legs, usually below the level of the tumor growth

* Changes in sensation (tingling, numbness) in the back, arms, or legs

* Changes in bowel and bladder function

Figure 2-6 shows an MRI scan of a tumor causing the spine to curve.

# From the CNS to the body

The brain and spinal cord communicate with the rest of the body via nerves, thin strings of tough fiber that extend throughout the body. The brainstem and spinal cord branch off into many nerves that carry information to and from every part of the body. Together, these nerves are known as the peripheral nervous system.

The peripheral nervous system carries commands from the central nervous system to various body parts and returns information gathered from your senses. For example, nerves close to the skin's surface are sensitive to touch and tell the brain if they notice

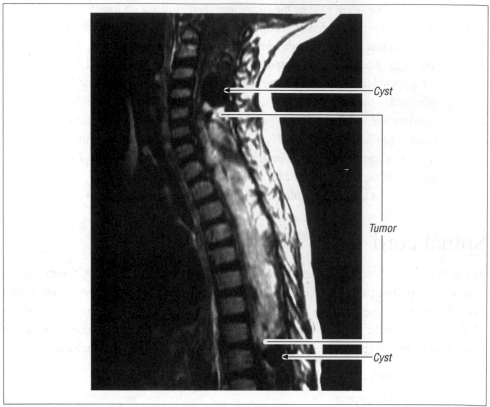

*Figure 2-6. MRI showing spinal cord tumor extending the full length of the spinal cord*

a crawling sensation. In response, your brain may trigger commands that cause you to absentmindedly brush a hand over the affected area, look at it, or scratch it.

Other nerves transmit information to and from the body's internal organs, including the heart, stomach, and intestines, as well as the sweat glands and the tiny muscles near the skin's surface whose contractions cause goosebumps. These nerves and the parts of the spinal cord and brain that control them are called the visceral or autonomic nervous system.

Most of the time the workings of the peripheral, autonomic, and central nervous systems go completely unnoticed. The majority of their interconnected activities concern basic physical functions: breathing, digesting food, producing hormones, pumping blood, and the like. Although it's possible to stop and purposefully make yourself aware of some of these processes, most people pay no attention as long as everything is working well. Brain and spinal cord tumors disrupt the normal, smooth workings of these nervous systems.

At the hospital a tall dark haired man met us in his office with a firm handshake. His kind brown eyes looked into mine. They held compassion and looked straight into you. They were willing eyes that held the horizon of the unknown. He was to be our neurosurgeon.

He showed us the scans from the MRI. It was like looking at a large negative. It is a picture of a slice from the body—as if you put a potato or an egg in a slicer and pulled out one slice to examine it. A foreign, alien feeling gripped me. From nothing wrong to brain tumor. This should not be happening. This was not normal. This is something that happens in someone else's life. Slow down. I wanted to say. Show me. Point with your finger to where it is. Tell me what is supposed to be in this picture and what is not?

That lemon-sized spot. That's not supposed to be there? Well, what is it? He explained that the best procedure would be to perform a craniotomy and surgically remove the tumor, find out what kind it was, and proceed from there. In just a few hours we went from suntanned vacationers to scared parents giving permission for someone to surgically explore our child's brain.

I wanted to slip away. I wanted to hold the picture in my hands and study it. I wanted to zoom in on the unwanted mass and understand why it was there. The mass, what does it mean. She's that sick. She's sitting in my lap. She can walk. She can smile. She looks normal. Can an intruder hide that well? The scans are removed. I didn't hold them. She's in my lap. I'm supposed to be strong.

We left the office and went to Admitting. It takes a long time to process the papers. Another opinion, yes, another opinion would be good. Yes, we probably should ask for a second opinion. We were at the best facility weren't we? We were with the best doctors. It was Friday night. Who would give us a second opinion tonight? She was being admitted. Should we wait? Could we wait? We risked a stroke, death, physical impairment.

I have learned since that the damage done in a rush surgery or by inexperienced hands results in handicaps that might have been prevented. I was lucky not to know this.

*At 4:30 P.M. a nurse called the waiting room. She was out of surgery and the neurosurgeon would be coming to talk with us. The man with the silent eyes approached. I rose, knowing that what he said would change me. If she had survived the surgery, what would her life be like? If she had not survived, how would I?*

*He approached the waiting room with a lightness in his step. Coming straight to the point he said, "Your daughter had an astrocytoma. Her surgery was longer than normal because the tumor was embedded in her brainstem. There is the possibility that some small part of the tumor is still remaining. This will be followed by future CT scans and MRIs."*

*I was seized by an incredible urgency to see her face. I needed to see her. To prove to myself that all of this had been real. And to prove she was still here. She was in recovery. I stood over her and reached for her hand. Her head was turned to one side and I tried to find her eyes. The room was cold and silent except for the beeps of the monitors. She looked small in the huge bed. There was a bandage around her head. It smelled like cold. It felt like cold. It was a place you would run from if you could. I stood there knowing she might not be okay. She might not ever run or laugh or play. This is the moment for prayers. And you hope.*

*She opened her eyes as if she came from heaven. Her eyes lighting a cathedral with a single candle.*

# CHAPTER 3

# Types of Tumors

TUMORS IN THE BRAIN or spinal cord (CNS tumors) are the second most common cancer in children. Symptoms vary depending on the location of the primary tumor. Tumors in the brain and spinal cord may languish for long periods with no growth, or they can dramatically increase in size in a just a few days. Recent advances in diagnosis and treatment have significantly improved the long-term survival rates for many children with CNS tumors.

This chapter begins with a discussion of the causes of brain tumors. It then describes the many types of CNS tumors, including their usual location, rate of growth, and treatment. It ends with a brief overview of treatments for CNS tumors.

## Who gets central nervous system tumors?

CNS tumors are the most common solid tumor in children. Approximately 2,200 children younger than age 20 are diagnosed with brain tumors in the US each year. Because there are many different kinds of brain tumors, the number of children diagnosed with each particular type is small. The incidence of brain tumors is higher in males than females, and higher among white children than any other group.

There has been a steady increase in the number of children diagnosed with CNS tumors over the last twenty years. This increase has been the focus of much research in an attempt to determine why CNS tumors are increasing in children. To learn more about the number of children who get cancer in the US, call (800) 4-CANCER and ask for a free copy of the book "Cancer Incidence and Survival among Children and Adolescents," written by the National Cancer Institute. This publication and additional information are available on the SEER web site at *http://www-seer.ims.nci.nih.gov.*

### Genetic factors

Most CNS tumors occur randomly and have no apparent cause. CNS tumors are, however, associated with several inherited syndromes. The most common inherited disorders are Von Recklinghausen neurofibromatosis, tuberous sclerosis, Turcot syndrome, and von Hippel-Lindau syndrome. Children with these genetic conditions have a greatly increased risk for developing brain tumors. Together, however, they account for less than 5 percent of childhood CNS tumors. Because of their high risk for tumors, children with these conditions should get periodic MRI scans to check for tumors.

## Environmental factors

Very little is known about environmental causes of brain or spinal cord tumors. The best-documented cause of brain tumors is previous radiation to the brain. CNS tumors can develop many years after radiation to the brain for treatment for leukemia or a previous brain tumor. The risk increases with the dose of radiation received.

Other environmental factors, such as electromagnetic radiation and pesticide exposure, have not been confirmed for CNS tumors. Many research studies have evaluated possible environmental causes, but no conclusive answers have yet been found.

# Types of CNS tumors

Tumors of the CNS are classified based on the cell from which they originate and by their rate of growth. CNS tumors develop from astrocytes or neuroglial cells (see Chapter 2, *The Brain and Spinal Cord*). Slower growing tumors are sometimes present for months or years and symptoms are subtle or picked up incidentally. Symptoms that develop over a short period of time usually indicate the presence of a fast-growing tumor.

After a sample of the tumor is obtained during surgery, a pathologist (doctor who specializes in examining body tissues) looks at the tumor under a microscope. He determines the type of tumor, depending upon the cell from which it develops and the rate of cell growth. Unfortunately, there is no uniform classification of brain tumors. Different pathologists may look at the same tumor and give it a different name. This can be very frustrating and confusing for parents. In this chapter, the most common types of tumors found in the CNS are described and alternatives names for the same tumors are provided.

Names for different types of CNS tumors include:

- Medulloblastoma
- Primitive neuroectodermal tumors (PNET)
- Astrocytomas
- Brainstem gliomas

- Ependymomas
- Optic pathway gliomas
- Craniopharyngiomas
- Germ cell tumors (pure germinomas and non-germinoma germ cell tumors)
- Choroid plexus tumors

## Malignant or benign tumor?

The terms malignant and benign are confusing when applied to many CNS tumors. Each tumor must be looked at in terms of rate of growth and location for classification.

All fast-growing tumors are considered malignant (and cancerous). Even if totally removed with surgery, these tumors will usually grow back without further treatment (radiation and/or chemotherapy). Malignant CNS tumors rarely spread to other parts of the body like breast or liver cancer, but most healthcare professionals still consider them to be a type of cancer. Thus, the following usually mean the same thing when used to describe CNS tumors: malignant, fast-growing, or cancer.

Slow-growing tumors are technically classified as benign. These tumors, if they are totally removed with surgery, rarely re-grow. Many slow-growing tumors, however, are found deep within the brain or brainstem, where aggressive surgery is not possible because of significant risk. In these cases other treatments (chemotherapy and/or radiation) are used in an attempt to shrink or halt further tumor growth. Thus, even if a tumor deep in the brain is slow-growing, it may require the same treatments as malignant brain tumors—and these treatments can cause the same long-term side effects. Some health care providers call this "malignant by location."

In this book, tumors are referred to as fast-growing or slow-growing. One must also consider the location of the tumor, along with its rate of growth, to understand the symptoms, likelihood of successful treatment, and possibility of late effects.

A discussion of the specific tumor types follows.

## Medulloblastoma

Medulloblastomas account for about 20 percent of all CNS tumors in children. The most important factors associated with this tumor are location and if the tumor has spread to other areas of the CNS. Medulloblastoma normally grows in the posterior fossa, starting in the cerebellum. As medulloblastomas grow, they sometimes extend into the cerebellar hemispheres, fourth ventricle, or brainstem. Figure 3-1 shows a medulloblastoma growing in the fourth ventricle. Because they can interfere with the

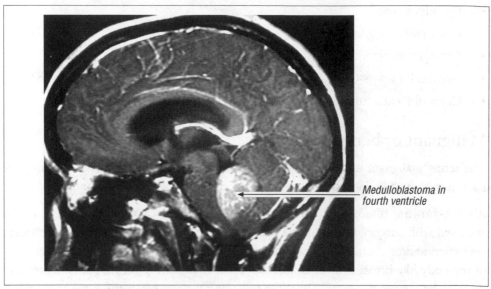

Medulloblastoma in
fourth ventricle

*Figure 3-1. MRI showing medulloblastoma growing in the fourth ventrical*

normal flow of cerebrospinal fluid, hydrocephalus (excess fluid in the brain) is often present at diagnosis. Medulloblastoma can also grow in the cerebral hemispheres. The name for a medulloblastoma-like tumor in the pineal gland is a pineoblastoma.

Unlike most other CNS tumors, medulloblastoma cells can spread throughout the brain and the spinal cord. Twenty five to forty percent of medulloblastoma tumors spread far from the primary tumor. For this reason children should have an MRI scan of the entire brain and spine at diagnosis to determine if the tumor has spread. An analysis of CSF (for presence of tumor cells) by lumbar puncture is also done.

Treatment plans vary depending upon the child's age at diagnosis, amount of tumor removed, and extent of tumor spread. Surgery (in one or several operations) is the first treatment for medulloblatoma. Total removal is the goal. This is sometimes difficult if the tumor has spread to the brainstem or the floor of the fourth ventricle. Medulloblastoma is very responsive to radiation therapy and to many chemotherapy drugs.

Medulloblastoma tumors are grouped into two broad categories: standard-risk and high-risk. A tumor that has been completely removed by surgery and has not spread to other areas of the CNS is called standard-risk. Children with standard-risk medulloblastoma receive craniospinal radiation and chemotherapy.

A medulloblastoma tumor is called high-risk if some tumor remains after surgery or if the tumor has spread to other areas of the CNS. Children less than 3 years old, regardless of the amount of tumor removed, are also classified as high-risk. High-risk medulloblastoma treatment plans include craniospinal radiation, aggressive chemo-therapy, and sometimes peripheral stem cell transplant. Radiation therapy is delayed for children less than 3 years old. (See Chapter 11, *Radiation Therapy*, Chapter 12, *Chemotherapy* and Chapter 14, *Bone Marrow and Stem Cell Transplantation*.)

## Primitive neuroectodermal tumors (PNET)

PNET and medulloblastoma were once considered the same type of tumor that arose in different locations in the brain. Historically, medulloblastoma was the name given to this tumor when it grew in the posterior fossa and PNET when it grew outside of the posterior fossa in the cerebral hemispheres. For many years, the two names were used interchangeably regardless of where the tumor grew. Recent research has shown that the two tumors are biologically distinct. However, they are usually treated the same, although some institutions are using high-dose chemotherapy with stem cell rescue to treat PNET.

## Astrocytomas

Astrocytomas (also called gliomas) are the most common type of CNS tumor in chil-dren. They may be slow-growing or very fast-growing and can arise anywhere in the brain and spinal cord. About 80 percent of astroctomas are slow-growing.

Common names of slow-growing astrocytomas or gliomas include:

• Juvenile pilocytic astrocytoma

• Oligodendroglioma

• Mixed glioma

• Ganglioglioma

Slow-growing astrocytomas in the brain arise in the cerebral hemispheres, the cere-bellum, or the spinal cord. Surgery is the primary treatment for slow-growing astrocy-tomas. This is possible in many areas of the cerebrum and always possible in the cer-ebellum. Multiple surgical procedures are needed if the neurosurgeon is unable to remove the entire tumor in the first surgery.

Chemotherapy and radiation are used for slow-growing tumors that are deep within the brain (hypothalamic or optic pathway glioma), where surgery is not possible, or when only part of the tumor is removed.

Slow-growing astrocytomas account for 75 percent of all spinal cord tumors in chil-dren. Surgery is the primary treatment, and multiple surgical procedures are usually needed to maintain tumor control. Radiation therapy is used for tumors that grow despite multiple surgical procedures. Chemotherapy is not usually given to children with slow-growing spinal cord tumors, so its effectiveness is unknown.

A small number of astrocytoma tumors grow rapidly. They usually grow in the cerebrum or brainstem, and are rarely found in the spinal cord. Types of rapid-growing astrocytomas are:

- High-grade anaplastic astrocytoma

- Glioblastoma multiforme

- Gliomatosis cerebri

High-grade astrocytomas are difficult to cure even with the most aggressive treatments. Surgery, followed by aggressive multi-drug chemotherapy, and radiation therapy are all used to treat these tumors. Chemotherapy for fast-growing astrocytomas may include high-dose chemotherapy with autologous marrow transplant (see Chapter 14).

## Brainstem gliomas

Astrocytomas that grow in the brainstem are called brainstem gliomas. They make up 10 to 15 percent of all pediatric brain tumors. Brainstem tumors can be fast-growing or slow-growing. Ninety percent of these tumors are fast-growing and cause rapidly developing symptoms. They involve multiple levels of the brainstem and have a diffuse appearance on the MRI scan. Surgery is not an option because aggressive surgery in the brainstem would result in severe neurological impairment. Radiation therapy, sometimes with chemotherapy, is the treatment.

About 10 percent of brainstem tumors are slow-growing brainstem gliomas. They usually are located in the medulla or midbrain, and symptoms develop over a long period of time. Treatment alternatives include surgery followed by observation, radiation, and/or chemotherapy.

## Optic pathway/hypothalamic gliomas

Approximately 5 percent of pediatric brain tumors are gliomas that grow around the optic nerves or hypothalamus. These slow-growing tumors sometimes are diagnosed in children with neurofibromatosis 1 (NF1 or Von Recklinghausen). Optic pathway/hypothalamic tumors may lie dormant for extended periods. Observation with careful clinical examination and serial MRI scans is the treatment of choice.

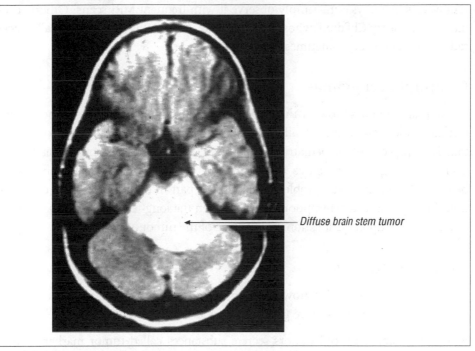

Figure 3-2. MRI showing diffuse brain stem tumor viewed from above

Additional treatment is given if the MRI shows tumor growth or if the child develops symptoms (usually visual or hormonal). The type of treatment depends upon the age of the child and the growth pattern of the tumor. Treatment may include surgery, but usually is chemotherapy (especially in children less than 10 years old). Radiation therapy is the third treatment option, but is rarely used in children under the age of 3. Most neuro-oncologists try to delay radiation therapy for these tumors for as long as possible.

## Ependymoma

Ependymomas make up 8 to 10 percent of childhood brain tumors. They arise from the cells that line the ventricles. About 70 percent of ependymomas occur in the posterior fossa, usually in the fourth ventricle. Ependymomas also occasionally grow in the cerebral hemispheres and in the spinal cord.

Surgery is the first treatment for ependymomas. It is difficult, however, to totally remove an ependymoma in the fourth ventricle because it is close to the brainstem. Treatment of ependymomas after surgery is controversial. If the tumor was totally removed, some physicians simply observe it with frequent MRI scans. Others recommend treatment. Children whose tumors were not totally removed usually receive radiation therapy and sometimes chemotherapy.

## Craniopharyngiomas

Craniopharyngiomas grow in the area of the brain that contains the hypothalamus, pituitary, and optic chiasm (called the supraseller area). They account for approximately 5 percent of all pediatric brain tumors. Treatment is controversial because aggressive surgery often cures the child, but can cause life-long memory, visual, behavioral, and hormonal problems. Taking out part of the tumor followed by radiation therapy is a treatment option that can lessen the long-term side effects. Treatment often depends upon the location and the size of the tumor.

## Germ cell tumors

Germ cell tumors typically grow in the pineal or suprasellar regions. There are two types of germ cell tumors: pure germinomas and non-germinoma germ cell tumors.

Non-germinoma germ cell tumors secrete substances called tumor markers. Doctors can diagnose these tumors by checking the blood or CSF for two markers, called alpha fetal protein and beta HCG. Therefore, diagnosis of a non-germinoma tumor does not require surgery. If the tumor is very large, however, part of it is removed (debulked) if the neurosurgeon feels it can be done with few to no side effects. Treatment for non-germinoma germ cell tumors includes chemotherapy followed by radiation.

Pure germinomas are diagnosed by a surgical biopsy. These tumors dramatically respond to radiation and chemotherapy. Radiation therapy is the gold standard of treatment. Recently, physicians have given chemotherapy following surgery with a reduction in the dose of radiation for those tumors that completely disappear with the chemotherapy. This is an attempt to reduce the dose of radiation needed, possibly reducing long-term side effects. If the tumor disappeared after chemotherapy, the radiation dose is usually reduced.

## Choroid plexus tumors

Choroid plexus papillomas (slow-growing) or choroid plexus carcinomas (fast-growing) arise from the choroid plexus located in the ventricles. The choroid plexus is the part of the brain that produces cerebrospinal fluid. These tumors account for 1 to 3 percent of all childhood brain tumors and most often occur in infants. The tumor is usually diagnosed simultaneously with hydrocephalus. Surgery is the treatment for choroid plexus papillomas. Surgery followed by chemotherapy and radiation is the treatment for choroid plexus carcinomas.

| Type of Tumor | Usual Location | Usual Treatment |
|---|---|---|
| Medulloblastoma PNET | Posterior fossa Cerebral hemispheres | Surgery, chemotherapy, and radiation therapy |
| Astrocytoma (glioma) slow-growing | Cerebral hemispheres and cerebellum Midbrain or brainstem | Total surgical removal, if necessary in stages Surgery, radiation, chemotherapy |
| Astrocytoma (glioma) fast-growing | Cerebral hemispheres | Surgery, chemotherapy, and radiation |
| Brainstem gliomas fast-growing | Brainstem (pons) | Radiation alone or with chemotherapy |
| Brainstem gliomas slow-growing | Brainstem (medulla) | Surgery, observation, radiation, chemotherapy |
| Optic pathway/ hypothalamic gliomas | Hypothalamus, optic nerves | Observation, then chemotherapy if tumor grows. Surgery and radiation therapy are sometimes used. |
| Ependymomas | Ventricular system, most commonly fourth ventricle. Rarely in cerebral hemispheres. | Surgery, radiation, chemotherapy |
| Craniopharyngiomas | Suprasellar region | Surgery alone if total removal, followed by observation If partial removal, follow with radiation |
| Non-germinoma germ cell tumors | Pineal region or suprasellar region | Positive tumor markers, possible surgery, chemotherapy followed by radiation |
| Pure germinomas | Pineal region or suprasellar region | Biopsy or conservative surgery, chemotherapy, and/or radiation |
| Choroid plexus papilloma slow-growing | Choroid plexus in the ventricles | Surgery |
| Choroid plexus carcinoma fast-growing | Choroid plexus in the ventricles | Surgery, chemotherapy, and radiation therapy |

# Treatment

At diagnosis, many parents do not know how to find the best doctors and treatments for their child. State-of-the-art care is available from physicians who participate in the Children's Oncology Group (COG). This study group, composed of pediatric surgeons and oncologists, neurologists, radiation oncologists, researchers, and nurses, develops the standard of care for patients worldwide and conducts new studies to discover better therapies and supportive care for children with all types of cancer. Some individual centers of excellence design their own trials. For further information, read Chapter 9, *Clinical Trials*.

Treatment of CNS tumors includes one or more of the following:

- Surgery
- Chemotherapy
- PBSCT (peripheral blood stem cell transplant)
- Radiation
- Observation

Research continues to evaluate new types of treatment. At the present time areas of exploration include new chemotherapy drugs and biological modifiers (drugs used in conjunction with chemotherapy and radiation therapy, which hopefully will improve responses to treatment). The next section provides a very brief overview of treatments. For more detailed information, refer to the chapters on chemotherapy, radiation, and stem cell transplants.

## Surgery

Surgery is the primary treatment for virtually all CNS tumors and has many important roles. It is used to establish the diagnosis and to remove as much of the tumor as possible. Figure 3-3 shows a low-grade astrocytoma that is usually treated only with surgery. Second-look surgeries are sometimes done after chemotherapy or radiation therapy to see how much tumor remains.

> *The surgery to remove the tumor took about four hours, and there were no major complications. Scott spent three hours in the recovery room before being ready to go to the ICU. His first words after waking were, "I love you, mom," which obviously touched Karen. While in the recovery room, we realized that Scott's stuffed Yoshi toy, who also went to the operating room, returned with a head bandage identical to Scott's. Someone had a sense of humor!*

· · · · ·

> *Kirsten's tumor had shrunk enough after four cycles of chemotherapy for a near total resection. However, the tumor was still considered active, and she went on to receive three further cycles.*

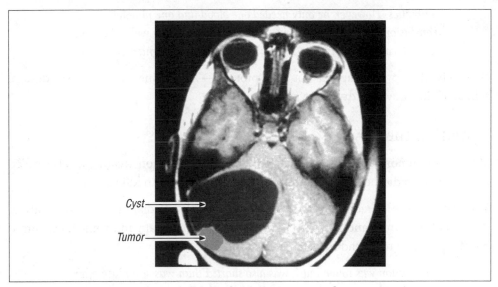

Cyst

Tumor

*Figure 3-3. MRI showing cystic cerebellar low-grade astrocytoma with an associated cyst*

## Chemotherapy

Chemotherapy (drugs that kill cancer cells) is given to many children with CNS tumors. It is used to treat all malignant CNS tumors and many benign tumors as well. Response rates have improved considerably by giving more than one chemotherapy drug at a time. The most commonly used chemotherapy drugs include vincristine, cisplatin, carboplatin, CCNU (lomustine), etoposide, and cyclophosphamide.

Some studies use only one drug at the beginning of therapy in a "window" study. This kind of study attempts to find out if the drug being studied has an effect on CNS tumors on its own. Chemotherapy is sometimes given simultaneously with radiation therapy in an attempt to increase radiation's effectiveness. In this case the chemotherapy is referred to as a radio-sensitizer.

> *Luke (2 years old) had side effects from his chemo protocol that were relatively minor compared to what other children experience. He did have nausea, but it usually consisted of one to three vomiting episodes over one or two days and was over quickly. Over the entire eight course cycle he did have numerous neutropenic bouts (low blood counts), with several visits to the emergency room for night-onset fevers resulting in short-term hospitalizations to get IV antibiotics. He did get two or three infections in his catheter which also required hospitalizations for*

*antibiotics. However, he only needed one blood and one platelet transfusion during the entire protocol. He ate incredibly well all during his protocol and even gained steadily in weight and height.*

Generally, therapy is mapped out in a protocol—an outline of the drugs, dosage, schedule, and ways the drugs are given.

## Radiation therapy

Many CNS tumors are very sensitive to radiation. Radiation treatment, also called irradiation or radiotherapy, is the use of high-energy x-rays to kill cancer cells.

The primary role of radiation is to destroy tumor cells. Radiation is given locally to the area of the tumor and may also be given to the entire brain and spine if the tumor has the potential to spread to other areas of the CNS.

> *Radiation was tough but it was also short. Ethan was still mute after surgery and pretty uncooperative throughout the six weeks, so we had no idea what he wanted to know. We opted to tell him everything: that he had cancer, that he needed radiation to treat the cancer, that they would be putting him to sleep everyday to do the radiation, and that he would lose all his hair, but through it all we would be with him.*
>
> *The radiation to the head and spine lasted 13 days and was the hardest part. Ethan was nauseated (despite ondansetron). He stopped eating completely at one point, and had odd cravings at others. We met with the pediatric oncology dietician and when we asked what we should do if Ethan would only ate French Fries her response was to take him to McDonalds three times a day. While we were shocked at the time, it really helped us readjust our expectations and priorities. Calories became king. Brownies for breakfast? So be it. We were so proud when he ate two instead of just one. These priorities continued into the year of chemotherapy and have served us well. It was a hard adjustment for our other kids (who did not get ice cream upon demand) but they managed.*

## Peripheral stem cell transplants

In the last decade, autologous bone marrow transplants (ABMT) and peripheral blood stem cell transplants (PBSCT) have been used with increasing frequency to treat children with malignant or relapsed CNS tumors. In these procedures, the child receives high-dose chemotherapy, with or without radiation. Normal marrow or stem cells are then infused into the child's veins. The marrow or stem cells migrate to the cavities inside the bones, where new, healthy blood cells are then produced.

> *Sean (18 months old) has now had two rounds of high-dose chemo with stem cell transplants. The first went off without a hitch, the second was a bit of a nightmare. He got a infection, colitis, and then a staph infection in his line. He was in hospital for about 10 days after the stem cell transplant (stinkies). The bad rounds are just part of the drama. I guess we have to expect it, but it never ceases to amaze me how difficult it is to watch him suffer. With Sean's diagnosis of atrypical teratoid/rhabdoid tumor (ATRT), we know that our time with him may be limited and we want to make sure we are focused on giving him the best shot at survival and, as important, the best shot at a joyful, loving life, however long.*

## Observation

Unlike many other cancers, brain tumors (especially slow-growing tumors) may have periods of little or no growth. For this reason, the physician may elect to follow the child with a CNS tumor by performing MRI scans at designated intervals. Observation may be the first treatment if the tumor was diagnosed by chance, is quite small, and causes no symptoms. A period of observation may follow partial removal of a deep, slow-growing tumor (especially in a young child) or in a spinal cord tumor. Lastly, observation occurs following completion of treatment for a malignant CNS tumor.

> *Brendon was diagnosed with a slow-growing tumor of the brainstem when he was 7 years old, after two years of confusing symptoms and dozens of doctor appointments. The first children's hospital told us, "We can't do chemo and we can't radiate it. It's too deep for surgery. Take him home, he has less than 6 months to live." We saw an article about a famous pediatric neurosurgeon in Reader's Digest, and called him. He called us right back and two days later he operated and took out about 90% of the tumor. The treatment was just observation then. We had MRIs every few months. When Brendon was 10 he started getting symptoms again—trouble swallowing, breathing problems, growing paralysis. The tumor was growing inward so surgery wasn't an option. So, we did chemo and it relieved many of the symptoms. Then we observed again. This has been the pattern for the last decade—treat, observe, treat, observe. Brendon is now 16.*

## Biologic modifiers and more

Many researchers are devoting their lives to unlocking the CNS tumor mystery by looking at ways to alter tumor growth. One method uses synthetic copies of proteins (antibodies) to attack foreign cells like cancer. Other substances (cytokines) trigger the body's immune system to halt tumor growth or interrupt cell movement. Tumor vaccine research attempts to reeducate the body to attack tumor cells. Although the research is still in the early stages, it focuses on new treatments that use the individual's immune system to attack CNS tumors.

Researchers also use biological modifiers to open up the blood brain barrier, thus allowing a larger amount of radiation and chemotherapy to penetrate the brain and kill more tumor cells. Although this research is in the early stages, it is hoped that it will improve responses (especially of fast-growing tumors) to current available treatments.

To learn about some of the newest treatments available, call (800) 4-CANCER and ask for the PDQ (physicians data query) for CNS tumors. These free statements, also available on the Internet at *http://cancernet.nci.nih.gov*, explain the disease, state-of-the-art treatments, and ongoing clinical trials. There are two versions available: one for patients, which uses simple language and contains no statistics; and one for professionals, which is technical, thorough, and includes citations to scientific literature. Both are available for free to the public.

*Our daughter was diagnosed with medulloblastoma in the cerebellum when she was 2 years old. We researched, took her to one of the top pediatric neurosurgeons in the country, and he totally resected it. We did more research on treatment options, since radiation at her age would be devastating. But, we also wanted to kill the cancer. We decided on a clinical trial that involved very high-dose chemotherapy with stem cell rescue. Those treatments were incredibly difficult.*

*Two years later, the tumor grew again at the same place, but we caught it early. It was again totally removed, and we again began a research effort on options for treatment. We chose a new type of radiation. It's now been two years, and the cancer has not reappeared. We, like many other families of kids with brain tumors, had to use many different treatment methods over time. We are so grateful that*

*new, and more effective, treatments had been developed to help our
daughter.*

*Our daughter is now 6 years old, goes to school, and loves to dance.
She plays with her younger sibs and has a good life. I do worry about her
future, but am so very glad she is here.*

# CHAPTER 4

# Coping with Procedures

THE PURPOSE OF THIS chapter is to prepare both child and parent for some common medical procedures by providing detailed descriptions of each. Because many of these procedures are repeated frequently during the treatment for childhood CNS tumors, it is important to establish a routine that is comfortable for your child. The procedure itself may cause discomfort, but a well prepared, calm child fares far better than a frightened one.

## Planning for procedures

Procedures are needed to make diagnoses, check for spread of disease, give treatment, and monitor response to treatment. Interventions range from figuring out the best way for your child to take numerous pills to having multiple and time-consuming body scans. Some procedures are pain-free, and the family merely needs clear explanations about what to expect. Others can cause both physical and psychological distress. In some instances, these reactions can be avoided or minimized by medication and good coping skills.

A family-centered approach works best when planning and implementing procedures. The procedures are often as frightening for parents as for children, or even more so. Memories of them can be long lasting. For this reason, children, parents, and staff should work together toward planning for and coping with procedures.

As soon as possible after your child's diagnosis, find out if the hospital has a child life program or other such team (of nurses, psychologists, social workers) that helps prepare families for procedures. The purpose of these programs is to minimize psychological trauma, promote optimal development, and maintain, as much as possible, normal living patterns during hospitalizations. They attempt to minimize the child's stress by giving the child developmentally appropriate explanations of the reasons for procedures and hospital routines. Smaller institutions may not have a child life program. In such cases, your child's nurses will often serve in this role.

*Our child life staff is available for inpatient stays, outpatient procedures, and in the oncology clinic. When Jamie had inpatient admissions during treatment, child life was there, talking to the kids, making cookies with them and running craft projects, and doing play therapy. Our first experience actually took place before treatment. Our pediatrician told us to contact a child life specialist to help James get over his dread of IVs. She pulled out play IV lines, and went through all the steps, and they practiced doing IVs on each other. At clinic, our child life person would come by, and try to distract him while his line was accessed.*

Many child life specialists or other team members accompany children to and provide support during procedures. They establish relationships with children based on warmth, respect, empathy, and understanding of developmental stages. They also communicate with the other members of the healthcare team about the psychosocial needs of children and their families.

Your response, as well as your child's, depends on temperament, age, previous medical or dental experiences, and other factors. Discuss with the child life professional, nurse, or social worker when and how to prepare your child for upcoming procedures. Usually, parents need to experiment with how much advance notice to give younger children about procedures. Some children do better with several days to prepare, while others worry themselves sick. Generally speaking, the younger the child the less the advance notice that is appropriate prior to procedures. Sometimes, needs change over the course of treatment, so good communication and flexibility are essential.

Another general rule is that children fare better with explanations about what sensations they will experience (e.g., see, taste, smell, hear, and feel) rather than giving lengthy technical explanations. Keep explanations short. Adults frequently speak in paragraphs when they should speak in sentences.

*I started giving my 4-year-old daughter two days notice before procedures. But she began to wake up every day worried that "something bad was going to happen soon." So we talked it over and decided to look at the calendar together every Sunday to review what would happen that week. She was a much happier child after that.*

Try to schedule procedures so that the same person does the same procedure each time. Although it may not always be possible, try to arrange for the same doctor or nurse practitioner to do each of your child's procedures, the same nurse to access the

Port-a-cath (See Chapter 10, *Venous Catheters*), and the same technician for blood work. Call ahead to check for unexpected changes to prevent any surprises. Although days off, illnesses, and vacations will interrupt this plan and are unavoidable, repetition can provide comfort and reassurance to children.

Parents can ask for the medical professional with the most experience to perform procedures, such as spinal taps. In the hospital hierarchy, attending physicians are above fellows and residents. However, at many large teaching facilities, attending physicians may not do these procedures very often. Many times, the fellow or resident (and in states where it is allowed, the nurse practitioner) is more skilled, because they do the vast majority of these procedures. It may be helpful to ask, "Who usually performs such procedures?" Parents should have a choice whether to be present or not during a medical procedure. Parents set the tone. A calm parent and a well-prepared child give the best chance for a quick, peaceful procedure. If you find that you are unable to be of help to your child during procedures, ask the child life specialist or other member of the healthcare team to be present solely to comfort your child.

Your job as a parent during the procedure should be one of support and positive distraction—not of restraint or inflicting discomfort. The best place to position yourself is at your child's head, at eye level and out of the field of the procedure. Speak calmly and supportively to your child. You may tell stories or read a favorite book. Praise your child for good behavior but do not reprimand or demean your child if problems occur. Pick a later time to address how things could have gone better and use play therapy to re-enact the experience.

> *We decided from the very beginning that, even though it's no fun to have a spinal, we were going to make something positive out of it. So we made it a party. We'd bring pizza, popcorn, or ice cream to the hospital. We helped Kristin think of the nurses as her friends. We'd celebrate after a procedure by going out to eat at one of the neat little restaurants near the hospital.*

Giving children some control over what happens helps tremendously, but give choices only when they truly exist.

> *Katy and I wrote down her requests for each procedure that first week in the hospital. For example, during spinal taps she wanted me (not a nurse) to hold her in position, she wanted lidocaine to be given with a needle, not the pneumatic gun, and she had a rigid sequence of songs that I sang.*

Oncology clinics usually have a special box full of toys for children who have had a procedure. It sometimes helps for the child to have a treat to look forward to afterward. Some parents occasionally bring a special gift to sneak into the box for their child to find.

# Pain management

The goal of pediatric pain management should be to minimize discomfort while performing the procedure. The two methods to achieve this goal are psychological (using the mind) and pharmacological (using drugs). These two methods can be used together to provide an integrated mind/body approach.

## Psychological method

Preparation for every procedure is essential. Unexpected stress is more difficult to cope with than anticipated stress. If children understand what is going to happen, where it will happen, who will be there, and what it will feel like, they will be less anxious and better able to cope. Methods to prepare children are:

- Verbally explain each step in the procedure.

- If possible, meet the person who will perform the procedure.

- Tour the room where the procedure will take place.

- Small children can "play" the procedure on dolls.

- Older children can observe a "demonstration" on a doll.

- Adolescents may observe a videotape describing the procedure.

- Encourage discussion and answer all questions.

> Ever since I was diagnosed with my brain tumor when I was sixteen, I have been doing research. When I go in for tests, I try and learn as much as possible about what this test will show, and how it is done. I think the research that I have done since I was diagnosed has greatly helped me. I feel like the things that are being done will one day help another person in my shoes. Because I am learning new information, it keeps the testing from getting too boring.

Hypnosis is a well documented method for reducing discomfort during painful procedures. If performed by a qualified healthcare professional (psychologist, physician, nurse, social worker, or child life specialist), hypnosis can help your child control painful sensations, release anxiety, and diminish pain. The professional helps guide children or teens into an altered state of consciousness that helps focus or narrow attention. To locate a qualified practitioner, visit the web page for the American Society of Clinical Hypnosis at *http://www.asch.net/find.htm* or call (630) 980-4740.

Imagery is a way to deliberately create a mental image of sights, sounds, tastes, smells, and feelings and is more commonly used than hypnosis. Imagery is an active process that helps children or teens feel as if they are actually entering the imagined place. Focusing on pleasant images allows the child to shift attention from the pain. It can also allow the child to actually alter the experience of pain, which simultaneously gives the child control and diminishes pain. Ask if the hospital has someone to teach your child this very effective technique.

The following description of the use of imagery was written by Jennifer Rohloff when she was 17 years old and is reprinted from the *Free to Be Yourself* newsletter of Cancer Services of Allen County, Indiana.

### My Special Place

*Many people had a special place when they were young—a special place that they still remember. This place could be an area that has a special meaning for them, or a place where they used to go when they wanted to be alone. My special place location is over the rainbow.*

*I discovered this place when I was twelve years old, during a relaxation session. These sessions were designed to reduce pain and stress brought on by chemotherapy. This was a place that I could visualize in my mind so that I could go there anytime that I wanted to—not only for pain, but when I was happy, mad, or sad.*

*It is surrounded by sand and tall, fanning palm trees everywhere. The blue sky is always clear, and the bright sun shines every day. It is usually quiet because I am alone, but often I can hear the sounds of birds flying by.*

*Every time I come to this place I like to lie down in the sand. As I lie there, I can feel the gritty sand beneath me. Once in a while I get up and go looking for seashells. I usually find some different shapes and sizes. The ones I like the best are the ones that you can hear the sound of the ocean in. After a while I get up and start to walk around. As I walk, I can feel the breeze going right through me, and I can smell the salt water. It reminds me of being at a beach in Florida. Whenever I start to feel sad or alone or if I am in pain, I usually go jump in the water because it is a soothing place for me. I like to float around in the water because it gives me a refreshing feeling that nobody can hurt me here. I could stay in this place all day because I do not worry about anything while I am here.*

*To me this place is like a home away from home. It is like heaven because you can do anything you want to do here. Even though this place may seem imaginary or like a fantasy world to some people, it is not to me. I think it is real because it is a place where I can go and be myself.*

Distraction is used successfully with all age groups, but it should never be used as a substitute for preparation. Babies are distracted by colorful, moving objects. Parents can help distract preschoolers by showing picture books or videos, telling stories, singing songs, or blowing bubbles. Many youngsters find comfort by hugging a favorite stuffed animal. School-age children can watch videos or TV or listen to music. Several institutions use interactive videos to help distract older children or teens.

Other adjuvant therapies that are used successfully to help deal with medical treatments include: relaxation techniques, biofeedback, massage, and acupuncture or acupressure. A physical therapy assistant shares this experience:

*Therapists use massage to decrease edema, improve circulation, decrease muscle spasm, and promote relaxation. This is such a nice part of physical therapy because it goes beyond traditional strengthening or range of motion, often helping to lessen emotional barriers so often present. One patient in particular comes to mind, a teenage boy with cancer. Initially in physical therapy, we focused on range of motion, bracing to support his feet, and strengthening. All too soon he began to spend more time as an inpatient than at home, so we focused on functional living skills. We played basketball, checkers, and even brought in weights to his room. He didn't want to talk with anyone. The only thing that he did request was massages to his "bald head" and his feet. Even a teenager with an attitude and a deadly tumor realized the benefits of massage.*

Children's hospitals are recognizing more and more the need to provide interventions like these for both child and parent. Ask the hospital's physical therapy staff, child life specialist, psychologist, or nurse to discuss these methods with you.

# Pharmacological method

Most pediatric oncology clinics offer the option of sedation and/or anesthesia for painful procedures or non-painful procedures that require that your child lie completely still (i.e., MRI scans). Sometimes anesthesia is available only for infants or overwhelmingly anxious children. If you find that your child is distressed by painful procedures or lengthy procedures that require your child to lie perfectly still, it is reasonable to explore all available options for pain relief.

The ideal pain relief drug for children should be easy to administer, be predictable in effect, provide adequate pain relief, have a short duration, and have minimal side effects. There are three topical anesthetics in wide use for pediatric procedures. EMLA cream is put on the skin one to two hours prior to the painful procedure. Numby Stuff also uses a cream anesthetic, but a mild electrical current helps it penetrate the skin in just a few minutes. Ethyl chloride spray is used immediately before the procedure to anesthetize the surface of the skin. Additionally, lidocaine may be injected under the skin to numb the skin and tissue under it. For more information, see Chapter 12, *Chemotherapy*.

Drugs for sedation and/or general anesthesia are given intravenously. Some facilities take the child into the operating room for the procedure; others use a preoperative area or clinic sedation room and allow the parent to be present the entire time. Drugs used for pediatric anesthesia during procedures include:

- **Valium or Versed plus morphine or fentanyl.** Valium and Versed are sedatives that are used with pain relievers such as morphine or fentanyl. These drugs can be given in the clinic, but the possibility of slowed breathing requires expert monitoring and the availability of emergency equipment. The combination of a sedative and a pain reliever will result in your child's being awake but sedated. The child may move or cry, but will not remember the procedure. Often, EMLA or lidocaine is also used to ensure that the procedure is pain-free.

- Propofol. A milky liquid given by IV, propofol has rapid onset with a rapid recovery. Administration and monitoring by an anesthesiologist (doctor who specializes in giving anesthetics) or an intensive care physician capable of maintaining your child's airway are required. Propofol, a general anesthetic, will cause your child to lose consciousness. It is frequently used as sedation for MRI scans or radiation treatments. At low doses, propofol prevents memory of the procedure, but may not relieve all pain, so it is often used with EMLA or lidocaine.

- **Ketamine.** Ketamine needs the expert monitoring of an anesthesiologist or intensive care physician. It has a much longer recovery time than the drugs listed above; upon awakening, up to 30 percent of children may become confused and/or hallucinate. For these reasons, ketamine is no longer in wide use for pediatric sedation for procedures.

There are many types of drugs and several methods used in administering them, from very temporary (ten minute) mild sedation to full general anesthesia in the operating room. Discuss with your oncologist and anesthesiologist which method will work best for your child.

> Let's face it, kids don't care about lab work or protocols, they just want to know if they are going to be hurt again. I think that one of our most important jobs is to advocate, strongly if necessary, for adequate pain control. If the dose doesn't work and the doctor just shrugs her shoulders, say you want a different dosage or drug used. If you encounter resistance, ask that an anesthesiologist be consulted. Remember that good pain control and/or amnesia will make a big difference in your child's state of mind during treatment.

Emotions may run high after a difficult procedure. Rather than engaging in a lengthy dissection of what went wrong, schedule an appointment time with your physician well in advance of the next scheduled procedure to air your concerns and problem-solve.

Because treatment for CNS tumors can take many months or years, some children build up a tolerance for sedatives and pain relievers. Often, over time, doses may need to be increased or drugs changed. If your child remembers the procedure or feels pain, advocate for a change in drug and/or dosage.

> My five-year-old has been very hard to sedate for medical procedures such as spinal taps. His oncologist experimented with the commonly used drugs, Versed and fentanyl, to find a combination that would work. For some recent procedures, he was premedicated with Ativan. Then he was given Versed and Pentobarb instead of fentanyl. I think we've got it right now, since the last sedation went very well. He still has a full 24 hours of vomiting and headache afterwards (even when he receives antinausea drugs), but at least we don't have to hold him down during spinal taps anymore.

. . . . .

*A new anesthesiologist suggested nitrous oxide before general anesthesia for my young daughter's MRIs. Life around MRIs has never been the same. She is actually excited about scans now as if it is some kind of holiday! The first time with laughing gas she started to go, "Wheeeee!!!!". I asked her if she was feeling like she was on a roller coaster, and she said, "No, I feel like I'm on the TILT-A-WHIRL!" The next day she said, "Mommy, I don't want to go to school today, I want to have ANOTHER SCAN!" I can't say I share her anticipation of a scan, but I am thankful for a good attitude and experience. I keep asking them to share the laughing gas, but they won't!*

All types of sedation require that your child not eat or drink for a number of hours prior to the procedure. Your child may eat or drink when she is alert and able to swallow. All sedation can result in complications, primarily to the airway. It is imperative that sedation be carried out under the care of trained, experienced personnel and that the child be monitored until fully recovered from the anesthesia.

# Procedures

Understanding what will occur during a procedure and what other parents do to prepare their children will arm you with essential information. Knowing what to expect will lower the anxiety level of both parent and child and lay the foundation for months of tolerable tests. The descriptions of procedures in the rest of the chapter may not exactly mirror your experience. Practices vary by hospital and practitioner, and this variability should be expected. What should be the same, however, is your comfort in asking questions and getting the support and help you need to prepare for and cope with your child's procedures.

## Questions to ask before procedures

Parents need information prior to procedures in order to prepare themselves and their child. Some suggested questions to ask the physician or nurse practitioner are:

- Why is this procedure necessary for my child and how will it affect her treatment?

- What information will it provide?

- Who will perform the procedure?

- Will it be an inpatient or outpatient procedure?

- Please explain the procedure in detail.

- Is there any literature available that describes it?

- Is there a child life specialist on staff who will help prepare my child for the procedure?

- If not, are there nurses, social workers, or parents who can come talk to me about how to prepare my child?

- Is the procedure painful?

- How long will the procedure take?

- What type of anesthetic or sedation is used?

- What are the risks, if any?

- What are the common and rare side effects?

- When will we get the results?

## Accessing catheters

The procedure that occurs most often during treatment, and can be the most or the least worrisome is accessing your child's central venous catheter. This is described in detail in Chapter 10.

> Mary Margaret had a terrible time having her port accessed. She would scream and cry (probably terrifying the other kids waiting outside the room for their turn!) and I became an expert at holding her down. I'd lie down next to her, holding down her hands, pressing my knee on her legs to keep her from kicking, and with my head on her forehead. It was horrible. I don't think it was particularly painful, just a terrible invasion for her, and she knew she'd feel badly after her treatment. We ended up meeting with the neuropsychologist on staff at the Hem-Onc office. The doctor was wonderful and warm, she talked to MM about why having her port accessed bothered her so much, and we talked about ways that she might cope. The doc made some good suggestions: listening to music, looking at a book, dreaming herself somewhere else, and then accompanied MM and me into the procedure room. MM was calm and completely still through the whole procedure, and never made a fuss again about having her port accessed. I'm very grateful.

## Angiogram

An angiogram is a special x-ray procedure to evaluate the circulation and blood supply in an area of tumor in either the brain or spinal cord. This procedure is performed in the radiology department and requires sedation or general anesthesia, depending on your child's age and temperament. No food or liquids are allowed for a period of time prior to the procedure. A catheter is put in a blood vessel in the groin, then threaded up to the area that needs to be evaluated. Dye is injected and doctors can see the blood supply to the tumor. After the procedure, your child will go to the recovery room until she is awake and then back to her room.

## Audiogram

Some of the chemotherapy drugs that children receive for treatment of CNS tumors can cause hearing loss. Additionally, some children with CNS tumors experience hearing loss as a result of injury to nerves caused by the tumor itself or from surgery. Your child's doctor may order a hearing test, called an audiogram, to monitor for possible hearing problems.

During the audiogram, your child is tested in a soundproof room to prevent outside noises from interfering. You can remain with your child during this procedure. Earphones are placed on her ears, through which sounds, such as beeps and tones, are relayed. Your child will be asked to signal when she has heard the sound by either raising her hand or pressing a button. Each ear is tested separately. The results of the audiogram are then usually displayed in the form of a graph. The amount of hearing loss is measured in decibels.

Audiograms are repeated throughout therapy to monitor your child's hearing if he is taking drugs that place him at risk.

> Matthew experienced some high-frequency hearing loss from the
> cisplatin. I think to Matthew, stepping into the soundproof booth and
> putting on his headset was somewhat like a game. The first few audiograms
> were done with me sitting in the booth beside him. Eventually, he reached
> a point where he felt he could do this test on his own.

## Brainstem auditory evoked response (BAER)

Auditory brainstem evoked studies use clicking sounds to evaluate the central auditory pathways of the brainstem. This test is used to evaluate children in whom standard audiometric testing is not possible, either because of age or inability to respond.

During the test, clicking noises or tone bursts are delivered through earphones. Your child's brain waves are measured by electrodes placed along the scalp and on each earlobe. The test is not painful and takes about 30 minutes to perform.

> *BAER was very easy, quick, and painless. They attach leads to Mary Margaret's head, very gently, and it didn't get tangled up in her hair or anything. Then they put earphones on, and the doctor told her she would hear a series of clicks in one ear, and a whooshing sound in the other, and to just sit still. So she did, and the little lines come out on the computer screen. The doctor duly recorded all the highest humps in the lines, and switched ears. Then they did the TV part, which I think is called VAER. MM stared at a small American flag in the center of a TV screen. She's good at staring at TV, so this was not difficult for her. The rest of the screen is small black and white squares, and they move around as the child stares at the flag in the center. I would say the test took about five minutes of sitting and staring.*

## Blood draws

Frequent blood draws are a part of life during radiation and chemotherapy. Blood specimens are employed for a number of purposes: to obtain a complete blood cell count (CBC), evaluate blood chemistries and anticonvulsant drug levels, or culture the blood to check for infection. A CBC measures the types and numbers of cells in the blood. It tells the physician how susceptible to infection the child is. The CBC also tells when a red blood cell or platelet transfusion is needed. Blood chemistries measure substances contained in the blood plasma to determine if the liver and kidneys are functioning properly and whether doses of chemotherapy need to be adjusted. Anticonvulsant levels in the blood tell your child's physician whether the dose of medication is therapeutic or whether it needs to be increased or decreased. Blood cultures help evaluate whether the child has developed a bacterial or fungal infection. For a list of normal blood counts, see Appendix A, *Blood Counts and What They Mean*.

If only a CBC is needed, a finger poke will provide enough blood. Blood chemistries, anticonvulsant levels, and cultures require one or more vials of blood obtained from a vein in the arm or the right atrial catheter.

Blood is usually drawn from the large vein on the inside of the elbow using a procedure similar to starting an IV, except that the needle is removed rather than left in the arm. The advice in the section "Starting an IV," later in this chapter, also applies to drawing blood from the arm.

Children with catheters usually have blood drawn from the catheter rather than the arm or finger. These procedures are described in Chapter 10.

## Blood transfusions

Chemotherapy and radiation can cause severe anemia (a low number of oxygen-carrying red blood cells). Many children require transfusions of red cells periodically throughout treatment.

> Whenever my son needed a transfusion, I brought along bags of coloring books, food, and toys. The number of VCRs at the clinic was limited, so I tried to make arrangements for one ahead of time. When anemic (hematocrit below 20 percent), he didn't have much energy, but by the end of the transfusion, his cheeks were rosy and he had tremendous vitality. It was hard to keep him still. After one unit (bag) of red cells, his hematocrit usually jumped up to around 30.

The volume of red blood cells to be given is based on your child's weight and current hemoglobin and/or hematocrit. The total transfusion takes three to four hours and is given through an intravenous line or your child's right atrial catheter. If your child develops chills and/or fever during a transfusion (signs of a transfusion reaction), the nurse should be notified so that the transfusion can be stopped immediately.

There are some risks of infection from red cell transfusions. Because new tests have been devised to detect the AIDS virus, the risk of exposure is minuscule, less than 1 in 450,000. Although there are excellent tests for the various types of hepatitis, exposure to this disease is still possible, although the risk is less than 1 in 4,000. The cytomegalovirus is also a concern. These risks are the reason transfusions are given only when absolutely necessary.

> My daughter received several transfusions at the clinic in Children's Hospital with no problems. After we traveled back to our home, she needed her first transfusion at the local hospital. Our pediatrician said to expect to be in the hospital at least eight hours. I asked why it would take so long when it only took four hours at Children's. He said he had worked out a formula and determined that she needed two units of packed cells. I mentioned that she only was given one unit each time at Children's. He called the oncologist, who said it was better to give only one unit. We went to the hospital where a unit of red cells was given. Then a nurse came in with another unit. I questioned why he

*was doing that and he said, "Doctor's orders." I asked him to verify
that order, as we had already discussed it with the doctor. He went
into another room to call the doctor, and came back and said the
pediatrician thought she needed 30 cc more packed cells. I called
Children's and they said she didn't need more, so I told them not to
give the second unit. It just wasn't worth the risk of hepatitis to get
30 cc of blood. Even though I was pleasant, the nurses were angry
at me for questioning the doctor.*

## Bone growth x-ray

A bone density test is a plain x-ray of your child's non-dominant hand and wrist. It is
performed to determine whether your child's growth is appropriate for her age. The
x-ray film is compared to a series of photographs of wrist films of children of all ages,
and the radiologist is able to define your child's "bone age" compared to her chrono-
logical age. This will help determine the need for further endocrinologic evaluation
and testing. This test takes only a few moments to perform and is not painful.

## Bone marrow aspiration/biopsy

Bone marrow aspirations or biopsies are done as part of the diagnostic workup for
several types of CNS tumor to see if the tumor has spread to the bone marrow. They
are also done prior to bone marrow or stem cell transplantation.

A bone marrow aspiration sucks bone marrow out of bone cavities with a needle. Bone
marrow biopsies remove a small piece of bone marrow with a special biopsy needle.

Unless sedated, many children and teens describe bone marrow aspirations as uncomfortable to unbearable. EMLA cream, a topical anesthetic, can be applied one to two
hours prior to the aspiration to help numb the area. Lidocaine is often injected under
the skin to numb the subcutaneous tissues and the outside layer of bone. Most institutions sedate children to do an aspiration or biopsy.

> *Melissa (age 5) has had several bone marrow aspirations since
> her diagnosis in 1995. We always use propofol (which I refer to as
> the "milk of human kindness," because of its milky appearance)
> before the procedure. After the aspiration is over, Melissa wakes up
> from a very deep sleep and has felt no pain whatsoever. She's usually
> hungry and ready to go ASAP. Propofol has worked exceptionally
> well for her.*

## Bone scan

A bone scan is a special test that is performed in the nuclear medicine department to evaluate a particular bone or the entire skeletal system. It is often used when the oncologist suspects spread of the tumor to bone. Although extremely rare in CNS tumors, such spread is possible.

Your child is given an injection of a radioactive material, called technetium, that travels through the blood to the bones. The injection is given through your child's right atrial catheter or an IV line. Approximately two hours later, your child will lie on a table and a large machine will move above her. It takes only a few minutes and there is no pain. You should be allowed to stay with your child during this procedure.

## Computed tomography (CT)

Computed tomography (CT) is also called "CAT" for computerized axial tomography. CT is a complex, computer enhanced procedure for obtaining x-ray images of the body. The machine looks very much like a big donut, and your child will be placed in the hole in the middle. Instead of having a fixed x-ray directed at one part of the body, during a CT scan an x-ray tube rotates around the body, generating hundreds of images as it moves. These images are called "slices," similar to slicing a loaf of bread.

CT imaging allows the doctor to see CNS structures in great detail. Development of the CT scan was a major step forward in the diagnosis, evaluation, and treatment of CNS tumors. It is used to look at the relationship between the tumor and bone. Although MRI is now the gold standard for evaluation of CNS tumors, CT is still a good screening tool.

Before the procedure begins, your child may need to receive a liquid dye, called a contrast agent. The contrast agent is given intravenously for CNS tumors. In the event that your child requires a CT scan of the abdomen or pelvis for another reason, oral contrast is given as well. The technologist will position your child in a manner so that the area being imaged will be inside the opening of the CT machine. The technologist does not stay in the room when the images are taken.

If you plan to remain with your child, you will need to wear a lead apron to protect your body from unnecessary exposure to radiation. Sometimes, if the site being imaged is the chest area, your child may be asked to breathe in and hold her breath for several seconds. It is important that your child remain still during the CT scanning process. Small children who are unable to remain motionless for several minutes at a time are sedated before the procedure. You are usually asked to stay in the department until the images have been reviewed by the technologist to ensure that they are adequate.

> *The first few scans, they used pentobarb to sedate our son. He was wobbly and sleepy for 24 hours after. Then they switched to propofol to sedate him. He went right to sleep and woke up after the scan without the after-effects. He is now 5 years out off treatment, and he no longer needs sedation for scans. But, one thing that I really appreciate is that the radiologist reviews the scans before we go home. We leave knowing that everything is okay. It breaks my heart that some families need to wait days to find out the results of scans.*

## Conventional x-ray

X-rays, a type of electromagnetic radiation, provide the doctor with a quick and simple method of viewing organs and structures inside your child's body. Pictures are taken and then displayed on a film or a computer screen X-rays are performed for many reasons during a child's treatment for a CNS tumor. Some of the most common reasons for taking x-rays are:

- Needed before operations

- Needed after your child's central venous catheter is placed to confirm that it is in the proper location

- Used to check cerebrospinal fluid shunt placement

- Used as part of a workup for fever to determine whether your child may have pneumonia

Your child is positioned by the technologist in a manner that will make it easiest to get the images that are needed. For chest x-rays, your child may be asked to breathe in, hold her breath, and remain perfectly still for a few seconds. The technologist leaves the room during the time that the x-rays are taken. As with CT scans, if you are planning to stay with your child, you need to wear a lead apron to protect you from radiation. Your child may also have to wear a lead apron or lead shield to protect specific areas of her body. Pregnant women should not be present in the room when x-rays are taken.

# Echocardiogram/EKG

Several drugs used to treat CNS tumors can damage the muscle of the heart, decreasing its ability to contract effectively. Many protocols require a baseline echocardiogram to measure the heart's ability to pump before any chemotherapy drugs are given. Echocardiograms are then given periodically during and after treatment to check for heart muscle damage.

An echocardiogram uses ultrasound waves to measure the amount of blood that leaves the heart each time it contracts. This percentage (blood ejected during a contraction compared to blood in the heart when it is relaxed) is called the ejection fraction.

A technician, nurse, or doctor administers the echocardiogram. The child or teen lies on a table and has conductive jelly applied to the chest. Then the technician puts a transducer (which emits the ultrasound waves) on the jelly and moves the device around on the chest to obtain different views of the heart. Pressure is applied on the transducer and can sometimes cause discomfort. The test results are displayed on videotape and photographed for later interpretation.

> *Meagan used to watch a video during the echocardiogram. Sometimes*
> *she would eat a sucker or a Popsicle. She found it to be boring, not painful.*

An EKG (electrocardiogram) measures the electrical impulses that the heart generates during the cardiac cycle. Prior to placing the electrodes, the technician will clean the area with alcohol and will apply a cool gel under the electrodes. The test is performed at the bedside, in the cardiologist's office or in the cardiac clinic or lab. Your child must lie quietly during the test and you may remain with him throughout the procedure, which generally takes less than ten minutes. Your child will feel nothing during the procedure other than the gel on the electrodes.

# Electroencephalogram (EEG)

The most widely used method for diagnosing any type of seizure disorder is the electroencephalogram, or EEG. During an EEG, measures of the electrical activity generated by the brain are taken. There is no health risk from an EEG, with the exception of several very specialized types of EEG (depth and subdural grid EEG), which are discussed below.

To prepare for an EEG, wash your child's hair before the test and avoid conditioner, creams, hairspray, oils, gels, and elaborate hairstyles. Your child should avoid caffeinated drinks for a day before the test. Although the test is not painful, a mild sedative is sometimes used before the test is performed.

For the most common type of EEG test, usually called a scalp EEG, the neurologist or EEG technician will apply 21 electrodes to your child's scalp with gooey, strong-smelling glue. Each disc is strategically placed to capture the brain wave activity from a different region of the brain, and each is attached to a wire called a lead. Because the heart's electrical activity can skew EEG results, it is usually monitored by a separate electrode placed on the chest. The loose end of each lead is attached to the EEG machine itself, which amplifies the tiny amount of sensed activity, making graphing possible. The EEG machine will represent the electrical output of your child's brain on a piece of paper, on a computer screen, or both. The basic type of EEG test lasts between half an hour and two hours. During the test, the neurologist or EEG technician may try some things that could provoke a seizure. Your child may be asked to look at a flashing light (photic stimulation) or breathe rapidly for several minutes (hyperventilation).

> Anna was about 3 and a half when she had one of her first EEGs. The technician we had told her the leads were like a rainbow. He told her the story of the rainbow, what it really means. He had a story for each of the colors, and talked in a very calm and soothing voice. He told her he was going to make her look very important, just like a rainbow. From that time on, she has referred to all her EEGs as "Rainbow Hair." The tech told us he would call it a "clown wig" for the boys. He was great!

Sleep-deprived EEGs are administered after a period of sleep deprivation. Sleep deprivation lowers the seizure threshold dramatically, and deep sleep is a time when some kinds of seizures are more likely to occur. For this test, your child must stay up all or most of the night and then have the scalp EEG performed in the morning. Once the electrodes are hooked up and the neurologist has reviewed the initial brain activity, your child will be allowed to go to sleep. The dual challenge of sleep deprivation and deep sleep often evokes seizure activity.

Videotaped EEG is performed while your child is simultaneously being videotaped. By comparing your child's visual symptoms and you or your child's reported symptoms with the EEG data, subtle correlations may be made.

The depth EEG requires surgery to temporarily put electrodes into your child's brain. Your child's head will be placed in a frame that is pinned to your child's skull. CT or MRI scanning will then help the doctor decide on positioning of the electrodes. The neurosurgeon will carefully drill through the skull and insert the electrodes into those parts of your child's brain where seizure activity is suspected. Because there are no nerve endings inside the skull, this is not painful; however, some people experience discomfort despite the use of local anesthetic. A post-procedure headache is a common occurrence; your child will have a bandage on her head and her scalp may be sore for up to four weeks. Depth (or subdural) electrodes are not used in highly sensitive areas of the brain, such as those affecting speech or movement.

Subdural grid EEG involves placing a grid or strip of electrodes on the surface of the brain. The electrodes do not penetrate the surface of the brain. This type of EEG is most frequently used when seizures occur in areas affecting language or movement. The grid is usually kept in place for two or more weeks before being removed during a second operation. As with the depth EEG, your child's head will be sore afterwards and will need time to heal thoroughly.

## Electromyogram (EMG)

An electromyogram measures the electrical activity of a specific skeletal muscle. The study is generally performed in an EMG laboratory. Your child's position for the examination is determined by the specific muscle being evaluated. Local anesthetic or topical analgesic agents (such as EMLA cream) are applied prior to the test. A fine small needle that acts as a recording electrode is inserted into the muscle. Additionally, a small skin electrode, such as that used in an electrocardiogram, is placed on the skin surface. Your child needs to lie still for a baseline reading and then contract the muscle repeatedly for several seconds. The neurologist and technician will then evaluate the monitor readings for evidence of abnormal or diminished function. Sedation is generally not used for this test, because your child's participation is necessary. Your child may experience some discomfort from the needle insertion (similar to an intramuscular injection). You may stay with your child throughout the procedure.

> Jessica (age 10) is having treatment for anaplastic astrocytoma, and has a lot of muscle weakness on one side. For the EMG, they put these circuits on her foot and then checked to get a reading while they put a little current there. They shocked her a little each time they did it. They did it on the foot and the knee on the left side, which is her weakest side, and also did a muscle check on her left arm and hand. The doctor was great and had her giggling much of the time. We got to hear what Jessica's muscle sounded like when she moved.

## Finger pokes

Finger pokes are different from blood draws in several ways. First, EMLA can be used successfully. Put a blob of EMLA on the tip of the middle finger. Cover the fingertip with plastic wrap, and tape it on the finger. Another method is to buy long, thin balloons with a diameter a bit wider than your child's finger. Cut off the open end, leaving only enough to cover the finger up to the first knuckle. Fill the tip of the balloon with EMLA and slide it on the fingertip. EMLA needs to be applied an hour before a finger poke to be effective. At the laboratory, remove the plastic wrap or balloon, wipe off the EMLA, and ask for a warm pack. Wrapping this heated pack around the finger for a few minutes opens the capillaries to allow the blood to flow out more readily. Now your child is ready for a pain-free finger poke.

The technician will hold the finger and quickly stick it with a small sharp instrument. Blood will be collected in narrow tubes or a small container. It is usually necessary for the technician to squeeze the fingertip to get enough blood. If EMLA is not used, the squeezing part is uncomfortable and the finger can ache for quite a while.

> Even though we use EMLA, Katy (5 years old) still becomes angry
> when she has to have a finger poke. I asked her why it was upsetting if
> there was no pain, and she replied, "It doesn't hurt my body anymore, but
> it still hurts my feelings."

## Gallium scan

Gallium scans are performed in the nuclear medicine department. Prior to the scan, your child will be injected with a radiopharmaceutical, called gallium citrate. Your child's right atrial catheter may be used for the injection, or you may apply EMLA cream to a peripheral vein site prior to the injection. Usually, the scan is performed 24 to 48 hours after the injection. Gallium localizes at sites of infection and malignancy. The procedure takes about 30 minutes. Your child needs to lie flat on an examination table while the machine scans above. The machine makes noise, but is not painful. You can stay with your child during this procedure.

## Gastrostomy

A gastrostomy is a feeding tube placed through the abdominal wall into the stomach. Gastrostomy tubes are often placed so that nutrition can be provided directly in a child's stomach. This is appropriate for children who cannot eat normally because of chronic swallowing problems or long-term pain in the mouth or throat or for children who have lost their normal appetite for a prolonged period because of disease or treatment. The stomach end of the feeding tube has a small balloon that prevents it from being accidentally pulled all the way out.

A skilled gastroenterologist or surgeon can perform the procedure in about ten minutes. Most children have general anesthesia for the procedure and remain in the hospital for one to two days postoperatively to receive pain medication and make sure that they tolerate feedings through the tube. Care of the tube is simple, and after two to three months the tube may be replaced with an unobtrusive skin-level device called a button. After a short recovery, children may play, bathe, and swim normally.

The tube is used for liquid feedings and medications as long as the child requires. If a child no longer requires the tube, it is removed and a bandage is placed over the site. The wound closes spontaneously in a day or two.

## Magnetic resonance imaging (MRI)

MRI uses a magnetic field to create two-dimensional images of a cross section of the brain or spinal cord. Your child may need to receive a liquid dye, called a contrast agent, prior to or during the scan. This can be administered through your child's central venous catheter or via a peripheral IV. The child lies on a platform that slides into a long tube. Inside the tube is a donut-shaped magnet. A special device, called a surface coil, is then placed around the area of the body that is to be imaged.

> From ages 2 to 5, our son was anesthetized for MRIs. Depending on what they used, he'd either come out acting like a little drunk, or be crabby all day, or sometimes have vomiting. At the children's hospital, they used IV sedation, versed and nembutol, which often made him sick. Our local hospital used liquid chloral hydrate, which he absolutely hated to take. When he turned five, the nurse asked me if I thought he could do the MRI without sedation; of course I thought no way. But she asked him, and he said, "I don't have to take the icky medicine? I can do that!" They told him when he could move a little and when he needed to lie perfectly still, and he did it!
>
> • • • • •
>
> Since the beginning, we've sent each of our MRIs to our pediatric neuro-oncologist for a second opinion. The radiologist will write "no change" on their report. Our neuro-oncologist provides tumor dimensions, mentions how much enhancement compares to last time, mentions structures that are looking the same or are looking different. It can be like night and day in terms of value of the information that you get for long-term follow-up.

The technologist does not stay in the room during the MRI. The MRI machine makes a loud knocking noise as the images are taken. Your child may need to wear special earplugs to help block out this sound. Young children, or any child with a fear of closed-in spaces (claustrophobia), may need to be sedated for the MRI procedure. MRI takes longer to perform than CT scans and requires that your child lie perfectly still to prevent motion artifact in the scan pictures. Although some centers now have open MRI scanners, this is not currently available in the majority of hospitals. Some doctors feel that magnet technology in open MRI scanners used by some facilities is not yet up to par with older closed machines, which may affect degree of detail, although this should improve over time. MRI is considered the gold standard for imaging of CNS tumors.

> We don't run around trying to get copies of scans after the fact (the ones made then aren't as clear anyway and cost money). We ask the technician for a second set of MRI scans to be made the same day it's taken. That way we always have sets to pull out for consults and other doctor visits. We've also learned that it appears to help with interpreting MRIs to use the same MRI machine, and we also try to get the same technician.

A medical oncologist offers this advice regarding MRI interpretations:

> A neuro-radiologist is usually the best person to notice small details or to give interpretations of unusual abnormalities in scans. Any "neuro doctor" who knows your case well—neurologist or neurosurgeon—is likely to be the best person to decide what a change in your scan means in your particular case. This is especially true if the doctor is someone who spends much of his or her time dealing with brain tumors.

## MUGA scan

A multiple-gated acquisition (MUGA) scan tests cardiac function. It is more sensitive than an echocardiogram and is generally ordered if the echocardiogram shows abnormality. Prior to having a MUGA scan, children are sometimes given a sedative to help them relax and stay perfectly still for the fifteen- to twenty-minute test. An injection of red cells or proteins tagged with a mildly radioactive substance (called technetium) is given through an IV. The child lies on a table with a large movable camera above. This special camera records sequential images of the technetium as it moves through the heart. These pictures of the heart's function allow doctors to determine how efficiently the heart muscle is pumping and if any damage to the heart has occurred.

> My three-year-old daughter had a MUGA scan before she started chemotherapy. They gave her an injection, and she fell asleep. They laid

*her on her back on a big table and moved a huge contraption around her*
*to take pictures of her heart beating. We watched on a screen, and they*
*printed out a copy on paper for the doctors.*

If either the echocardiogram or MUGA scan shows heart damage, the oncologist may reduce the dosage or remove the drug causing the damage from your child's protocol.

## Needle aspiration biopsy

Needle aspiration biopsies are sometimes used to obtain a sample of cells from a mass in an accessible area. Prior to the biopsy, children need to fast for several hours. The doctor will first use ultrasound, CT, or fluoroscopy images to determine the exact location of the mass. Once your child has been anesthetized, a needle is guided into the mass and a sample is removed. The sample is then sent to a pathologist, who will view the cells under a microscope. Your child will need to stay in bed for the next several hours with vital signs closely monitored to ensure there is no bleeding.

## Neuropsychological testing

Neuropsychological testing encompasses a broad category of oral, written, and performance tests that help to define and describe your child's level of functioning. If your child's condition allows, it is best to perform such tests prior to surgery, but sometimes this is impossible. Postoperative and post-therapy testing performed every few years is important to document cognitive function and to assist with planning educational and rehabilitative interventions for your child. For more information on neuropsychological testing, see Chapter 20, *School*.

## Platelet transfusions

Platelets are an important component of the blood. They help form clots and stop bleeding by repairing breaks in the walls of blood vessels. A normal platelet count for a healthy child is $150,000/mm^3$ to $420,000/mm^3$. Chemotherapy severely depresses the platelet count for most children. If a transfusion is not given, uncontrollable bleeding can result. Many centers require a transfusion when the child's platelet count goes below 10,000 to $20,000/mm^3$, and sometimes repeat transfusions are required every two or three days until the marrow recovers. In some cases, the platelet count may need to be higher for patient safety. For patients with CNS tumors, such situations include recent surgery and radiation therapy. In these situations, your physician may want the platelet count to be above 50,000.

*Justin had a platelet reaction which caused profuse sweating and difficulty breathing. They stopped the transfusion immediately, and he got over it.*

• • • • •

*Three-year-old Matthew had countless platelet transfusions, and only once did he have a reaction. It was an awful thing to watch, but the nurse that was monitoring him was very calm and professional, which helped both of us. Matthew was always premedicated for his platelet transfusions with Benadryl, which made him very drowsy. Most often he would sleep through the entire transfusion.*

Infections transmitted by platelets are identical to those of other blood products: hepatitis, cytomegalovirus, and HIV (the virus that causes AIDS). The chance of contracting these infections is very small. Because uncontrollable bleeding can be life threatening, prevention is paramount. Platelet transfusions require less time to administer than red blood cell transfusions. Generally one hour is needed to complete such a transfusion.

## Pulmonary function tests

Some of the chemotherapy drugs that children receive can damage the lungs. Your child's doctor may order a pulmonary function test to evaluate her respiratory status. The basic pulmonary function test is called a spirogram. Your child will blow into the machine to measure the amount of air that she can inhale and exhale. The respiratory technician who administers the test will coach and instruct your child throughout the procedure to ensure that she is giving her maximum effort. The test is administered at least three times to ensure that the results are reliable. You can stay with your child while this test is done.

Your child cannot take this test if she is agitated, is in pain, or is too young to cooperate with the procedure. Your child should not take any bronchodilators or use an inhaler for six hours prior to the procedure. Also, be sure to have a list of medications your child is currently taking with you, because this is necessary for proper test interpretation.

*Our son didn't like having pulmonary function tests. On the outside, it looks so simple. But blowing into the spirogram was hard for him. He was usually a little tired after the test was complete. We would always make a trip to the hospital gift shop afterwards, because we felt he deserved a special treat for working so hard.*

## SPECT scan

A single photon emission tomography (SPECT) scan is a new test used to measure uptake of various metabolites within the brain. It is used to differentiate between brain cells, tumor cells, and scars. It uses a machine similar to an MRI. Sedation or short-term general anesthesia may be necessary if your child is unable to lie still and, in that case, your child will have to refrain from eating or drinking before the procedure. You can usually remain in the room with your child.

## Spinal tap (lumbar puncture or LP)

Due to the blood-brain barrier, systemic chemotherapy sometimes cannot destroy tumor cells present in the central nervous system (brain and spinal cord). Chemotherapy drugs may have to be directly injected into the cerebrospinal fluid in order to kill any tumor cells present. For certain diseases (i.e., medulloblastoma, ependymoma), spinal taps are used to monitor response to treatment. Spinal taps are diagnostic (done to obtain a specimen of fluid for analysis) or therapeutic (done to inject chemotherapy).

Some hospitals routinely sedate children for spinal taps, and others do not. As with other intrusive procedures, your child's age and temperament will influence whether the procedure requires this. Additionally, this procedure is sometimes performed at the time your child is undergoing a general anesthesia for another reason, such as central venous catheter placement. If the child is not sedated, EMLA cream is usually prescribed. This anesthetic cream is applied to the spinal tap site one to two hours prior to the procedure to anesthetize deep into the tissue and prevent some or all of the pain associated with the procedure. For more information about EMLA, see "Starting an IV." Have your physician or nurse practitioner show you where to apply the cream. To perform a spinal tap, the physician or nurse practitioner will ask the child to lie on her side with her head tucked close to the chest and knees drawn up. A nurse or parent usually helps hold the child in this position.

> During spinals, Brent listens to rock and roll on his Walkman, but he
> keeps the volume low enough so that he can still hear what is going on.
> He likes me to lift up the earpiece and tell him when each part of the
> procedure is finished and what's coming next.

It is essential that your child hold very still for the rest of the procedure. The doctor will push a fine, hollow needle between two vertebrae into the space where cerebrospinal fluid (CSF) is found. The CSF will begin to drip out of the hollow needle into a container. After a small amount is collected, a syringe is attached to the needle in the back and the medicine is slowly injected, causing a sensation of coldness or pressure down the leg. The needle is then removed and the spot bandaged. Occasionally, older children and teenagers get severe headaches from spinal taps. Lying flat for up to an hour after the procedure can sometimes prevent these.

If your child develops a persistent severe headache following the procedure that abates while he lies flat, but throbs when he sits up, notify your physician or nurse, keep your child lying flat, and offer high-caffeine beverages, such as Mountain Dew. If these measures fail to give your child relief, an anesthesiologist sometimes does a procedure called a "blood patch." Your child lies in the same position as for the spinal tap. The anesthesiologist will draw a small amount of blood from your child's arm or central line. She will then inject it at the site of the prior spinal tap where CSF may be slowly leaking from the canal into the tissues. If this is the cause of the headache, the relief is immediate. This procedure is generally performed in the recovery room, emergency room, clinic, or inpatient unit. You can stay with your child during the procedure.

## Starting an IV

Many pediatric hospitals have teams of technicians who specialize in starting IVs and drawing blood. In other situations, the nurses or physician caring for your child will start the IV. The IV technician will generally use a vein in the lower arm or hand. First, a constricting band is put above the site to make the veins larger and easier to see and feel. The vein is felt by the technician, the area is cleaned, and the needle is inserted. Sometimes a needle is left in place and sometimes it is withdrawn, leaving only a thin plastic tube in the vein. The technician will make sure that the needle (or tube) is in the proper place, then will cover the site with a clear dressing and secure it with tape.

Some methods that help when having an IV started are:

- **Stay calm.** The body reacts to fear by constricting the blood vessels near the skin surface. Small children are usually calmer with a parent present; teenagers may or may not desire privacy. Listening to music, visualizing a tranquil scene (mountains covered with snow, floating in a pool), or using the same technician each time can help.

- **Use EMLA cream or Numby Stuff.** EMLA—a cream anesthetic—is applied to the skin one to two hours prior to the procedure to prevent pain. In some cases, it can constrict the veins, so experiment to see if it works for your child. Numby Stuff—a needle-free anesthetic—delivers a cream anesthetic through the skin using a mild, low-level electric current. EMLA cream and Numby Stuff are not recommended when giving medications that can burn the skin if leakage occurs (for example, vincristine).

- **Keep warm.** Cold temperatures cause the surface blood vessels to constrict. Wrapping your child in a blanket and putting a hot water bottle or heating pad on the arm can enlarge the veins.

- **Drink lots of fluids.** Dehydration decreases the fluid in the veins, so encourage lots of drinking.

- **Let gravity help.** If your child is lying in bed or sitting on your lap, have her hang her arm down over the side to increase the size of the vessels in the arm and hand.

- **Let your child have control as appropriate.** If your child has a preference, let him pick the arm to be stuck. If he is a veteran of many IVs, let him point out the best vein. Good technicians know that patients are quite aware of their best bet for a good vein.

- **Stop if problems develop.** The art of treating children is spending lots of time on preparation and not much time on procedures. If a conflict arises between your child and technician, take a time-out and regroup. Children can be remarkably cooperative if their needs are respected and they are given some control over the situation.

> You'll think I'm crazy, but I'll tell you this story anyway. After getting stuck constantly for a year, my daughter (5 years old) lost it one day when she needed an IV. She started screaming and crying, just flew into a rage. I told the tech, "Let's let her calm down. Why don't you stick me for a change?" She was a sport and started a line in my arm. I told my daughter that I had forgotten how much it hurt and I could understand why she was upset. I told her to let us know when she was ready. She just walked over and held out her arm.

· · · · ·

> Even though our 6-year-old son seemed okay with IVs and port access during treatment, afterwards he showed lots of aggression, including sticking people really hard with pointy objects, and pinching people's arms. It's gotten better off treatment with some counseling sessions.

# Subcutaneous injections

Some children require medications given by subcutaneous injection (shot under the skin) during their treatment. For example, Neupogen (G-CSF) a colony-stimulating factor that is often used to boost the white blood cell count, is usually given by subcutaneous injection. To minimize pain caused by subcutaneous injections, apply EMLA cream one to two hours before administration. Parents can also reduce pain by rubbing ice over the site to numb the area prior to injection.

> We always used EMLA cream before our son needed a subcutaneous injection. I think part of the benefit to him was pharmacological, and part of it was psychological. He just seemed to be more at ease with the injections when he knew the EMLA was applied a few hours before the needle was given.

· · · · ·

> I would give Florence her growth hormone injections with a needleless injector into her bottom. She would lie on the floor on her tummy watching a distracting program on TV and wear a walkman playing a tape so that she couldn't hear the bang. We got this all set up and found it worked. Soon Florence didn't mind the injections at all. I tried as hard as possible not to make bruises although this was not possible much of the time. Sometimes the bruises were black and deep and lasted a long time. We often had to ring the nurses to get advice on the pressure settings to try and minimize this.

· · · · ·

> We eventually gave Matt his Neupogen shots while he was asleep. At the time, Matt was around 3 years old and we had a night nurse anyway for monitoring his trach and I could not bear the thought of giving him his shots. It is just one of those things that I had to draw the line on. We had the nurse try all different times/ways/techniques to give the shots. He hated everything about it, which triggered other, more difficult problems (turning blue and passing out). Sometimes Matt would sleep through the shot and other times he would wake up. Once treatment was over, Matt had great difficulty with going to sleep at all. Fought it till the bitter end. The night nurse was here anyway (trach, again) so he stayed up with her. It took a long time to develop a new safe bedtime/wake-up routine and I often wonder if sneaking the Neupogen in on him was more traumatic than we realized.

## Swallowing tests

Swallowing tests are necessary if your child is unable to swallow or does not have an adequate gag reflex. Swallowing tests are performed in the radiology department; your child cannot eat or drink anything prior to the procedure, but will be given a barium-containing "meal" during the test. X-rays are taken and examined to evaluate swallowing. Swallowing tests help determine whether your child can begin to eat and drink more normally following surgery or whether a gastrostomy tube, nasogastric tube, or intravenous nutrition is necessary for a period or time. You can stay with your child during the procedure.

## Taking pills

Over the course of your child's treatment, it will be necessary to administer pills and/ or liquid medications on a regular basis. When giving oral medications, it is essential to get off to a good start and establish cooperation early.

> To teach Brent (6 years old) to swallow pills, when we were eating corn for dinner I encouraged him to swallow one kernel whole. Luckily, it went right down and he got over his fear of pills.

· · · · ·

> I wanted Katy (3 years old) to feel like we were a team right from the first night. So I made a big deal out of tasting each of her medications and pronouncing it good. Thank goodness I did because the prednisone was nauseating—bitter, metallic, with a lingering aftertaste. I asked the nurse for some small gel caps, and packed them with the pills which I had broken in half. I gave Katy her choice of drinks to take her pills with and taught her to swallow gel caps with a large sip of liquid.

Gel caps come in many sizes. Number 4s are small enough for a 3- or 4-year-old child to swallow. Many pills can be chewed or swallowed whole without taste problems. Steroid medications (prednisone, decadron, etc.) should not be chewed, because they have a bitter aftertaste and may cause your child to develop an aversion to all oral medications. Just remember that children develop different taste preferences and aversions to medications, and gel caps are useful for any medication that bothers them.

> After much trial and error with medications, Meagan's method became chewing up pills with chocolate chips. She's kept this up for the long haul.

· · · · ·

> *I always give choices such as, "Do you want the white pill or the six*
> *yellow pills first?" It gives her a little control in her chaotic world.*

For younger children, many parents crush the pills in a small amount of pudding, applesauce, jam, frozen juice concentrate, or other favorite food. Chocolate syrup masks the bitter aftertaste of steroid medications extremely well. It is important, however, to make sure that the medication may be safely crushed and that the act of doing this does not alter the stability of the medication. Check with your pharmacist if you have questions in this area.

> *Jeremy was 4 when he was diagnosed, and we used to crush up the pills*
> *and mix them with ice cream. This worked well for us.*
>
> • • • • •
>
> *Carrie Beth was 2 when diagnosed. She hated the taste of the pills, so I*
> *would submerge them in teaspoonfuls of pure maple syrup. The next year*
> *when she just decided she didn't want to cooperate about taking pills, I'd*
> *say to her and her two older sisters, "Strawberry gum for everybody as*
> *soon as Carrie Beth finishes her pills." Then I would leave, and the older*
> *kids encouraged her to swallow the pills.*

Many children receiving treatment take SMZ-TMP (sulfamethoxazole and trimethoprim), Bactrim, or Septra two to three times a week to prevent a specific type of pneumonia that can develop in patients whose immune systems are suppressed. It comes in liquid or pill form, and is produced by several different manufacturers. Ask your pharmacist for a kid taste test. Letting your child choose a medicine that appeals to him encourages compliance.

> *Whenever my son had to take a liquid medicine, such as antibiotics, he*
> *enjoyed taking it from a small syringe, especially if it was bitter. I would*
> *draw up the proper amount, then he would put it in his mouth and push*
> *the plunger. Smaller doses at a time worked best.*

For teenagers, issues about taking pills are completely different from those of young children. The problems with teens revolve around autonomy, control, and feelings of invulnerability. It is normal for teenagers to be noncompliant. Teenagers cannot be forced to take pills if they choose to not cooperate. Trying to coerce teens fuels conflict and tends to frustrate everyone. If you need help, ask for an assessment by the psychosocial team at the hospital to work out a plan for adherence to treatment. Everyone will need to be flexible to reach a favorable outcome.

*I think the main problem with teens is making sure that they take the meds. Joel (15 years old) has been very responsible about taking his nightly pills. I've tried to make it easy for him by having an index card for the week and he marks off the med as he takes it. I also put the meds on a dry erase board on the fridge as a reminder. As he takes the med, he erases it. That way it's easy for him (and me) to see at a glance if he's taken his stuff. The index card alone wasn't working because he couldn't find a pen or forgot to mark it off.*

## Taking a temperature

During the period in which your child is undergoing treatment, fever becomes an enemy because it is often the first sign of infection. Parents take hundreds of temperatures, especially when their child is not feeling well. Temperatures can be taken under the tongue, under the arm, or in the ear using a special type of thermometer. Rectal temperatures are not recommended due to the risk of tears and infection. Here are a few suggestions that might help, especially when blood counts are depressed.

- Use a glass thermometer under the tongue.

- Digital thermometers can be purchased at any drug store. Some have an alarm that beeps when it is time to remove the thermometer.

- Tympanic thermometers measure infrared waves and are very easy to use. They are quite accurate, but can't be used if your child has tympanostomy tubes in place.

> *When my in-laws asked at diagnosis if there was anything that we needed, I asked them to try to buy a tympanic (ear) thermometer. The device cost over a hundred dollars then, but it worked beautifully. It takes only one second to obtain a temperature. You can even use it when she is asleep without waking her. They are now sold at pharmacies and drug stores, and cost much less.*

Before you leave the hospital, you should know when to call the clinic because of fever. Usually, parents are told not to give any medication for fever and to call if the fever goes above 101°F (38.5°C). This allows the doctors to make a judgment on whether it is an infection that requires treatment. It is especially important for parents of children with implanted catheters to know when to call the clinic, as an untreated infection can be life threatening. It is also very helpful to have a copy of your child's most recent blood counts when you call to notify your physician about fever issues.

## Urine collections

Timed urine collections are sometimes needed at various times during your child's treatment. Such collections are useful in evaluating your child's kidney function prior to receiving chemotherapy drugs that can cause damage to the kidneys or to measure the production of certain substances in the blood, such as epinephrine and other hormones. If your child is toilet trained, the collection is done by saving all the urine your child produces in a defined period of hours. If your child is not yet toilet trained, a foley catheter (catheter that goes up the urethra into the bladder) will need to be placed for a period of time.

## Urine specimens

Chemotherapy requires frequent urine specimens. Some chemotherapy drugs may cause blood, protein, or glucose to be excreted in the urine. One way to help obtain a sample is to encourage lots of drinking the hour before or ask the nurse to increase the drip rate on the IV. Explain to your child why the test is necessary. Ask the nurse to show how the dip sticks work (they change color, so they are quite popular with preschoolers). Use a "hat" under the toilet seat. This is a shallow plastic bucket that fits under the seat and catches the urine.

> Turn on the water while the child sits on the toilet. I don't know why it works, but it does.

As all parents learn, eating and elimination are areas that the child controls. If she just can't or won't urinate in the hat, go out, buy her the largest drink you can find, and wait.

If infection is suspected, then a clean catch urine specimen will be ordered. Your child's perineal area will need to be gently cleansed with soap or an antiseptic towelette, and she will need to urinate in a small sterile container. Urinary tract infections are much more common in girls than boys, because the female urethra is much shorter.

Occasionally, your physician will order a urinary catheterization if a clean specimen can't be obtained or your child is unable to urinate. This procedure can be quite stressful because it involves placing a sterile rubber tube up the urethra and into the bladder. It is quite appropriate to ask for a mild sedative or muscle relaxant before the procedure if your child is anxious. It is also perfectly acceptable to request that the most skilled person available perform the procedure. In skilled nursing hands, the procedure takes less than five minutes to perform.

## Visual acuity testing

Visual acuity testing is important if your child's CNS tumor involves the optic nerve pathways or an area of the brain, such as the occipital lobes, that controls vision. These children are routinely followed by a neuro-ophthalmologist or, in some cases, a pediatric ophthalmologist because vision loss can be a symptom and indicator of tumor growth. When done by an expert, such testing is accurate and fun for your child. Most ophthalmologists who specialize in the care of children employ technology that presents visual stimuli to your child in the form of toys and mechanical games. They usually understand that patience helps produce valid test results. Baseline testing is important prior to surgery and at specified periods throughout treatment.

> *Jamie's eye exams, which happen every three to six months, involve multiple stops at the children's eye clinic: first, visual field testing with our specialist who checks his fields using handheld toys and a machine with two different size light points. Then we go to our ophthalmologist for acuity testing and eye drops for optic nerve checking. Then one more check with an orthoptist. It used to take most of a day when he was two, but now that he's a little older, it can be done in one morning.*

## Wada test

The Wada test (intracarotid sodium amobarbitol test) is sometimes used to help locate speech and memory centers within the brain. Sodium amobarbitol is injected into the carotid artery in the neck in such a way that half of the brain is temporarily put to sleep. This allows your child's physician to perform tests of speech, memory, and other functions while your child can use only one side of his brain. Sometimes an EEG is performed during this procedure. The Wada test is particularly crucial before surgery, to ensure that these areas are well-defined and protected from injury.

> *Six-year-old Ethan's introduction to procedures started the day he presented with crossed eyes. The MRI that afternoon was no problem for him; our usually perpetual-motion machine was nearly comatose from the increased pressure in his brain. Getting through that scan was difficult only for my peace of mind. His next scan was a day later; now near-manic from steroids, he lay still, occasionally giggling, for the MRI while watching 'Men in Black' through special MRI-safe video goggles. Though*

*he was under anesthesia for his third scan (at that time he was mute, paralyzed on one side, and NOT capable of cooperating with testing), when he regained his power of speech and communication, scans became a not-so-hard routine. Reminded to lie still, he often fell asleep through the jackhammer-like din of the MRI magnet.*

*Getting to Ethan's blood was, at first, a bit more challenging. After his port was placed, we at first had to hold Ethan down while accessing it. We were told it shouldn't hurt after being anesthetized with EMLA, but the sight of the needle was scary. The breakthrough came when a child life specialist (what a great addition to pediatrics!!) distracted him and he found that it really did not hurt.*

*Since that time, with my suggestions, he has devised (often-changing) routines; for accessing the port, he is sitting semi-upright, clutching his left ear with his left hand and holding a parent with his right. For receiving daily GCSF shots, the special Band-Aid that looks like a tattoo needs to be open on the table; the appropriate site (left or right thigh) agreed upon, pinched, and alcohol-swabbed; a sibling holding one hand and he pinching an ear with the other; on the count of three the QUICK injection, followed as nearly-instantaneously as possible by the Band-Aid. Simple, really, when you know how. No fear and no tears. Audiometry, psychological/academic testing, and vision checks are just games which he enjoys. Now if we can only get by the hurdle of the eye-drops which sting like the devil . . .*

# CHAPTER 5

# Your Child's Hospitalization

THERE ARE FEW THINGS in life more uncomfortable than arising from a lumpy pullout couch to face another day of your child's hospitalization for cancer. Hospitals are huge, noisy bureaucracies on a time schedule all their own. For a child, being hospitalized means being separated from parents, brothers, sisters, friends, pets, and the comfort and familiarity of home. A child's hospitalization can rob both the parent and child of a sense of control, leaving them feeling helpless. There are ways, however, to wrest back a sense of control while adding a great deal of cheerfulness to the proceedings.

This chapter provides you with useful information about coping during your child's stay in the hospital and suggestions about things you can do to make the experience as pleasant as possible.

## The room

Hospital rooms are often painted an institutional shade of gray or green, and somehow most of the windows seem to look out over the power plant. Covering the walls with big bright posters (Disney characters, sports figures, rock groups) can liven up the room immensely.

> *The first thing we put up in Meagan's room was a huge poster of the Little Engine That Could saying, "I think I can, I think I can."*
>
> • • • • •
>
> *We were away from home for surgery, and I wanted to be sure to have lots of family pictures around for Anthony to see when he woke up. We covered the walls with them.*

Cards can be displayed on the walls, hanging from strings like a mobile or taped around the windowsills. Put up pictures of the child engaged in her favorite activity, and add photos of friends, too. Most hospitals don't allow flowers on oncology floors, because they can grow a fungus that can make children sick, but it's fun to have bouquets of balloons bobbing in the corners. Younger children derive great comfort from having a favorite stuffed animal, blanket, or quilt on their bed. If it doesn't bother your child, make the room smell good with potpourri or aromatherapy oils.

To personalize the visit of each member of the medical staff, some parents bring a guest book to sign. Others put up a visitor sign-in poster, which must be signed before examinations begin or vital signs are taken. Another variation of the sign-in poster is to have each staff member outline his hand and write within the print. If your budget allows, an instant camera can help identify the many staff members involved in your child's care and can provide a fun activity for your child.

> In my position as a parent consultant, I suggest that a journal be kept in the child's room for any visitor, family member, or medical care giver to write in at any time. Leaving a message if the child is sleeping or out of the room for procedures can be a nice surprise. Later, a surviving child and her family, or the family of a child who has died, have a memory book of those who have touched their lives.

Some children who have undergone surgery for a CNS tumor have problems communicating for a period of time after surgery. If your child loses the ability to speak, you should request a communication board (a felt or plastic board with pictures and movable figures) so that your child can tell you his needs and wishes until his speech is more understandable.

> My son Alex was diagnosed in 1999 with medulloblastoma when he was six years old. He came out of surgery speaking and then two days later couldn't say a word. He was mute for about two months and then very slowly he could pronounce things again. His voice and his muscle movements (swallowing and coughing) were okay, but he just couldn't say anything. All he would do is shake his head for yes and no or he would cry. It was so frustrating for him. He couldn't laugh. He would just stare into space. You know what brought him around, the show "America's Funniest Home Videos"! He had such a belly laugh and after that he started saying words again. My husband and I would practice words with Alex after he made an effort to talk, and before that we just had a system where he would squeeze our hands for yes or no. We also used flashcards for "hungry," "bathroom," "lights on/off," and for different kinds of food.

Bringing music will help block out some of the hospital noise as well as help everyone relax. A small cassette player, Walkman with earphones, or CD boom box is portable and useful.

*My daughter's preschool teacher sent a care package. She made a felt board with dozens of cutout characters and designs that provided hours of quiet entertainment. She also included games, drawings from each classmate, coloring books, markers, get well cards, and a child's tape player with ear phones. Because we had run out of our house with just the clothes on our backs, all of these toys were very, very welcome.*

Although many hospitals provide brightly colored smocks for the patients, most children and teens prefer to wear their own clothing if at all possible. This can pose a laundry problem, so check to see if the floor has washers available for families to use.

As soon as possible after admission, ask for a "floor tour." Find out if a microwave and refrigerator are available, learn what the approved parent sleeping arrangements are, and ask about showers and bathtubs for both patients and parents. Obtain a hospital handbook if one is available. These booklets often include information on billing, parking, discounts, cafeteria and gift shop hours, and other helpful items.

Many children's hospitals have in-room or portable VCRs available. Sign up for a convenient time and bring in or rent a favorite funny video. Ask if the floor has a sign-out video library and review the list for your child's favorite movies or cartoons. Bring in age-appropriate games, puzzles, and books. Humor helps, so joke books and things that make kids laugh (silly string, funny movies) are great items to pack.

*A friend brought in a bag full of fun stuff from the local dime store. He included a water pistol (good for unwelcome visitors or unfriendly interns), play dough, Slinky, checkers, dominos, bubbles, a book of corny jokes, and puzzles.*

If your child is hospitalized during a holiday season, check with the staff to find out if there are any restrictions on decorations in rooms and then brighten up the rooms with colorful decorations for the season. It may provide a fun diversion for both you and your child.

# Food

Buying meals day after day in the hospital cafeteria is expensive. Check with the hospital social worker to find out if the hospital has food discount cards or free meal trays for parents. In addition, many of the food items available in the cafeteria deserve the notorious reputation of "hospital food." Check to see if the floor has a refrigerator for parent's food and stock it from home. Remember to put your name in a prominent place on your containers.

*Our hospital provides vouchers for the cafeteria that can be used instead of ordering food for the room. For us, they have been a godsend. The food on the tray is much worse than what is in the cafeteria. Also, oncology patients have no spending cap on the vouchers, so we can get a few extras. When our son is not up to going to the cafeteria, we go down and bring it up.*

Many hospitals have cooking facilities for families where they can cook or microwave favorite meals. Ask family and friends to bring food in when they visit, and consider ordering extra items to come up on your child's tray.

Ordering out for dinner can also be a nice change of pace for you and your child. As long as there are no medical restrictions, there's no reason why pizza can't be delivered to the hospital. Ask the nurses if they have menus from local restaurants. One important thing to remember, however, is to remove old food trays and unused portions of food. Such items can add to room clutter, contribute to your child's anorexia or nausea, or attract unwanted insect visitors to the room.

*Just the smell of food nauseated my daughter. I'll never forget taking the tray out in the hall, and gobbling it down myself. I always felt so guilty, and thought that staff viewed me as that parent who ate her kid's food. But it saved money and prevented her meals from going to waste. I also did not want to leave her side for the few minutes it took to go to the cafeteria, although in hindsight, the walk would have done me some good.*

# Parking

Many parents of children with cancer have unpleasant memories of driving around in endless loops looking for a parking space while their child is throwing up in a bucket in the back seat (or even worse when the bucket was left at home). Learn about both long- and short-term parking arrangements. Ask the hospital social worker if parking passes are available and ask other parents where the cheapest parking is located. Some hospitals have valet parking, which may be as cheap as self-parking for a one- to two-hour visit or appointment.

*I had no idea that the hospital gave out free parking passes to their frequent customers. Now I tell every new parent to check as soon as possible to see if they can get a parking pass. It will save them lots of money that they would have spent on meters and parking tickets, and*

*time they would have spent running out to move the car out of the*
*emergency parking spot.*

# The endless waiting

Parents need to become experts in learning how to wait without losing their minds. You need to expect long waits for everything from blood draws to procedures. Many parents find themselves getting nervous or angry while waiting for the doctors to appear during "rounds" each morning, when the attendings (senior physicians), residents, and interns move from room to room in a large group, then feel let down when the visit lasts only a few moments.

If you have questions to ask the doctors, write them down and tell the doctors when they come in that you would like a few moments to discuss concerns or ask questions. Keeping a pad and pencil available in your child's room at all times is an absolute necessity. You may find that the most important questions and concerns come to mind at 2:00 A.M. when no one is around to address them.

It helps for both caregiver and child to come prepared for long waits each time that you go to the hospital. Some progressive (and well-supported) institutions have VCRs, toys, and games available, but usually you need to bring your own things. Have your child pick out favorite card games, board games, computer games, drawing materials, and books. Remember to bring food and drinks. Some children will take comfort from taking a favorite blanket or pillow along with them for a day in the clinic or a lengthy hospitalization. If your child is scheduled for surgery, bring a good book, a jigsaw puzzle that multiple people can work on together, your holiday card list, or a recipe file that needs revision. Such pre-planning helps pass the time and will also give you a feeling of accomplishment.

> *I remember when my son was newly diagnosed, and soon after had*
> *a partial resection. I waited in the surgery family room, fearful and*
> *numb. Across from me was a man who was reading the newspaper,*
> *and a woman crocheting. I had to ask them, "How can you be so*
> *calm?" The mother said that their daughter had a recurring deformity*
> *from a rare congenital condition, and she had had twenty major*
> *surgeries so far. This surgery would take over fifteen hours, just like*
> *all the other times. I couldn't imagine back then doing anything*
> *productive, other than praying, while I was waiting.*

# Befriending the staff

Hospitals are staffed by many wonderful and some not so wonderful people. Many parents find that their heightened stress makes them less tolerant of inefficiency or confusion. As discussed in Chapter 7, *Forming a Partnership with the Medical Team*, working together, rather than becoming adversaries, will provide your child with a sense of security. Doing things like helping change soiled bedding, taking out food trays, and giving baths frees up overworked nurses to take care of medicines and IVs. Nurses usually appreciate the help. A pediatric oncology nurse and child life specialist offer these comments:

> Parents should not have to worry about helping the staff or whether the staff is stressed. They have enough on their plate to worry about. But families often feel like they're so helpless, and they think, "What can I do, how can I get in control of this situation?" Many parents find comfort in changing the bed; they very often feel so completely overwhelmed, because they can't give the medicines, and they can't make the cancer go away. So they do what they can do for their child. Look at the staff as a team. You are part of that team. And no, oftentimes you can't give the chemotherapy, and you can't do a spinal tap, but no one can be that child's parent but you.

· · · · ·

> Your parental role doesn't stop when you walk in the door of the hospital. You can touch your child, you can talk to her, you can help her through a bath, brush her hair, do her teeth, and all the things that you would do at home. You are the one who knows what works best for your child and for your family, so if there's something that you do at home, let us know, and the nurses will find a way for you to do it here, too.

As soon as possible, learn about the shift changes on the oncology floor. If you need to leave, don't leave a request with one nurse if another will be coming on duty soon. If you have a request or reminder, you can post it on the child's door, the wall above the bed, or on the chart. Such communication efforts on your part will be well received by the staff and they will quickly identify you as a helpful team player in your child's care.

> We made sure we knew the exact doses Megan (age 21 months) should be getting for everything. We received good advice from another mom to

*check every drug Megan was given, so I had our doctor write in the chart*
*that we wanted to verify every med, including chemotherapy, that was*
*administered to Megan, no matter what time of day or night it was. With*
*this double-checking, there was only one time that we found an antibiotic*
*dose dispensed at one and half times the dose required.*

It sometimes helps to make a list for yourself of the various members of the multidisciplinary team who are involved in your child's care. This might include physicians, nurse practitioners, primary staff nurses, therapists, and social workers. It is also very helpful to determine who is the primary physician in charge of your child's care for each hospital admission. For example, the neurosurgeons are in charge during your child's hospital stay for surgery, but the oncologists are in charge during an admission for fever following a course of chemotherapy.

# Being an advocate for your child

Hospitals can be frightening places for children. Parents need to provide comfort, protection, and advocacy for their vulnerable child. To fulfill these roles, parents need to be present.

> *We were in for one of our post-chemo/fever admissions, and the*
> *children's floor was full. During the night, a little newborn was given the*
> *space next to ours, and put under bili lights. They lit up the room! I had*
> *to call the nurse back in, and ask if the baby's bassinet could be turned, so*
> *we didn't have lights glaring in our direction the whole night. Even with*
> *all the curtains closed, the room was hot. In the morning, I spoke to one of*
> *the nursing supervisors. Next time, no lights, please.*

Most pediatric hospitals are quite aware of how much better children do if a parent is allowed to sleep in the room. Sometimes small couches convert into beds, or parents can use a cot provided by the hospital. Additionally, many hospitals allow parents to go into the operating room prior to anesthesia or to remain with their child during scans and some procedures. Ask for clarification of hospital procedures and rules early on, so that you can discuss your wishes about this important area with your physicians and nurses.

> *Whenever my husband couldn't be at the hospital at bedtime, he would*
> *bring in homemade tapes of him reading bedtime stories. Our son would*
> *drift off to sleep hearing his daddy's voice.*

*Sometimes you can create your own fun with just a little imagination.*
*On one particular occasion, Matthew was feeling especially bored. With a*
*little ingenuity, we soon discovered that four unused IV poles and as many*
*blankets as we could "steal" from the linen cart made for one pretty cool*
*tent. We then used the mattress from a roll-away cot, and spent the night*
*"camping" in his hospital room. He had a wonderful time.*

If hospital policy requires the parent to leave, insist on staying. Geralyn Gaes tells a
story in *You Don't Have to Die* about a confrontation at her local community hospital:

*One night a nurse came into Jason's room and curtly informed me that*
*I would have to leave, since it was past visiting hours. With my son pale*
*and retching from chemotherapy, I was not about to go anywhere.*
*Looking her in the eye, I said "You can send security after me if you like,*
*but I'm not leaving here." No one disturbed me again.*

Of course, sometimes it isn't possible to stay with your child if you are a single parent
or if both parents work full time. Many families have grandparents or close friends
who stay with the hospitalized child when the parents cannot be present. Older children and teenagers may not want a parent in the room at night, but they need an
advocate there during the day just as much as the preschoolers.

*Our hospital did not allow parents into the MRI suite. We worked with*
*the head of that department, and now it is permitted for all families. This*
*avoided the use of general anesthesia, so it as good for everyone involved.*
*You don't need to take "no" for an answer.*

Whenever a family member cannot be present, children who are old enough should
be taught to use the telephone. Tape a phone number nearby where a parent can be
reached and have the child call if anyone tries to do procedures that are unexpected.
The hospital staff should be informed that any changes in treatment (except emergencies) need to be authorized by a parent.

Having cancer strips children of control over their bodies. To help reverse this process, parents can take over most nursing care. Children may prefer parents to help
them to the bathroom or to clean up diarrhea or vomit.

*I was embarrassed to have the nurse change the sheets when I had an*
*accident in the bed. I couldn't help it when I was taking the cytoxan, but I*
*was still embarrassed.*

Making the bed, keeping the room tidy, changing dressings, and giving backrubs help your child feel more comfortable and lighten the burden on nurses. However, some children may do better with the nurses. Parents should allow the child to express his needs, even if it feels like rejection. Parents should discuss these issues with the nursing staff as soon as possible and establish a workable plan about who should do what.

Parents can also help out by checking for mistakes. People who work in hospitals are human, so they sometimes make errors. It helps to have a written copy of the protocol. If you weren't given one, ask. If your child is enrolled in a clinical trial, you may have the short roadmap that describes dates, drugs, and tests. However, you also have a right to get a copy of the full trial protocol if you would like one. For more information, see Chapter 9, *Clinical Trials*. Parents can be the last line of defense against mistakes.

> Know every drug your child takes. Write down the name of the drug
> and the dosage. Watch that the name on the drug matches what YOU
> are expecting them to get, and ask if it isn't anything you recognize.
> Watch that the name on the blood matches up with the child's name
> band. Watch everything.

Parents can help their child regain some control by encouraging choices whenever possible. Older children should be actively involved in discussions about their treatment, while younger children can decide when to take a bath, which arm to use for an IV, what to order for meals, what position for procedures, what clothes to wear, and how to decorate the room. Some children request a hug or a handshake after all treatments or procedures.

> Our son is almost six. He prefers to talk first with the nurse or
> technician about fun stuff, like his trains, before he allows any kind
> of IV or blood draw. Most good techs don't mind, they try to do that
> anyway. He definitely prefers it when I step back, stay quiet, and let
> him lead.

Hospitals work on schedules that are not based on the convenience of patients and families. It helps to establish a schedule that is appropriate for your child's age, developmental level, usual activities, and illness. One adolescent patient coped with lengthy chemotherapy treatments by setting up a daily schedule that allowed her time to visit with the nurses in the morning, do school work, eat lunch, watch a movie, take a nap, and then be ready to go home late in the afternoon. Structuring her time in this fashion not only helped her pass the time but also gave her some control over her environment.

# Where do the kids play?

Children need to play and teens need to socialize, especially when hospitalized. Ask whether the hospital has a recreation therapy department. Often, a large room is devoted to toys, books, dolls, and crafts and is staffed by specialists who really know how to play with children. These rooms provide many therapeutic activities, such as medical play with dolls that help children to express fears or concerns about what is happening to them. By encouraging contact with other children in similar circumstances, recreation therapy helps children feel less alone, less different from other children.

Recreation therapy rooms are a cheerful change from lying in a hospital bed and are full of fun-filled activities and smiling staff people. If the child is too ill or his counts are too low to go to the play area, arrangements can be made for a recreational therapist to bring a bundle of toys, games, and books to the room. This can give the parent time to go out to eat or take a walk.

> When I wanted to have a conference with the oncologist about Katy's protocol, I called recreation therapy and they sent two wonderful ladies to the clinic. The doctor and I were able to talk privately for an hour, and Katy had a great time making herself a gold crown and decorating her wheelchair with streamers and jewels.

Find out if there are support groups for teens. Visiting restrictions vary from institution to institution, but most are liberal these days regarding adolescent visitation. You might also try to bend the rules a bit to allow your teen to have friends in as much as possible.

Exercise is important, too. For kids strong enough to walk, exploring the hospital can be fun. Plan a daily excursion to the gift shop or the cafeteria. Go outside and walk the entire perimeter of the hospital if weather and the neighborhood permit. Don't feel limited by an IV pole; it can be pushed or pulled and will feel normal after a while. Many children have been seen standing on the base of the IV pole with a parent pushing them down the hall at a good clip.

Check to see if the hospital has a swimming pool for you to swim in (your child probably can't use it) or a gym. Ask if there is an outdoor playground for patients and parents and make use of it whenever your child feels well enough to go outside. Your child will probably sleep much better at night in the hospital if he can get some daily fresh air and exercise. Also, the physical therapy department may have an exercise program in which you can participate.

Many children and teens feel refreshed by going up on the roof just to feel the wind on their faces and have the sun warm their skin. Some hospitals even grant passes to young patients whose white counts are high enough. Be sure to check before requesting a pass whether your insurance plan allows this. Over the last five or so years, third party payers have begun to frown on this practice and may not pay for that day of hospitalization.

> Tori was in the hospital recently for fever and positive blood cultures. She has a great time in the hospital. I had been trying to get her out on a pass as she was to have Grandparent's Day at school. We only would have been gone for a couple hours but no go. We came up with a plan to videotape the school part and have her do it with the tape for her grandparents at the hospital. In addition, child life got another videotape and we made a video for the school about the hospital at the same time. She was able to go all over the hospital (the play room, PT and OT gym, McDonalds). It was great and I think I am going to treasure the copy.

> Tori and I also went reverse trick or treating. She had wanted to do it Halloween week but we were not in clinic. We were inpatient, but I had promised, so we did it anyway. I brought in her witch costume and she ran around the hospital giving out candy to her therapists, nurses, and doctors. It was fabulous. She looked so cute. People in the halls did think it was a little weird but everyone from oncology understood that you do what makes you happy. Just call November 16th Halloween and everyone just pretends it is.

Any action that parents, family members, and friends take to support and advocate for the youngster with cancer buoys up the spirit. Remember: courage is contagious.

> It becomes second nature. Step, shuffle, shuffle. Step, shuffle, shuffle. Sometime between two and five o'clock in the morning—somewhere between the nurse's station and the bathrooms—your gait, pulse, and breath synchronize into a rhythm of surprising calm. Step, shuffle, shuffle.

> The Walk. That's what we call it. It's a milestone of sorts. A sign of acceptance and perseverance. A notice to the rest of the Club that you have put in sufficient hours of hospital vigil to find solace in simple

movement. Hurried paces, strident races to the pay phones are far behind you. Tearful staggers and despairing stumbles are also long gone. Long stretches of hospital hallway lay before you, endless miles to be traversed while waiting and watching. Step, shuffle, shuffle: the comforting drag of the bottom of your feet against industrial linoleum.

I round the corner and modify my slide to catch up with the woman in front of me. "Hey, Susan."

"Hey, Gigi." Her Walk is smooth and practiced. I suspect it follows her home. We move down the corridor together, clutching empty water pitchers, cutting a path through beeps, moans, and rustles that issue from the doors on each side. Each of us is only partly in the space our body inhabits—our essential selves are back in our assigned rooms watching over little boys in huddled sleep.

I am in the Club. I am allowed direct questions. "How's Matthew doing?"

"Shunt infection, I.V. antibiotics, you know."

I nod. My son has a shunt, too. It drains excess fluid from the brain.

"Heparin for the clot in his leg," she continues. "Feeding tube still in. And they want to increase the steroids." Too many complications for such a little guy. My heart gets tight and I am fervently glad not to be Susan. An instant later, I am ashamed of my thoughts and blurt out some hopeful babble. "But he's sleeping okay?"

Susan raises her eyes to mine. The Look is there, much more developed than mine—she's had four months longer to perfect it. It is calm (with a dead-hold over hysteria), it is knowledgeable (endless hours of research masterfully synthesized and assimilated), it is forgiving (of COURSE you don't want to be me). Look to Look, my shame fades away. She smiles and squeezes my arm. "Yeah. He's sleeping okay."

We stop briefly in front of the water dispenser and then head back the way we came. The tan plastic pitchers sweat coldness over our hands, but we don't hurry. That's one thing about the Walk. It buys you time—alone time, out-of-the-room time. A chance to look at something other than the disease that is breaking your heart.

"And Ben?" she asks as we reach my corridor.

*"Pretty good. This chemo cycle doesn't seem as rough on him."*

*"Great!" She means it. Good news for any one in the Club is good news for all of us. Small victories add up.*

*I veer off to the left. "See ya."*

*"See ya," she calls back. Step, shuffle, shuffle. Step, shuffle, shuffle. Our feet take us quietly back to battle.*

# CHAPTER 6

# Family and Friends

THE INTERACTIONS BETWEEN the parents of a child with a CNS tumor and their extended family and friends are complex. Potential exists for loving support and generous help, as well as for bitter disappointment and disputes. The diagnosis of cancer creates a ripple effect—first touching the immediate family, then extended family, friends, coworkers, schoolmates, church members, and the entire community. Parents are often surprised at the diversity of coping abilities exhibited by relatives and friends.

This chapter discusses some of the experiences the family might encounter, as well as scores of ideas for helpful things that family and friends can do. To prevent possible misunderstandings between family members and friends, veteran parents also share ideas on things that do not help.

## The extended family

Extended family—aunts, uncles, cousins, grandparents—can cushion the shock of a cancer diagnosis by loving words and actions. Extended family members sometimes drop their own lives to rush to the side of the child with a tumor, often remaining steadfast for the years of treatment. Regrettably, some family members may not be helpful, either from ignorance of what is helpful or simply because they are overwhelmed by events in their own lives. The following sections explore how some families notified extended family members, kept the lines of communication open, and dealt with grandparents.

### Notifying the family

Notifying relatives is one of the first painful jobs for the parent of a child diagnosed with a tumor. In times of crisis, family is refuge, and the news is usually quickly shared.

> *I called my sister and asked her to take care of telling everyone. She called my other sister, and together they told my frail mother.*

· · · · ·

*We approached each grandmother differently and got totally unexpected responses. We thought the first grandmother, who knew the most about the symptoms we were investigating, could take the news over the phone, but it was too much for her. The other grandmom had heart problems, and we sent my brother to her house to tell her. When he got there, she wanted to know why we didn't call right away. She said, "Don't worry about me, just worry about this little one."*

Paradoxically, the family members who potentially may provide the greatest support may also be sources of added stress. Some extended families and even entire communities rally around the stricken family, while support never materializes for others. Several factors affect the strength of support: well-established community ties, good communication within extended family, physical proximity to extended family, and clear exchange of information on needs of the affected family. If any of these elements are missing, support may evaporate.

*Except for one good friend, none of my friends called when I was home. It seemed that after the initial three-month crisis, family and friends removed themselves from the situation, as often happens.*

## Staying in touch

The most important first step for families is to set up clear communication over what truly will help. Sometimes, the child is too sick or too fatigued for company, and this needs to be expressed. When visits are welcome, make them brief and cheerful. Not only do long visits distress sick children, but they can also overtax a tired parent. Establishing a telephone chain is a good way to keep family informed of the child's progress. One family member can be delegated as communicator, and this person will relay the information to another person, who will then phone another. Some families leave updates on their telephone answering machines or web sites.

*There were many days I wanted to hide in bed and pull the covers over my head. I know everyone was well meaning and genuinely cared, but the constant stream of people through the house and phone ringing added to the stress we were already under. We already had a home care nurse coming five days a week, a physical therapist coming three days a week, in addition to constant phone calls to follow up on blood work and tests, appointments to schedule, and family members to keep track of. Bubba, our dog, loved all the commotion, but the rest of us tired quickly.*

It's okay not to answer your phone when you are home from the hospital to shower or pick up clothes. You can delegate the communication to someone else, take the phone off the hook, and enjoy the peace and quiet.

## Helpful things for family to do

Families differ in what is truly helpful for them. The suggestions in this chapter are snapshots of what some families appreciated. True listening and working on maintaining the relationship are paramount. Connections can be made in many different, unique, and personally meaningful ways.

- Be sensitive to the emotional state of both child and parent. Sometimes parents want to talk about the illness; sometimes they just need a hand to hold.

- Encourage all members of the family to keep in touch through visits, calls, mail, videotapes, audiotapes, or pictures.

- Be understanding if the parents do not want phone calls in the hospital. Remember that the child can hear all phone conversations when parents talk on the phone in the room.

- A cheerful hospital room really boosts a child's spirits. Encourage sending balloon bouquets, funny cards, posters, toys, fancy pajamas and slippers, or humorous books. Be aware that some hospitals do not allow rubber balloons, only mylar. Rubber balloons can be a choking hazard. Flowers are also not allowed in children's rooms, because they can increase risk of infection.

  *We plastered the walls with pictures of family and friends and so many people sent balloons that the ceiling was covered. It was a lovely sight.*

- Laughter helps heal the mind and body, so send funny videotapes or arrive with a good joke if you think it's appropriate.

  *I was diagnosed in 1997, at the age of 16, with a low-grade astrocytoma. I've had seven surgeries, which include shunt revisions, and radiation. I have a large family, and I have a lot of little cousins. When I was diagnosed, I explained everything to them, and they seemed to take it pretty well. Kids can deal with issues like this, better than most adults. My youngest cousin was five years old. She has really grown up learning about brain tumors and knowing that her cousin has a brain tumor. She has coped with it, and understands what I have to do to fight this monster. She tells her friends that I'm her favorite cousin and she wants to be just like me! It has drawn us much closer since I was diagnosed, and I believe it is because we did not hide anything from her. We answered the questions she had, and tried to explain everything to her. She knows almost everything that we know about brain tumors, and explains to others the importance of having your brain checked. The way she deals with it makes me laugh a lot of times, and that is what I need. I need a way to let go of all the stress of the brain tumor, and just get a laugh every so often.*

• Puzzles, games, picture books, coloring books, age-appropriate computer games, and crafts are welcome. Remember that attention spans are sometimes shortened by treatment, so keep it simple.

> *A friend who was a nurse came to my son's room shortly before Christmas and brought an entire gingerbread house kit, including confectioner's sugar for the icing. We had a very good time putting it together.*

• Offer to give the parent a break from the hospital room. A walk outside, shopping trip, haircut, dinner with a spouse, or just a long shower can be very refreshing.

• Donate frequent flyer miles to distant family members who have the time but not the money to help.

• If you don't hear from a family member, call. Often silence means that she doesn't know what to do or say.

• Offer to drive or accompany the parent and child to outpatient appointments (radiation, physical therapy, or doctor's appointments). This provides company for the parent, help with the ill child, or simply relief from the stress of driving.

• Donate blood. Your blood may not be used specifically for the ill child, but it will replenish the general supply, which is depleted by children with cancer.

> *Our family friend John is terrified of needles. John always avoided giving blood. John doesn't like going to the doctor. But John showed up to donate platelets once, early on, and we found that he was a great platelet match for Deli. So he kept returning to that awful two-needle machine that you stay hooked onto for three hours at a time, probably a couple dozen times, because we needed him. Then we had Beth, who was one of my professional acquaintances. Beth was always pretty nice to us, but she found out that she too was a good "sticky" platelet donor. Probably at least a dozen times she took hours out of her workday and donated*

*platelets whenever Deli needed some. We concentrated on the few "star"*
*friends and relatives, the one or two people whose attitude and abilities*
*and circumstances allowed them to be the most helpful.*

- Join the bone marrow registry. This requires only giving a small sample of blood.

## Grandparents

Grandparents grieve deeply when a grandchild is diagnosed with a tumor. They are concerned not only for their grandchild, but for their own child (the parent) as well. Cancer wreaks havoc with grandparents' expectations, reversing the natural order of life and death. Grandparents frequently say, "Why not me? I'm the one who is old." Parents express anguish at having to tell the grandparents the grim news. A brain or spinal cord tumor in a grandchild is a major shock to bear.

Many parents reported that the grandparents responded to the crisis with tremendous emotional, physical, and financial support.

> *Our parents did a lot of care taking. They helped with meals, baby-*
> *sitting, cleaning, washing clothes, etc. They also stayed with Jeremy in the*
> *hospital when we were not able to.*

· · · · ·

> *John is Grampa's only grandchild. He's always there to play a board*
> *game, tell jokes, or watch his favorite video with him for the 1000th time.*
> *I wish he'd hide his fears a little better, but that may be too much to*
> *expect from a truly loving grandfather.*

Some parents express tremendous gratitude for the role played by the grandparents in providing much-needed stability to the family rocked by cancer. Caring for the siblings and running the household allow the parents to care for the sick child and return to work.

Other families are not so fortunate. Many grandparents are too old, too ill, or just unable to cope with a crisis of this magnitude. Some simply fall apart.

> *My mother became hysterical when my daughter was diagnosed. She*
> *called every day, sobbing. Luckily, she lived far away and this minimized*
> *the disruption. We had to ask her not to come because we couldn't handle*
> *the catastrophe at home and her neediness too. It hurt her feelings, but we*
> *just couldn't cope with it.*

Other grandparents allow pre-existing problems with their adult child to color their perceptions of what the family needs. Sometimes cancer allows grandparents to renew criticism of the way grandchildren are being raised.

> *While we stayed at the hospital the grandparents moved into our house*
> *to care for our eight-year-old daughter. They decided that this was their*
> *chance to "whip her into shape, teach her some manners, and get her*
> *room cleaned up." Our daughter was in tears, and we ended up saying,*
> *"We appreciate your help, but we will take over."*

Sometimes grandparents try to blame the parents for the tumor or make other kinds of hurtful comments. Disagreements can also arise if grandparents try to take charge. Criticizing parents' choice of doctors, hospitals, or treatment can be very disruptive and further stress the family's resources. Some grandparents simply cannot cope and withdraw from the situation.

> *I will never, ever be able to forget how my mother let me and my son*
> *down. She never came to the hospital, saying, "He's too sick for company."*
> *I told her he would love to see her; that his little face just would light up*
> *when he had visitors. But she never came. She never offered to help at*
> *home when he was so ill. She just disappeared.*

It is hard to predict how anyone will react to the diagnosis of childhood cancer. Grandparents are no exception. Some respond with the wisdom gleaned from decades of living, others become needy, and some withdraw. It is natural in a time of grave crisis to look to your parents for support and help, but it is important to remember that grandparents' ability to respond also depends on events in their own lives. If problems develop, help can be obtained from hospital social workers or through individual counseling.

# Friends

Like family, friends can cushion the shock of diagnosis, ease the difficulties of treatment with their words and actions, and provide balance when the timing is right.

## Notifying friends

The easiest way to notify friends is to delegate one person to do the job. Calling and asking one neighbor or close friend to do this prevents numerous tearful conversations. Most parents are at their child's bedside and want to avoid more emotional upheaval, especially in front of the child. Parents need to recognize that friends' emotions will mirror their own shock, fear, worry, or helplessness. Because most friends want to help but don't know what to do or say, giving cues of what would be helpful is welcome.

## Helpful things for friends to do

It is a given that the family of a newly diagnosed child is overwhelmed. The list of helpful things to do is endless, but here are some suggestions from veteran parents.

### Household

- Provide meals.

   > We found that the most helpful thing was when people brought us food to eat while in the hospital (where food is scarce for everyone but the patient), and also while recuperating at home. Often feeding ourselves took a back seat to caring for Ayla. This is not conducive to garnering energy to care for someone else!

- Take care of pets or livestock.

- Mow grass, shovel snow, rake leaves, weed gardens.

   > We came home from the hospital one evening right before Christmas, and found a freshly cut, fragrant Christmas tree leaning next to our door. I'll never forget that kindness.

- Clean house.

   > My husband's cousin sent her cleaning lady over to our house. It was so neat and such a luxury to come home to find the stove and windows sparkling clean.

- Grocery shop (especially when the family is due home from the hospital).

- Do laundry or drop off and pick up dry cleaning.

- Provide a place to stay near the hospital.

   > One of the ladies from the school where I worked came up to the ICU waiting room where we were sleeping and pressed her house key into my hand. She lived five minutes from the hospital. She said, "My basement is made up, there's a futon, there's a TV, you are coming and staying at my house." I hardly knew her, but we accepted. Every day when we came in from the hospital, there was some cute little treat waiting for us like a

*bowl of cookies, or two packages of hot chocolate and a thermos of hot milk.*

A child life specialist shared the following:

> *For many of the families I work with, allowing acquaintances into the home to clean and cook is just too personal and uncomfortable to allow during such a private time in their lives. It's just too intrusive. However, these families have shared many stories of anonymous giving. For instance, the following were very welcome: restaurant/fast food certificate, baskets of beauty products mysteriously left on the doorstep, journals, phone cards, movie rental cards, gas cards, and Polaroid film and camera left at the doorstep. The anonymity helped prevent the family from feeling indebted.*

## Siblings

It takes an entire chapter to deal with the complex feelings that siblings confront when their brother or sister has cancer. Chapter 16, *Siblings,* provides an in-depth examination of the issues from the perspective of both siblings and parents. Below is a list of suggestions on how family and friends can help with siblings.

- Babysit whenever parents go to clinic, to the emergency room, or for a prolonged hospital stay.

- When parents are home with a sick child, take sibling(s) to the park, sports event, or a movie.

- Invite sibling(s) over for meals.

- If you bring a gift for the sick child, bring something for the sibling(s), too.

- Offer to help sibling(s) with homework.

- Drive sibling(s) to lessons, games, or school.

- Listen to how they are feeling and coping. Siblings' lives have been disrupted, they have limited time with their parents, and they need support and care.

## Psychological support

There is much that can be done to help the family keep on an even emotional keel.

- Call frequently, and be open to listening if the parents want to talk about their feelings.

> *What I wished for most was that friends and family had been able*
> *to call more often to see how we were doing; that someone could have*
> *handled my confidence on the good days and my tears on the bad days.*
> *It somehow took too much emotional energy to make a call myself, but*
> *I valued any phone call I received.*

- Call to talk about topics that are not related to cancer.

- If one parent has to leave work for an extended time to stay in the hospital with the sick child, coworkers can send messages by mail or tape.

- If you think the family might be interested, call Candlelighters (contact information is in Appendix B, *Resources*) or the social worker at the local hospital to find out if there are support groups for parents and/or kids in your area.

- Offer to take the children to the support groups, or go with the parents. For most families, the parent support group becomes a second family with ties of shared experience as deep and strong as blood relations.

- Drive parents and child to clinic visits.

- Buy books (uplifting ones) for the family if they are readers.

- Send cards or letters.

- Baby-sit the sick child so that the parents can go out to eat, exercise, take a walk, or just get out of the hospital or house.

> *Constance and Michael and their son Byron were the only friends who*
> *always said, "Whenever you'd like us to watch Jamie, you just let us*
> *know," but because Jamie's seizures weren't controlled, we hesitated. It*
> *was literally two years later that we finally took them up on their offer.*

- If you have medical training, are knowledgeable about surfing the Internet, or can understand medical terminology, offer to do research. Don't assume that the family wants this information. Many can handle only certain things at certain times.

> *There were some friends and family that did research for us (Internet,*
> *books, finding doctors to consult) to help streamline our efforts and to*
> *assist us in focusing on important questions to ask doctors, and in*
> *knowing the latest research results. However, it was important for these*
> *researchers to give all the information and not filter out bad news.*
> *Strength and wisdom comes from information, whether good or bad.*

- Send the family a gift certificate for professional photographs.

*My daughter wanted her picture taken several months into treatment. She was bald, sick, and frightened of strangers. I called Donnette Studio, asked to speak to the photographer who was best with kids, and explained the situation. I told him that how the pictures looked didn't matter, I wanted it to be a fun experience. He scheduled one and one half hours for the appointment, and he played with her the majority of that time. They did puppets, chased each other around, and just had a ball. She had a glorious smile on her face for the pictures, and we go back every six months to see Donny.*

- Ask, "What needs to be done?" and then do it.

  *A close friend called and asked what she could do. So I asked if she could drive our second car the 100 miles to the hospital so that my husband could return in it to work. She came with her family to the Ronald McDonald House with two big bags containing the following: snack foods, a large box of stationery, envelopes, stamps, books to read, a book handmade by her 3-year-old daughter containing dozens of cut-out pictures of children's clothing pasted on construction paper (which my daughter adored looking at), and a beautiful, new, handmade, lace-trimmed dress for my daughter. It was full length and baggy enough to cover all bandages and tubing. She wore it almost every day for a year. It was a wonderful thing for my friend to do.*

- Give lots of hugs.

## Financial support

Helping families avoid financial disaster can be the next greatest gift after the life of the child and the strength of the family. It is estimated that even fully insured families spend 25 percent or more of their income on co-payments, travel, motels, meals, and other uncovered items. Uninsured or under-insured families may lose their savings or even their house. Even families with full health insurance, such as those in Canada, have additional expenses that are not covered. Most families need financial help. Here are some suggestions:

- Start a support fund.

- Share leave. Governments and some companies have leave banks that permit persons who are ill or taking care of someone who is ill to use other coworkers' leave so they won't have their pay docked.

*My husband's coworkers didn't collect money, they did something even more valuable. They donated sick leave hours, so that he was able to be at the hospital frequently during those first few months without losing a paycheck.*

- Job share. Some families work out job-share arrangements in which a co-worker donates time to perform part of one job to enable one parent to spend time at the hospital. Job sharing allows the job to get done, keeps peace at the job site, and prevents financial losses for the family. Another possibility would be for one or more friends with similar skills (e.g., word processing, filing, sales) to rotate through the job on a volunteer basis to cover for the parent of the ill child.

- Collect money at church or work to give informally.

  *After our son was diagnosed, my workplace collected over $1500. We were shocked. It really helped to cover hotel and travel expenses during our stay out of town for surgery.*

  • • • • •

  *Finances were a main concern for us because I wanted to cut back on work to be at home with Meagan. Sometimes my coworkers would pool money and present it with a card saying, "Here's a couple of days' work that you won't have to worry about."*

- Collect money by organizing a bake sale, dance, or raffle.

- Keeping track of medical records and medical bills is time-consuming, frustrating, and exhausting. If you are a close relative or friend, you could offer to review, organize, and file (or enter into a computer) the voluminous paperwork. Making the calls and writing the letters over contested insurance claims or errors in hospital billing are very helpful. See Chapter 18, *Record Keeping and Finances,* for further information.

  *I am the one handling all of the administrative duties for the family. We have learned when Kevin gets his MRI to ask the techs to make a copy for us right then and there. I have to keep copies of everything regarding Kevin's treatment and surgery, including pathology reports, second opinion consults, lab reports, etc. I now have copies of all MRI films, all of the hospital records, every report that was ever written, and all of the radiological reports. I make tons of copies of these in case they're ever needed.*

*Talking to insurance people really hits a sore spot with me; right from the beginning of the call, there is a menu with many options to choose from, and it can take ten minutes if you are lucky to get a real live person on the phone. I have, many times, asked for supervisors, demanded and insisted that expediency is necessary. I have learned to take the person's name, their title, and write down time and date on every conversation I have. It is a time-consuming job.*

## Help from schoolmates and school staff

Friends and social life primarily revolve around school. Trying to maintain ties with school, teachers, and friends will help the child make a smooth transition back as soon as he is able.

- Encourage visits (if appropriate), cards, and phone calls from classmates.

    *Our son had a rough time with fever and seizures during chemo, and he was really missing his routine. His preschool teachers, Kate and Ellie, surprised him one time with a homemade book. They had all the kids pose for an instant picture for the cover, and each one drew a picture for the inside. He loved it.*

- Classmates can sign a brightly colored banner to send to the hospital.

- Ask the teacher to send the school newspaper and other news along with assignments, and express your concern that they keep in touch with your child during prolonged absences from school.

    *On a Thursday, our second grade son Christopher was diagnosed with a pilocytic astrocytoma of the cerebellum the size of an orange. By Friday morning, Christopher's classroom, Room 35 at Carpenter Avenue Elementary School, was already making Get Well Pizza cards for him. One of his teachers sat down with the kids and talked about what it would be like in the hospital, and an appointed person from the school community called us regularly for updates and passed on prayers and loving regards from families and staff. We had amazingly touching responses from many school parents, teachers, coaches, and even our principal.*

    *The PTA president came to visit and brought a huge card signed by all of Christopher's classmates, teachers, and other Carpenter friends. She had also lined up parents from Room 35 to bring dinners to my husband Jim and I for the entire upcoming week. As the weeks went on, the love and support just escalated. Christopher found his greatest joy throughout the whole hospital ordeal was receiving more incredible Beanie Babies than he could have ever imagined getting.*

*Our whole family has a view of Carpenter Avenue Elementary School that has changed us forever. They are an extraordinary community of families that I wish every family in need can experience.*

- School friends and civic groups can show their support by doing volunteer work at their local hospital or by participating in or organizing cancer and brain tumor awareness events.

*I have recently been so impressed with some 12- to 13-year-old Girl Scouts in our area. They saw our web site for the Hem/Onc clinic and decided to do a drive for the things on our clinic wish list. They are coming into the outpatient clinic with gifts in hand and plan to spend a morning doing crafts with our young patients. We are getting some TV media coverage for it because it is such a positive community service.*

## Religious support

For families who have religious affiliations, here are a few suggestions:

- Ask the family if they would like you to contact clergy.

- Arrange for the pastor, rabbi, priest, minister, or church members to visit the hospital, if that is what the family wants.

- Arrange prayer or healing services for the sick child and the family.

*The day our son was diagnosed, we raced next door to ask our wonderful neighbors to take care of our dog. The news of his diagnosis quickly spread, and we found out later that five neighborhood families gathered that very night to pray for Brent.*

- Have the child's religious class send pictures, posters, letters, balloons, or tapes to the sick child.

- Involve the church or synagogue in fundraising or awareness events.

## Accepting help

It is often very difficult to accept help in a crisis. Even harder is telling people what you need.

One father's thoughts on accepting help:

> *I had always been considered the provider in our family. I think I did a very good job with that, too. But nothing prepared me for the nightmare that Matthew's cancer brought into our lives. It took me some time to realize it, but I came to the conclusion that it was impossible for me to do this on my own.*

One mother's thoughts on accepting help:

> *The most important advice I received as the parent of a child newly diagnosed with cancer came from a hospital nurse whom I turned to when I was overwhelmed with all the advice being offered by family and friends. This wise nurse said, "Don't discount anything. You're going to need all the help you can get." I think it is very important for families to remain open and accept the help that is offered. It often comes when least expected and from unlikely sources. I was totally unprepared at diagnosis for how much help I would need, and I'm glad that I remained open to offers of kindness. This is not the time to show the world how strong you are.*

## Giving gifts

When a child is diagnosed with cancer, many families' first response is to buy the biggest, brightest toy in the store. Appropriate gifts can often be beneficial to a child's well-being, but parents may want to control the flow of incoming gifts.

> *One January afternoon, I am at the hospital with a devastating CT scan in my hands that shows my son has medulloblastoma. I call my husband at work: "Come here. Now." When he arrives, we try to be brave in front of Ben, our 5-year-old son, but finally I ask my husband if he will take Ben home in his car, so I can be alone. As I drive home alone in my van, I sob, scream and have to pull over to the side of the road a few times to calm down.*
>
> *I arrive at our home first and wait for them. And wait. And wait. I begin to worry that my husband was too distraught himself to drive safely. Just when I am considering making official inquiries, they walk in the door—with a train set. From the age of two, Ben has wanted a real train set, with tracks and engines and smoke, but our house is very small and space a premium. My husband is sheepish, and I say, "Oh well, what the heck." They immediately set it up in the living room. Ben plays with it all evening,*

*and wants to sleep in a sleeping bag on the floor next to it that night. The next morning he goes to the hospital for surgery.*

*Word gets out. Every visitor who comes to see Ben, every well-wisher, every relative from another state, bosses, coworkers, family friends, bring or send additions to the train set. I learn that the local train store has registered my son like a bride.*

*When my seriously incapacitated son arrives home from the hospital, we expand the train set to lure him out of his depression. When he takes his first stumbling steps with a walker and nearly trips on the track, we push the setup to the side of the room. When it becomes clear that the train set is Ben's joy, the one thing this kid can have complete control over, we decide it needs to be a permanent fixture. So. The stereo goes in the dining room, the couch is pushed up next to the heater, the floor-length blinds are chopped in half, all so Grandpa can build a ten-by-six foot train table in the living room.*

*Ben's big sister has her own train, hubby has his special engine that he keeps in a box and won't let anyone touch, and one day each weekend is "train day," where they visit the three local train stores, or go to a train show, or build a table, or enlarge the table, or add some trestles. Yes, we are crowded, but we have one happy little boy, let me tell you.*

A child life worker cautions that gift giving can create problems:

*Many parents tell me that they want to tone down the gift giving. Kids shouldn't learn to expect something every time someone walks through the door. After months or years of treatment, the house can look like a toy store. Many parents have difficulty setting limits, expectations, and discipline for their child. Non-stop gifts don't help. If you feel you must bring something, try to bring stickers, crayons, videos or music, or a craft project that you can do with the child.*

## What to say

The following are some suggestions for family and friends on what to say and how to offer help. Of course, much depends on the type of relationship that already exists, but a specific offer can always be accepted or graciously declined.

- I am so sorry.
- I didn't call earlier because I didn't know what to say.

- Our family would like to do your yard work. It will make us feel as if we are helping in a small way.

- We want to clean your house for you once a week. What day would be convenient?

- Would it help if we took care of your dog (or cat, or bird)? We would love to do it.

- I walk my dog three times a day. May I walk yours, too?

- The church is setting up a system to deliver meals to your house. When is the best time to drop them off?

- I will take care of Jimmy whenever you need to take John to the hospital. Call us anytime, day or night, and we will come pick him up.

## Things that do not help

Sometimes people say hurtful things to parents of children with cancer. If you are a family member or friend of a parent in this situation, please do not say any of the following:

- "God only gives people what they can handle." (Some people cannot handle the stress of having a child with a CNS tumor.)

- "I know just how you feel." (Unless you have a child with cancer, you simply don't know.)

- "They are doing such wonderful things to save children with tumors these days." (Yes, the prognosis may be good, but what parents and children are going through is not wonderful.)

- "Well, we're all going to die one day." (True, but parents do not need to be reminded of this fact.)

- "It's God's will." (For many families, this is just not a helpful thing to hear.)

- "At least you have other kids," or "Thank goodness you are still young enough to have other children." (A child cannot be replaced.)

    *A woman whom I worked with, but did not know well, came up to me one day and out of the blue said, "When Erica gets to heaven to be with Jesus, He will love her." All I could think to say was, "Well, I'm sorry, but Jesus can't have her right now."*

Parents also make the following suggestions of things to avoid doing:

- Do not say, "Let us know if there is anything we can do." It is far better to make a specific suggestion.

> *Many well-wishing friends always said, "Let me know what I can do." I wish they had just "done," instead of asking for direction. It took too much energy to decide, call them, make arrangements, etc. I wish someone had said, "When is your clinic day? I'll bring dinner," or "I'll baby sit Sunday afternoon so you two can go out to lunch."*

- Do not make personal comments in front of the child: when will his hair grow back in, she's lost so much weight, he's so pale, etc.

> *When in the mall or other public place, strangers had no qualms about staring at Ayla (age 3) who had an eye patch, tubes that sometimes snuck out from under her shirt, and no hair. We combated this by telling her that she was so absolutely stunningly beautiful that people just could not help but stare at her. We really played this up and tied it in to her belief in Snow White, Cinderella, etc. Many times we let her and her sister Jasmine wear their princess costumes out in public. Then they really got a kick out of people staring. I also did not hesitate to tell people that she had cancer when they asked what was wrong with her. I never minimized what she was going through. We talk about cancer freely and how doctors are there to fix you up if you get this.*

- Do not do things that require the parent to support you (for example, repeatedly call up crying).

- Do not talk continually about the cancer; some normal conversations are welcome.

- Do not ask "what if" questions: What if he can't go to school? What if your insurance won't cover it? What if she dies? The present is really all the parents can deal with.

- Refrain from saying, "I don't know how you do it," or "You're so strong."

> *Whenever someone says: "You're so strong" or "I don't know how you do it," answer: "I don't do it alone," or "With lots of help" or (if it's true) "I'm pretty close to losing it completely." There's a thin line between being honest about your situation and being oppressive, for want of a better word. In my more cynical moments, I am convinced the world wants us (i.e., the cancer kids/families) to valiantly triumph over hardship with the Movie-of-the-Week-attitude. Well if that gets them to wash my floors, it's a small price!*

> *I think some of the most supported families I've seen on treatment had a knack at keeping people informed about the current situation. I updated the outgoing message on our answering machine every couple of days and*

*people could call our home for current news (a hospice nurse/neighbor gave
me that idea). Other friends from the hospital used newsletters, phone
chains, announcements in church, etc. Again, my cynical side recognizes
that you're opening up your most personal moments to the public (anyone
who called my house and heard the message the day after my son's stroke
probably felt like an intruder) but it's a way to help people feel invested in
your family.*

- Stories of children you know who have survived cancer and are doing fine are welcome.

## Losing friends

It is an unfortunate reality that most parents of children with tumors lose friends. For a variety of reasons, some friends just can't cope and either suddenly disappear or gradually fade away. Many times this can be prevented by calling them to keep them involved, but sometimes they just can't handle the stress.

> *My daughter Lauren was diagnosed with a very rare and aggressive
> cancer. We finished treatment in April of this year, and since that time
> I have been feeling an overwhelming series of emotions, most of which lie at
> the bottom of the happiness scale. This past weekend, I finally met with my
> best friend, who had her first baby in March. Needless to say, I have not
> been overly involved with her life of late. My own was often more than I
> could hack. This friend did prove to be a true friend throughout the cancer
> trip as she visited us often at the hospital. She confessed to me that she
> missed me so much, and that she sometimes mistook my silence for
> indifference. I didn't take offense, as I might have, but rather, this seemed
> to be the "invite" that I needed to re-enter the world that I had left when
> Lauren was diagnosed. The fact that I had value as a friend, and not just
> as a caregiver, was a wake-up call. Throughout the past year, I had isolated
> myself from everyone from my old life, and was starting to think that
> maybe I would never make it back. Maybe now I can pull back the cobwebs
> and struggle back.*

# Restructuring family life

Benign or malignant tumors do not strike only families with brave children and heroic parents. In the United States, the popular press has responded to people's fear of cancer by churning out story after story of people who faced the diagnosis with almost superhuman hope and strength. Families rally round, the community cheers, and human will triumphs over the evil of cancer. This simply is not always the case. CNS tumors strike all types of families: single-parent families, those with two parents in the home, financially secure families, those with no insurance, families with strong community ties, those who have just moved to a new community: families of every size, type, and color. Most parents do find unexpected reserves of strength to deal with the crisis. They survive the years of stress and pain, emerging different and sometimes stronger. Still, expectations of heroism are not appropriate.

## Keeping the household functioning

Every family of a child with cancer needs massive assistance. It is important for families to recognize this early and learn not only to accept aid gracefully, but also to ask for help when needed. As discussed earlier in the chapter, most family members, friends, neighbors, and church members want to help, but they need direction from the family on what is helpful but not intrusive.

In families where both parents are employed, decisions must be made about the jobs. It is better, if possible, to use all available sick leave and vacation days prior to deciding whether one parent needs to terminate employment. Parents need to be able to evaluate their financial situation and insurance availability. This requires time and clarity of thought, both of which are in short supply in the weeks following diagnosis.

## Family and Medical Leave Act

In August 1993, the Family and Medical Leave Act (FMLA) became federal law in the US. FMLA protects job security of workers in large companies who must take a leave of absence to care for a seriously ill immediate family member. It also covers employees who are unable to work because of their own medical condition, as well as when a child is born, adopted, or placed in foster care. The Family and Medical Leave Act:

- Applies to employers with 50 or more employees who work for at least twenty work weeks within a 75-mile radius.

- Provides twelve weeks of unpaid leave during any twelve-month period to care for a seriously ill spouse, child, or parent. In certain instances, the employee may take intermittent leave by reducing his or her normal work schedule's hours or taking leave in blocks of time.

- Requires employer to continue to provide benefits, including health insurance, during the leave period.

- Requires employer to return employee to the same or equivalent position upon return from the leave. Some benefits, such as seniority, need not accrue during periods of unpaid FMLA leave.

- Requires employee to give 30-day notice of the need to take FMLA leave when the need is foreseeable.

- Is enforced by complaints to the Wage and Hour Division, US Department of Labor, or by private lawsuit. The nearest office of the Wage and Hour Division may be located by looking in the US Government pages of your telephone directory.

In Canada, a parent may be entitled to benefits under the Employment Insurance Act. Consideration is provided in the act for a parent having to leave work to provide care for an ill child. Entitlement to benefits is made on a case-by-case basis. Should a parent qualify, benefits are determined by the number of hours the parent has worked prior to making the claim. For further information, parents should contact the nearest Human Resources Development Canada office listed in the Government of Canada pages of the telephone directory.

## Marriage

Cancer treatment places enormous pressure on a marriage. Couples may be separated for long periods of time, emotions are high, and coping styles differ. Initially, family life is shattered. Couples must simply survive the first few overwhelming weeks, then work together to rearrange the pieces in a new pattern. Following are parents' suggestions and stories about how they managed.

- Share medical decisions.

    *My husband and I shared decision-making by keeping a joint medical journal. The days that my husband stayed at the hospital, he would write down all medicines given, side effects, fever, vital signs, food consumed, sleep patterns, and any questions that needed to be asked at the next rounds. This way, I knew exactly what had been happening. Decisions were made as we traded shifts at our son's bedside.*

· · · · ·

    *I made most of the medical decisions. My husband did not know what a protocol was, nor did he ever learn the names of the medicines. He came with me to medical conferences, however, and his presence gave me strength.*

- Take turns staying in the hospital with the ill child.

*We took turns going in with our son for painful procedures. The doctors loved to see my husband come in because he's a friendly, easygoing person who never asked them any medical questions. We shared hospital duty, also. I would be there during any crisis because I was the person better able to be a strong advocate, but he went when our son was feeling better and needed entertaining company. It worked out well.*

• • • • •

*My wife took care of most of the medical information gathering because she had a scientific background. But my work schedule was more flexible, so I took my son for almost all of his treatments and hospitalizations. I cherish my memories of those long hours in the car and waiting room, because we were always so very close.*

• Share responsibility for home care.

*My husband worked long hours, and therefore I had to do almost all of the home care. It was very hard on me, especially in the beginning when she was so ill and needed so many medications. I felt like I was doing all the horrible things to her; I wish that he could have done some of it.*

• • • • •

*We both worked full time, so we staggered our shifts. He worked 7 to 3, I worked 3 to 11. He did every single dressing change for the Hickman catheter—584 changes, we counted them up. Wherever I left off during the day, he took over. He was great, and it really worked out well for us. We shared it all.*

• • • • •

*My husband really didn't help at all. I couldn't even go out because he wouldn't give the pills. He kept saying that he was afraid that he would make a mistake.*

• • • • •

*My husband does about 75 percent of the hospital/clinic/radiation visits. In fact, he does all of them when he is in town. I take care of the rest of the children and float in when I get a chance. I keep in touch with the doctors via email.*

• Accept differences in coping styles.

*We both coped differently, but we learned to work around it. I didn't want to deal with "what if" questions, but he was a pessimist and constantly asked the fellow questions about things that might happen. I felt that it was a waste of energy to worry about things that might never*

*happen. I didn't want to hear it and felt that it just added to my burden.*
*It was all I could do to survive every day. We worked it out by going to*
*conferences together, but I would ask my questions and then leave. He*
*stayed behind to ask all of his questions.*

. . . . .

*My husband didn't have the desire to read as much as I did. However,*
*whenever I read something that I felt he should read, he always took the*
*time to do so and then we discussed it.*

. . . . .

*My husband and I have always been a team. We complement the*
*strengths and weaknesses of each other and I think that was the reason*
*we managed to hold everything together. When I was down, he would*
*bring me up. When he was down, I would do the same for him. With*
*the exception of the initial trauma when our son was diagnosed, we*
*handled things in that manner throughout treatment.*

- Seek counseling.

  *I went for counseling because I couldn't sleep. At night, I got stuck*
  *thinking the same things over and over and worrying. I ended up*
  *spending two years on antidepressants, which I think really saved my life.*
  *They helped me sleep and kept me on an even keel. I'm off them now, my*
  *son is off treatment, and everything is looking up.*

  . . . . .

  *My husband and I went to counseling to try to work out a way to split*
  *up the child rearing and household duties because I was overwhelmed and*
  *resenting it. I guess it helped a little bit, but the best thing that came out of*
  *it was that I kept seeing the counselor by myself. My son wanted to go to*
  *the "feelings doctor," too. I received a lot of very helpful, practical advice*
  *on the many behavior problems my son developed. And my son had an*
  *objective, safe person to talk things over with.*

Some marriages survive and some don't. It is usually marriages with serious pre-existing problems that are further strained by cancer treatment.

*My husband had a lot of problems that really brought my daughter and*
*me down. The cancer really opened my eyes to what was important in*
*life. We stayed together through treatment, but we divorced after the bone*
*marrow transplant. I just realized that life is too short to spend it in a bad*
*relationship.*

. . . . .

*My husband went to work rather than with us to Children's when our*
*son was diagnosed. It went downhill from there. He started using drugs*
*and mistreating us, so we divorced.*

## Deciding to have more children

Once a life-threatening illness enters the family scene, the decision to have more children is never easy.

*Andy was our first baby. We looked forward to having him, and we were*
*prepared to become a family. We were not prepared for a brain tumor!*
*Our focus now is 100 percent on making him well, and although at one*
*time I thought I'd like to have more children, that's definitely changed.*

· · · · ·

*You know the scenario: ICU vigils, living through each decision we make*
*about treatment, procedures that cause pain and permanent damage "all*
*for his own good," wondering if our young son would be better off without*
*all this, convincing him that clinic is "fun," that tubies are his friends, that*
*medicine will make him better. I lose the life I have carefully crafted for*
*myself. Writing? I can barely manage a grocery list. Marriage? We can't*
*bear each other's pain so we withdraw from each other, until, that one*
*night, when the grief breaks through and we comfort each other.*

*Boom ... I'm pregnant. A baby is not such a bad idea, but I am afraid to*
*be made vulnerable, all over again. The thought of loving another child*
*who could be hurt is more than I can bear. A child conceived in grief. A*
*new life forming while another is in jeopardy, I can hardly get my thoughts*
*around it. I'm fighting for my son's life and have no energy to spare for the*
*other. I whisper my misgivings only to myself*

*I know that we will welcome this child and love it and bear it no ill will,*
*and that it is probably well-timed in many ways, and may be even more*
*cherished for all these odd circumstances. It will quicken and grow and a*
*relationship will form. Soon enough.*

## Blended families

Many children diagnosed with tumors live in blended families. Parents may be separated or divorced, remarried, or living as single parents. There may be foster parents, biological parents, stepparents, or legal guardians. Communication between involved adults may be open and amiable or stressed and uncooperative. It is best for the child when all parents involved put their differences aside and work together to provide an environment focused on curing the ill child.

> *My son has been treated off and on for ten years for a brainstem tumor.*
> *He is now paralyzed and on a respirator in a care facility. In the*
> *beginning, my ex-husband was overseas, so my husband and I made all*
> *the appointments, took turns in the hospital, and tucked Brendon in at*
> *night. Over the years, my ex-husband has become more and more part of*
> *our family care network. He goes to the care facility every day after work*
> *and on weekends. I stay with Brendon the days my husband has off, and*
> *my husband stays two evenings a week. My ex-husband will babysit my*
> *three other children so my husband and I can go to see Brendon together.*
> *His mother also helps out enormously with visiting at the care facility and*
> *babysitting the three younger children. It's become a community effort.*
> *It works out well because we all love our son and we've chosen to work it*
> *out rather than bicker.*

If the child with cancer has two homes due to a blended family, it often helps to have a journal that goes with the child to each set of parents. It keeps everyone involved up-to-date. It can contain meds given, dose changes, doctor appointments, blood test results, and current symptoms.

Unfortunately, the diagnosis of cancer in a child can make strained family relations even worse. It is important that all parents with a legal right to information about all aspects of the illness receive that information and are able to participate in the decision-making process. In some situations a social worker, nurse practitioner, primary physician, or psychologist will work with all parties to set up family meetings (whether together as one group or separately, based upon family dynamics) with healthcare providers to make this possible.

> *Telling your friends about cancer is difficult, but not as hard as keeping*
> *it a secret would be. Fighting this cancer has been a family effort and*
> *frequently an effort involving our larger circle of friends. The more people*
> *we've been able to call on for support, the better. We've had to keep in*
> *mind that we've had an opportunity to adjust. But, the news is brand-new*

to our friends, and it can be a shock. People often don't know what to do or say when they've been told that someone they care about has cancer.

After we've given them some time, and when they ask what they can do, we tell them something constructive: mow the lawn, take back the recyclables, go to the store, bring over a pizza on Friday night, whatever would help.

Before my son was diagnosed, I had no idea what this experience was like, and I try to remember that my friends don't really know either unless I tell them. They can't know the sleepless nights, the anxiety over tests, the fear when your child says he doesn't feel well, or the numbing fear that we might lose our precious child. Some of us have found great support and others none. I hope your family and friends come to your side.

I want to say that I hope that cancer does not become your life. For us, it used to be an "elephant in the living room," and now it's maybe a "zebra in the kitchen." There are times when it demands everything you can give, no doubt, but there will be moments when there is time for the rest of your life.

# CHAPTER 7

# Forming a Partnership with the Medical Team

IT IS VITALLY IMPORTANT THAT parents and the healthcare team establish and maintain a relationship based on excellent medical care, good communication, and caring. In this partnership, trust is paramount. Physicians rely on parents to make and keep appointments, give the proper medicines at the appropriate times, prepare the child for procedures, and be vigilant in noticing any illness or drug side effect. Parents rely on physicians for medical knowledge, expertise in performing procedures, good judgment, and clear communication.

Unlike many other diseases, children with CNS tumors spend months or years being treated on an inpatient and outpatient basis. In addition, the treatment of CNS tumors in children requires a multidisciplinary approach involving many teams of medical, surgical, and rehabilitative specialists. At various points of the diagnosis and treatment journey, the primary responsibility of providing treatment for the child with a CNS tumor shifts from one group of physicians to another.

At diagnosis and in the initial stages of treatment, the pediatric neurosurgeon is usually the captain of the multidisciplinary team. This leadership shifts after surgery to the neuro-oncologist, oncologist, neurologist, radiation oncologist, or physical therapy specialist to coordinate the next phase of treatment. Once treatment is finished, the neuro-oncologist or a primary care pediatrician may assume leadership of the necessary long-term follow-up. It is the parents, however, who bear the responsibility for coordinating the care and communication between members of the multidisciplinary team.

A climate of cooperation and respect between the multidisciplinary healthcare team and parents allows children to thrive. This chapter explores ways to create and maintain that environment.

# The hospital

Children who are diagnosed with a CNS tumor are usually sent to the nearest academic medical center or children's hospital. It is in those large centers that one will find the multidisciplinary team needed for state-of-the-art treatment. Most of these centers combine their efforts by participating in clinical studies with other institutions across the country.

If you are sent to a local hospital or to an oncologist, rather than a multidisciplinary team that includes pediatric neuro-oncologists and pediatric neurosurgeons, you should consider fighting that referral. Recent research showed that children treated at major brain tumor centers did significantly better than those treated at local hospitals.

Because most CNS tumors require several phases of treatment, you may need to go to different hospitals at different times. For example, your child may get radiation at one hospital and chemotherapy at another. The neuro-oncologist may see your child in a clinic separate from the hospital.

> We consider our pediatrician and local pediatric oncologist as
> co-directors of our son's care. At the same time, we make frequent visits
> to specialists for acuity and visual field testing, endocrine follow-up, and
> day-to-day seizure management. We've enrolled our child in a post-
> treatment study at the National Cancer Institute, in Bethesda,
> Maryland, so we go there twice a year, and we also see a pediatric
> neuro-oncologist for long-term brain tumor management.

After admission to the hospital, a steady parade of anonymous faces enters the life of a child with a CNS tumor. To understand who is responsible for your child's treatment, an explanation of the various members of the healthcare team is necessary.

## The multidisciplinary team

The first step of treatment for most children with CNS tumors involves surgery. It is vital that a pediatric neurosurgeon perform the surgery. A pediatric neurosurgeon is a physician who has either done a pediatric fellowship (an extra year of training in pediatrics after neurosurgical residency) or devotes at least half of his time to operating on children. Most pediatric neurosurgeons are in large teaching hospitals or in children's hospitals in large cities. A list of pediatric neurosurgeons is provided in Appendix D, *List of Pediatric Neurosurgeons*.

After surgery, the responsibility for care of most children with CNS tumors shifts to a pediatric neuro-oncologist. Neuro-oncologists are doctors who specialize in the nonsurgical treatment of brain tumors. Smaller clinics may not have a neuro-oncologist on staff. In these cases, a pediatric oncologist or pediatric neurologist is responsible for medical treatment and long-term follow-up.

Along with neurosurgeons and neuro-oncologists, children with CNS tumors may also see one or more of the following physicians:

- **Radiologist.** Doctor who interprets scans at diagnosis and throughout treatment.

- **Pathologist.** Doctor who determines the type of brain tumor after surgery by analyzing cells under a microscope.

- **Radiation oncologist.** Doctor who designs and manages the administration of radiation therapy.

- **Ophthalmologist.** Doctor who specializes in the eye.

- **Endocrinologist.** Doctor who monitors hormonal or growth problems.

- **Pediatric surgeon.** Surgeon who inserts catheters used for chemotherapy.

- **Pediatric neurologist.** Doctor who treats seizures.

- **Neuropsychologist/psychologist.** A medical specialist who assesses children at various stages of treatment to identify any learning problems that may arise from the CNS tumor or treatment.

- **Pediatrician.** Doctor who cares for children in their hometown or hospital.

- **Physiatrist.** Doctor who coordinates all physical, occupational, and speech therapy known as "rehab."

- **Orthopedic surgeon.** Doctor who monitors the spine for any curves (i.e., scoliosis) or changes resulting from surgery or treatment of a CNS tumor.

- **Psychiatrist.** Physician who diagnoses and treats mental or psychological problems.

> I'd strongly recommend that a neuro-oncologist be involved, even if he/
> she is advising from a distant major brain tumor center. Too often the
> local oncologists and neurologists are just not that experienced with pedi
> brain tumors, nor are they up to speed on the newest treatments, trials,
> drug combos, etc. Having a pedi BT specialist involved is in your child's
> best interest.

# The doctors

At large hospitals, there are doctors at all levels of training, from first year medical students to experienced professors of medicine. It is often hard to sort them all out in the early days after diagnosis. The following section describes each type of doctor you might meet at a training hospital.

A medical student is a college graduate who is attending medical school. Medical students often wear white coats, but do not have MD after the name on their nametags. They are not doctors.

An intern (also called a first year resident) is a graduate of medical school who is in his first year of postgraduate training.

A resident is a graduate of medical school in his second year or beyond of postgraduate training. Upon completion of their residencies, each doctor will be a specialist in their particular field; for example, a neurosurgeon, neuro-oncologist, or pediatrician. Length of residency varies, depending upon the specialty: neurosurgery is seven years, neuro-oncology is four to five years, pediatrics is three years.

After residency, if the physician wishes to further specialize, she applies for a fellowship. Fellows work only at academic centers with fellowship programs, not at all pediatric centers. A fellow who treats children with CNS tumors is a doctor who has completed four years of medical school, one year of internship, and two to seven years of residency in her field and is taking additional specialty training.

Above fellows in the hospital hierarchy are attending physicians (called simply "attendings"). These well-established doctors are hired by the medical center to provide and oversee medical care and to train interns, residents, and fellows. They are frequently also professors on the staff of the medical school.

> Our medical team was wonderful. They always answered our questions
> and spent the time with us that we needed. We had a group of doctors
> who were all working together for the patients. I always felt that we were
> known by each doctor, and that they were on top of Paige's treatment.

The physician in charge of your child's care should be board certified or have equivalent medical credentials. This means that he has taken rigorous written and/or oral tests by a board of examiners in his specialty and meets a high standard of competence. You can call the American Board of Medical Specialties at (866) ASK-ABMS to find out if your child's physician is board certified.

While an inpatient, your child will see a large number of other doctors. Residents usually rotate to different services every four weeks, so they are an ever-changing group. If questions arise about your child's illness or treatment that the resident cannot answer, you should ask the fellow or attending assigned to your child.

If your family is insured by a health maintenance organization (HMO), you probably will be sent to the affiliated hospital, which will have one or more pediatric neurosurgeons and pediatric neuro-oncologists on staff.

## The nurses

An essential part of the hospital hierarchy is the nursing staff. The following explanations will help you understand which type of nurse is caring for your child.

An LPN is a licensed practical nurse. LPNs complete a vocational training program and have a narrow scope of practice; for example, they usually do not start IVs or give IV medications.

An RN is a registered nurse who obtained an associate or bachelor's degree in nursing and then passed a licensing examination. These medical professionals give medicines, take vital signs (heart rate, breathing rate, blood pressure), monitor IV machines, change bandages, and care for patients in hospitals, clinics, and doctors' offices.

> At our hospital, each of our nurses is different, but each is wonderful. They simply love the kids. They throw parties, set up dream trips, act as counselor, best friend, stern parent. They hug moms and dads. They cry. I have come to respect them so much because they have such a hard job to do, and they do it so well.

The head or charge nurse is the supervisor of all the nurses on the floor for one shift. If you have any problems with a nurse, your first step in resolving them would be to talk to the nurse involved. If this does not work, a discussion with the charge nurse is necessary.

The clinical nurse manager is the administrator for an entire unit, such as a surgical or medical floor or outpatient clinic. She is in charge of all of the nurses on the unit.

A nurse practitioner or clinical nurse specialist is a registered nurse who has completed an educational program that has taught her advanced skills. For example, in some hospitals and clinics, nurse practitioners perform procedures such as spinal taps. Nurse practitioners or clinical nurse specialists are often the liaison between the medical teams and patients and families. They help parents keep all the different multidisciplinary team "players" straight and help interpret medical jargon.

## The tumor board

Many facilities utilize a committee to review MRI scans and discuss potential treatment plans for patients. This committee is called the tumor board. Members consist of representatives from the patient's multi-disciplinary team and other senior specialists who deal with CNS tumors. Very often, the consensus opinion from the tumor board is the treatment offered to the family.

# Finding a surgeon and neuro-oncologist

Sometimes parents do not have the luxury of time in choosing a pediatric neurosurgeon or pediatric neuro-oncologist. At diagnosis, the family is usually referred to the nearest pediatric center of excellence. The young patient may be assigned the attending or fellow who happens to be on call at the time of diagnosis.

> A medical oncologist sees patients with a wide variety of cancers and blood diseases. Through his doors march people with any number of cancer types, leukemias, and HIV/AIDS. It will necessarily have taken him much longer to accumulate respectable clinical experience with brain tumors than would a neuro-oncologist, who sees brain tumor patients exclusively and on a daily basis. What a neuro-oncologist would learn in a single year of practice might take a medical oncologist a decade to grasp. When a situation arises, you want the doctor who calls to mind a hundred similar cases he has seen recently, not the doctor who will rack his brain trying to remember the dozen cases he may have seen or merely read about long ago.
>
> A neuro-oncologist, because of his understanding of the entire brain tumor experience (not just the chemo part), can address questions related to cognitive changes, family tensions, etc., and will have a better handle on interactions among drugs the brain tumor patient is likely to be taking simultaneously. He is also more likely to have the tact and sensitivity needed to deal with the very specific needs of the brain tumor patient and family. The difference between our oncologist and neuro-oncologist was amazing. We considered the original guy fine (and he was), but then someone came in and turned on the light. It was like that moment when Dorothy from the Wizard of Oz steps out of the house and the world's in color.

During treatment, your child will see a myriad of doctors. It is essential that you are comfortable with your surgeon and neuro-oncologist and that the family finds the doctors competent, caring, and easy to communicate with. When choosing your child's pediatric neurosurgeon and/or neuro-oncologist, here are several traits to look for:

- Board certified in the field

- Establishes good rapport with child

- Communicates clearly and compassionately

- Skillful in performing procedures

- Uses the latest surgical tools and techniques

- Answers all questions

- Consults with other doctors on complex problems

- Uses language that is easy to understand

- Makes the results of all tests available

- Acknowledges parents' right to make decisions

- Respects parents' values

- Able to deliver the truth with hope

If you don't develop a good rapport with your physicians, ask to be assigned to a different physician whom you have met on rounds or during clinic visits. Most parents are accommodated, for hospitals realize the importance of good communication and rapport between family and physician. You will, however, still see different physicians, because many institutions have rotating physicians on call.

> The neurosurgeon told us that everything looked great on Janet's MRI and to come back and see him in three months. He also gave me $10.00 and said if we get down to Biloxi again to play #22 on roulette for him. I asked, "Why 22?," and he said that was the date that he met an individual that helped change his perspective on life, which in turn has allowed him to treat his patients better. He then handed me Janet's chart and pointed to our first appointment date: Sept. 22, 2000.

• • • • •

> For two months, we were dealing with a doctor who said there was only a "vanishingly small" chance at a cure—NO clinical trials, NO other options, NO, NO, NO. I did my own research, and ended up with a doctor new to our hospital, who gives Danny a "real chance." Not only

does his attitude make a difference to my own attitude (it's actually pleasant to be in the same room and talk to him) but I believe he is actively searching out treatment options and in fact has a whole list of things to try. The first doctor came at it from a much more conservative vantage point—if something didn't have a tried and true track record he wouldn't recommend it. The problem in our case was that Danny has an incredibly rare brain tumor so there is no track record. One final note, every doctor I spoke with, except of course our first one, said that there are always exceptions. They've seen patients ten years ago who they said would never make it, and they're doing great. I need a doctor who helps me keep my head attuned to the positive.

· · · · ·

Good rapport and communication is optimal and should be encouraged. However, sometimes the manner in which the medical professional is approached can set the tone. I have often found that doctors that do not have the best "bedside manner" become easier to deal with if they feel they are respected. If the parent has been courteous and respectful in their dealings and the physician is still uncompromising in their manner, then switching would be advisable. My comment stems from commentary given by parents who view the doctors as hired help that they will fire if they so choose. The communication game is a two way street.

## Choosing a hospital

At diagnosis, if your family is not initially referred to a specific hospital or if there are several excellent pediatric hospitals in the area to choose from, it may be necessary to choose where you would like your child to be treated. Parents can obtain a free referral to an accredited center from either the National Cancer Institute, (800) 4-CANCER, or:

**Children's Oncology Group**
440 East Huntington Drive #300
Arcadia, CA 91006
(626) 447-0064
(800) 458-6223 (US and Canada)
http://www.childrensoncologygroup.org

# Types of relationships

There are primarily three types of relationships that develop between physicians and parents:

- **Paternal.** In a paternal relationship, the parent is submissive, and the doctor assumes a parental role. The problem with this dynamic is that, although medical personnel never intend harm, they are human, and mistakes occur. If parents are not monitoring drugs and treatments, these mistakes may go unnoticed. In addition, parents are the experts on their own child and her reactions to drugs and treatments. A surprising number of parents are intimidated by doctors and express the fear that if they question the doctors their child will suffer. This type of behavior robs the child of an adult advocate who speaks up when something seems wrong.

  > *I once asked a fellow about my daughter's blood work. She literally patted me on the head and said it was her job to worry about that, not mine. I said in a nice voice that I thought it was a reasonable question and would appreciate an answer.*

- **Adversarial.** Some parents adopt an "us against them" attitude that is counterproductive. They seem to feel that the disease and treatment are the fault of medical staff, and they blame staff for any setbacks that occur. This attitude undermines the child's confidence in his doctor, a crucial component for healing.

  > *I knew one family who just hated the children's hospital. They called it the "house of horrors" or the "torture chamber" in front of their children. Small wonder that their children were terrified.*

- **Collegial.** This is a true partnership in which parents and doctors are all on the same footing and they respect each other's domains and expertise. Here the doctor recognizes that the parents are the experts on their own child and are essential in ensuring that the protocol is followed. The parents respect the physician's expertise and feel comfortable discussing various treatment options or concerns that arise. Honest communication is necessary for this partnership to work, but the effort is well worth it. The child has confidence in his doctor, the parents have reduced their stress by creating a supportive relationship with the physician, and the physician feels comfortable that the family will comply with the treatment plan, giving the child the best chance for a cure.

  > *We had a wonderful relationship with the oncologist assigned to us. He blended perfectly the science and the art of medicine. His manner with*

*our daughter was warm, he was extremely well qualified professionally, and he was very easy to talk to. I could bring in articles to discuss with him, and he welcomed the discussion. Although he was busy, he never rushed us. I laughed when I saw that he had written in the chart, "Mother asks innumerable appropriate questions."*

Another mother relates a different experience:

*We tried very hard to form a partnership with the medical team but failed. The staff seemed very guarded and distant, almost wary of a parent wanting to participate in the decisions made for the child. I learned to use the medical library and took research reports in to them to get some help for side effects and get some drug dosages reduced. Things improved, but I was never considered a partner in the healthcare team; I was viewed as a problem.*

A pediatric oncologist shares her perspective:

*All parents are different and have different coping styles. Some deal best with a lot of information (lab results, meds, study options) up front, while others are overwhelmed and want the information a little bit at a time. There is no way for the doctor to know the parents' coping styles at the beginning (even the parents may not yet know!). So if they let the doctor know how much information they want or don't want, it is very helpful.*

# Communication

Clear and frequent communication is the lifeblood of a positive doctor/parent relationship. Doctors need to be able to explain clearly and listen well, and parents need to feel comfortable asking questions and expressing concerns before they grow into grievances. Nurses and doctors cannot read parents' minds, nor can a parent prepare his child for a procedure unless it has been explained well. The following are parent suggestions on how to establish and maintain good communication:

- Tell the staff how much you would like to know.

  *I told them the first day to treat me like a medical student. I asked them to share all information, current studies, lab results, everything, with me. I told them, in advance, that I hoped they wouldn't be offended by lots of questions, because knowledge was comfort to me.*

- Inform staff of your child's temperament, likes, and dislikes. You know your child better than anyone so don't hesitate to tell the clinic staff about what works best.

  > Whenever my daughter was hospitalized, I made a point of kindly reminding doctors and nurses that she was extremely sensitive and would benefit from quiet voices and soothing explanations of anything that was about to occur, such as taking temperatures, vital signs, or adjustments to her IV.

- Encourage a close relationship between doctor, nurse, and child. Insist that all medical personnel respect the young person's dignity. Do not let anyone talk in front of the child as if she is not there. The relationship between the child and the medical staff is important. If a problem persists, you have the right to ask the offending person to leave. Marina Rozen observes in *Advice to Doctors and Other Big People:*

  > The best part about the doctor is when he gives me bubble gum. The worst part is when he's in the room with me and my mom and he only talks to my mom. I've told him I don't like that, but he doesn't listen.

- Many children's hospitals assign each patient a primary nurse who oversees all care. Try to form a close relationship with your child's nurse. Nurses usually possess vast knowledge and experience about both medical and practical aspects of cancer treatment. Often, the nurse can rectify misunderstandings between doctor and parents.

  > Michael was assigned to two nurses, but because of scheduling, we never seemed to see them on our admissions. I later learned that some parents would ask right on admission for a particular nurse that their child worked best with, and for the most part their requests were approved.

- Children and teenagers should be included as part of the team. They should be consulted about treatments and procedures and be given age-appropriate choices.

- Cooperate. If your hometown pediatrician will handle all of your child's outpatient treatment, find ways to facilitate communication between neuro-oncologist and pediatrician.

  > Leeann's doctor here in town has been great. She doesn't usually treat children, but knows how to talk to them without talking down to them. She would take the time during her hospital rounds to help Leeann with her homework and laugh at all of our stupid jokes. A good sense of humor was a must for all of us.

- Go to all appointments with a written list of questions. This prevents the exhausted parents from forgetting something important and saves the staff from numerous follow-up phone calls.

- Ask for definitions of unfamiliar terms. Repeat back the information to ensure that it was understood correctly. Writing down answers or tape recording conferences are both common practices.

- Some parents want to read their child's medical chart to obtain more details on their child's condition and to help in formulating questions for the medical team. Often, the doctor or nurse will let the parents read it in the child's hospital room or in the waiting room at the clinic. Most states/provinces have laws that allow patient access to all records. However, you may have to write to the doctor asking to review the chart and pay any photocopy costs.

- If you have questions or concerns, discuss them with the physician or the nurse practitioner. If he is unable to provide satisfactory answers, ask the child's assigned fellow or attending physician.

    *We found that sitting down and talking things over with the nurses helped immensely. They were very familiar with each drug and its side effects. They told us many stories about children who had been through the same thing and were doing well years later. They always seemed to have time to give encouragement, a smile, or a hug.*

- The medical team includes many specialists: doctors, nurses, physical therapists, nutritionists, x-ray technicians, radiation therapists, and more. At training hospitals, many of these persons are in the early stages of their training. If a procedure is not going well, you have the right to tell the person to stop and to request a more skilled person to do the job.

    *At our hospital, family practice residents rotate through, and are often assigned to do procedures. Once, the resident tried for an hour to do a spinal tap, and just couldn't do it. Later, I requested a conference with the oncologist and asked him to perform all the procedures in the future. He agreed, but I didn't intervene that first time and I felt very guilty.*

- Know your rights. Legally, your child cannot be treated without your permission. If a procedure is proposed that you do not feel comfortable with, keep asking questions until you feel fully informed. You have the legal right to refuse the procedure if you do not think that it is necessary. However, if the hospital feels that you are wrongfully withholding permission for treatment (i.e., you reject standard treatment in favor of an unproven remedy, or you are so concerned about side effects that you are endangering the child's chance for cure), they can take you to court. The child is the important person in this equation, and both the hospital and the parents have input once you step into the legal arena.

• Don't let problems build up into a long laundry list of grievances.

• Use "I" statements. For example, "I feel upset when you won't answer my questions" rather than, "You never listen to me."

> One time we had a doctor who was reluctant to answer questions for us. After making sure that it wasn't a case of trying to spare us worrying, but only someone who didn't want to spend the time, my wife, who is a nurse practitioner, quietly told the doctor that she understood that perhaps these questions were a little too hard for him, and would he be good enough to send in one of his partners who could answer them for us? That was the end of that problem!

• If it helps you feel more comfortable, keep track of your child's treatments to check for mistakes.

> Few children were on the same protocol at the time my daughter was being treated. The attendings always knew exactly what was supposed to be done, but the fellows sometimes made mistakes. I was embarrassed to correct them, but I just kept reminding myself that they had dozens of protocols to keep track of, and I had only one.

> • • • • •

> It was important for us to make sure that we were educated about all aspects of this disease without fear. The more we read and researched the better equipped we were to make decisions. It's important to know the bad news also. An added benefit to constant research was that I stumbled upon more and more survivors of PNET and medulloblastoma. This gave us hope and it only came from continuous research. In our family, I left my job and became the main researcher and home/care coordinator, while my husband continued to work.

• Be specific and not confrontational when describing problems. Allow room for the staff to save face. For example, "My son gets very nervous the longer we wait for our appointment. We have waited over two hours for our last two appointments. Could we call ahead next time to see if the doctor is on schedule?" rather than "Do you think your time is more valuable than mine?"

*Noah was 5 months old and receiving radiation treatment for a small tumor located adjacent to the optic nerve. I felt very strongly that an infant should be able to wake up to his mother (and that not having the mother present was emotionally damaging to the baby). I was upset that the anesthesia team was not honoring this concern, and I was simply told, "He won't remember." I made the point that "He may not remember here," pointing to my head, but that "He does remember here," pointing to my heart. I arranged to be called to the treatment room shortly before he awakened from anesthesia.*

- If you have something to discuss with the doctor that will take some time, request a conference. These are routinely scheduled between parents and physicians, and should allow enough time for a thorough discussion. Grabbing a busy doctor in the hallway is not fair to her, and may not result in a satisfactory answer for you.

*One technique I use to keep from forgetting what I want to say at the doctor's appointment is to type out an agenda for the appointment. I make a brief list, and I also make a copy for the doctor. This helps me stay calm and focused on the agenda, and it gives me and my doctor a written record of what our concerns were, and what was discussed during the appointment.*

- Do not be afraid to make waves if you are right or to apologize if you are wrong.

- Show appreciation.

*My 6 year-old daughter Tori is being treated for medulloblastoma. I wanted to give her medical team some recognition. So, I thought maybe I could get half a sheet cake and have "The Best Team" put on it and all the names. Well, it ended up having 23 names. There was a red border and green holly with berries in the corner. Her three primary people were highlighted in red gel and the others were in black. It was spectacular! I took it in and the response was just as I hoped. I had included the docs, nurses, social workers, registration, office manager, and nurse practitioner. It was funny, a lot of people wanted the piece with their own name.*

• • • • •

*Early in my daughter's treatment, we changed pediatricians. The first was aloof and patronizing, and the second was smart, warm, funny, and caring. He was a constant bright spot in our lives through some dark times. So every Christmas Eve during my daughter's treatment, she*

*and her younger sister put on their Santa hats and brought homemade*
*cookies to her pediatrician and nurse. This year was the first time she was*
*able to walk in, and she looked them in the eye and sang, "We Wish You a*
*Merry Christmas." Her nurse went in the back room and cried, and her*
*doctor got misty-eyed. I'll always be thankful for their care.*

The National Coalition for Cancer Survivorship (NCCS) produces an audio resource program called the *Cancer Survival Toolbox,* which is available free by request. Its goal is to "help develop practical tools in daily life" to deal with a cancer diagnosis and treatment. Audiotapes include the topics: Communicating, Finding Information, Making Decisions, Solving Problems, Negotiating, Standing Up for Your Rights, and Finding Ways to Pay for Care. Call the NCCS at: (877) 622-7937, or email your request to: *info@cansearch.org.*

# Getting a second opinion

Conscientious doctors welcome consultations and encourage second opinions. Because there are many gray areas in the treatment of CNS tumors where judgment and experience are as important as knowledge, consultations are frequent. Many insurance companies require second opinions. If, after discussions with the doctor, you are still uneasy about any aspect of your child's medical care, you should not hesitate to seek another opinion.

There are two ways to get a second opinion: see another specialist or ask the child's physician to arrange a multidisciplinary second opinion. Many parents seek a second or third opinion at the time of diagnosis. Do not do this in secret. Explain to your child's surgeon or neuro-oncologist that, before proceeding, you would like additional viewpoints. To allow for a thorough analysis, arrange to have copies of all records, scans, and pathology slides sent ahead to the physician(s) who will give the additional opinions. It is often helpful to get an opinion from a neuro-oncologist and one from a neurosurgeon.

> *Personally, I feel there is nothing wrong with getting a second opinion*
> *from another major center. If you like and feel comfortable with your*
> *current team, that's great, but I definitely do not like when a doctor tells*
> *the patient there's "no reason" to go elsewhere, "they can't do anything*
> *we don't do," and so forth. Many people choose to go elsewhere and*
> *have great results when a first doctor may have told them "no surgery,"*
> *"it's hopeless," whatever the case may be. Many people travel great*

*distances to get treatment at another facility whose treatment
philosophy they prefer. And, granted, that is their choice. We chose
to take our son to a top neurosurgeon about three hours away and,
let me tell you, it has been the best thing that we have done for him.
Now, your second opinion doctor may look at your child's MRIs and
say, "Your team is doing exactly the right things; stick with them,"
or they may tell you something totally different and then you can
make your own decision on what to do. It is always wise to get
more than one opinion when dealing with something as serious as
a brain tumor.*

Multidisciplinary second opinions incorporate the views of several different specialists. Parents who would like to get various viewpoints can ask to have the child's
situation discussed at a tumor board, which usually meets weekly at major medical
centers. These boards include medical, surgical, and radiation oncologists, as well as
fellows and residents. Your child's surgeon or neuro-oncologist will present the facts
of your child's case for discussion. Ask him to tell you what was said at the meeting.

Doctors informally seek second opinions all the time. Residents confer with their
fellow for complicated situations; fellows confer with the attending when unusual
drug reactions or responses to treatment occur. Neuro-oncologists confer with the
surgeons at various stages of treatment for their opinions about additional surgery.
Parents should feel free to ask their physician if he has conferred with other staff
members to gain additional viewpoints.

*Brent developed a seizure disorder so he was on anticonvulsant
medications as well as chemotherapy for two years. We were worried
about the interaction of all the drugs, as well as the advisability of his
continuing on the more aggressive arm of the protocol. We asked the
fellow to arrange a care conference, and she met with the clinic director
as well as Brent's neurologist to discuss how to best manage his care.*

Parents often fear seeking a second opinion because they are afraid of offending the
doctor or creating antagonism. Conscientious doctors do not resent a parent seeking
a second opinion. If she does resist, consider changing doctors. CNS tumors are life or
death, and you won't have a second chance.

Two opinions that agree are all that parents need before proceeding. Treatment usually begins within days of diagnosis, after all questions have been answered and other
opinions have been obtained. Needless delay in treatment should be avoided.

# Conflict resolution

Conflict is a part of life. In a situation where a child's life is threatened, such as in childhood CNS tumors, the heightened emotions and constant involvement with the medical bureaucracy guarantee conflict. Clashes are inevitable, and resolving them is of paramount importance. As Henry Ford once said, "Don't find fault, find a remedy."

Following are some suggestions from parents on how to resolve problems:

- Treat the doctors with respect and expect respect from them.

  *I always wanted to be treated as an intelligent adult, not someone of lesser status. So I would ask each medical person what they wished to be called. We would either both go by first names or both go by titles. I did not want to be called mom.*

- Expect a reasonable amount of sensitivity from the staff.

  *During our little boy's first MRI, I was very emotional, and wondered out loud if he could feel or hear what was going on even though he was sedated. The MRI nurse caught me completely off-guard by banging loudly on the side of the transport bed without getting any reaction from him. "See, he's out," she said. I was too startled then, but I wished I had told her how much that bothered me.*

- Treat the staff with sensitivity. Recognize that you are under enormous stress, and so are the doctors and nurses. Do not blame them for the disease or explode in anger. Be an advocate, not an adversary.

  *Doctors must deal with this disease over and over again. They can never really escape unless they change their careers. And, many many times they lose yet another patient. Our treatment for PNET/ medulloblastoma lasted less than a year. While our subconscious is still filled with fear, at least the actual act of going to the hospital and receiving treatment is finite. If we lose our child, that also is a finite act. The doctors must deal with pain over and over again. In some ways it is so dreadful for them because they are the ones we look to for a cure. So, doctors now hold a very special place in my heart!*

- If a problem develops, state the issue clearly, without accusations, and then suggest a solution.

  *I found out late in my daughter's treatment that short-acting, safe sedatives were being used for many children at the clinic to prevent pain and anxiety during treatments. Only parents who knew about it and requested it received this service. I felt that my daughter's life would have been incredibly improved if we had been able to remove the trauma of procedures. I was angry. But I also realized that although I thought that they were wrong not to offer the service, I was partially at fault for not expressing more clearly how much difficulty she had the week before and after a procedure. I called the director of the clinic and carefully explained that I thought that poor staff/parent communication was creating hardships for the children. I suggested that the entire staff meet with a panel of parents to try to improve communication and to educate the doctors on the impact of pain on the children's daily life. They were very supportive and scheduled the conference. This is a classic example of how something good can come out of a disagreement, if both parties are receptive to solving the problem.*

- Recognize that it is hard to speak up, especially if you have never had to be assertive before. But it is very important to solve the problem before it grows and poisons the relationship.

- Most large medical centers have social workers and psychologists on staff to help families. One of their major duties is to serve as mediators between staff and parents. Ask their advice on problem solving.

- Monitor your own feelings of anger and fear. Be careful not to dump on staff inappropriately. On the other hand, do not let a physician or nurse behave unprofessionally toward you or your child. We all have bad days, but we should not take it out on each other.

- Do not fear reprisal for speaking up. It is possible to be assertive without aggression or argument.

- There are times when no resolution is possible, but expressing one's feelings can be a great release.

*My son and I waited in an exam room for over an hour for a painful procedure. When I went out to ask the receptionist what had caused the delay, she said that a parent had brought in a child without an appointment. This parent frequently failed to bring in her child for treatment, and consequently, whenever she appeared, the doctors dropped everything to take care of the child. When the doctor finally came in, one and one half hours later, my son was in tears. The doctor did not explain the delay or apologize, he just silently started the procedure.*

*After it was finished, I went out of the room, found the doctor, and said, "I am so angry. You just left us in here for hours and traumatized my son. Our time is valuable, too." He told me that I should have more compassion for the other mother because her life was very difficult. I replied that he encouraged her to not make appointments by dropping everything whenever she appeared. I added that it wasn't fair to those parents who played by the rules; she was being rewarded for her irresponsibility. After we had each stated our position, we left without resolution.*

# Changing doctors

Changing doctors is not a step to be taken lightly, but it can be a great relief if the relationship has deteriorated beyond repair. It is a good policy to exhaust all possible remedies prior to separating, or the same problems may arise with the new doctor. Communication, verbal or written, and mediation, using the social service staff, can sometimes resolve the issues and prevent the disruption of changing doctors.

Although there are many reasons for changing doctors, some of the most common are:

- Not the most qualified person

- Grave medical error(s) made

- Inability to communicate well or refuses to answer questions

- Serious clash of philosophy—for example, a paternalistic doctor and a parent who wishes to be informed and share in the decision-making

It is one of life's great struggles to face CNS tumors. If you have a physician whom you trust, can rely on for the best medical treatment, feel comfortable with, communicate freely with, and can count on for advice and support, the struggle is greatly eased. If, on the other hand, the doctor adds to your discomfort rather than reducing it, change.

*It was late on a Friday night when our 2-year-old son was diagnosed with medulloblastoma at a local hospital in NYC. We were told that we had to move quickly on surgery, although we were not comfortable with the neurosurgeon on their staff. He had a pompous demeanor and wasn't a very good communicator. One of our friends (a pediatrician) took us aside and recommended the best pediatric neurosurgeon in the city. We called the doctor's office and he arranged for a neurosurgery fellow to*

*meet us first thing on Sunday morning to review the scans. It was that*
*Sunday afternoon that the neurosurgeon called us from his home to*
*discuss our son's case. He was warm and caring and, we later found out,*
*one of the top people in the country. We arranged for the transfer to his*
*hospital on Monday and were greeted by an experienced neurology and*
*neurosurgery team. We were lucky to find this out so soon after diagnosis*
*since those first days were such a blur.*

Do not change doctors because you're searching for a better diagnosis. If two reputable physicians, or a tumor board, have agreed on the diagnosis and treatment, it is best for the child to immediately begin treatment.

Many parents choose to continue with a physician in whom they have no confidence, due to fears of reprisals. Children may actually suffer more from the additional family stress caused by a poor doctor/parent relationship than from changing doctors. If you do change doctors, there may be lingering bitterness or anger between parents and doctors, but your child will continue to benefit from the best-known treatment.

Once the decision is made, parents must be candid. Either verbally or in writing, an explanation should be given for the change and a formal request made to transfer records to the new physician. Physicians are legally required to transfer all records upon written request.

*We've had wonderful docs, mediocre docs, and one who made a terrible*
*mistake. We've had warm compassionate docs, ho-hum docs (on a good*
*day they're nice, on a bad day they're neutral), and we've met some*
*world-class jerks. Sounds pretty much like a slice of humanity, right?*

*We hold doctors to a different standard since the stakes are so high—*
*our kids' lives. But the reality is they are usually overworked, exhausted,*
*and deal with newly diagnosed families on an almost daily basis, day*
*after day, week after week, year after year. I can't even begin to imagine*
*the emotional toll that must take.*

*I tell my kids all human relationships are like a goodwill bank. If you*
*make lots of deposits, an occasional withdrawal won't be so noticeable. I*
*tell my docs and my kids' docs whenever things go right. I like to write, so*
*I send many thank you notes. When our pediatrician went on sabbatical,*

*he took me into his office and showed me every mushy Christmas card I'd sent him lined up on the back of his messy desk. I also have been known to bring in brownies for the office staff. We did this on my daughter's last day of radiation and several people broke down and cried when they saw the thank you note she drew—a picture of herself holding a Snow White and the seven dwarves audiotape. She listened to that every session because I'd promised it would be over before the dwarves appeared.*

*I recently asked one of my favorite doctors (a pediatric oncologist who has world class compassion) how many thank you notes she had received from parents over the years. She said she could count them on one hand. I asked how many complaints, and she said, "You wouldn't want to know."*

*So, while I think docs should be called on for bad behavior and bad medicine, I also think we should acknowledge good medicine and good behavior. I'd like to encourage the good ones to stick around—new little innocents keep getting cancer every day.*

# CHAPTER 8

# Surgery

SURGERY HAS A CENTRAL ROLE IN THE TREATMENT OF CNS TUMORS. At each new treatment stage, surgery is considered as an option. Surgery is used to remove all of or debulk a tumor, biopsy a suspicious area where aggressive surgery is dangerous, insert a shunt to treat hydrocephalus, or insert a central line for treatment. Surgery is a vital part of treatment to try to make your child well again.

This chapter describes the importance of consulting a pediatric neurosurgeon to obtain an opinion about surgical options for your child's tumor. Next, it explains the advances in technology that have improved the surgical treatment of children with CNS tumors. Information is provided on the evaluation before surgery and what happens in the operating room. Finally, caring for your child after surgery is discussed.

## The neurosurgeon

Pediatric neurosurgery developed as a subspecialty in the 1980s. Generally, neurosurgeons who operate 50 percent of the time or more on children are considered pediatric neurosurgeons. Today most pediatric neurosurgeons complete one year of fellowship with an established pediatric neurosurgeon in a program approved by the American Board of Pediatric Neurological Surgery. There are approximately 110 pediatric neurosurgeons in the United States. Surgeons who devote the majority of their practice to children usually provide the most aggressive surgical approach to the tumor to try to cure the child.

Results of the most recent research indicate that the amount of tumor removed by the surgeons directly impacts the chances of survival and cure. Research has also confirmed that children operated on by pediatric neurosurgeons have more tumor removed than those operated on by adult neurosurgeons. Therefore, it is probably best to have your child's surgery performed by a pediatric neurosurgeon with extensive experience operating on children with cancer. Appendix D, *List of Pediatric Neurosurgeons*, lists names and contact information for more than 150 pediatric neurosurgeons in the US. The American Society of Pediatric Neurosurgeons maintains a current list of pediatric neurosurgeons at *http://www.aspn.org*.

A senior pediatric neurosurgeon suggests:

> *The most important advice I would offer to a family is logical but not necessarily widely accepted. Quite simply, this is to be certain that your child is cared for by a surgeon who is experienced in caring for children. Children are not simply "little adults." There is no rationale in assuming that the surgeon who cares largely for adults is equally qualified to look after a newborn baby or young child. This has nothing to do with intelligence, but is simply a logical extension of the meaning of experience in any facet of life. A carpenter who builds bookshelves will probably do it better than a carpenter that has spent his life building houses. A pilot of a space shuttle is not trained to be an airline pilot.*

Surgical treatment is only one aspect of overall care. Therefore, when a major surgical procedure is planned, it is essential that it be carried out in a facility that has a team approach. Pediatricians, pediatric anesthesiologists, pediatric radiologists, and pediatric nurses are all part of an integrated group that is devoted to a single goal: the recovery of a child.

# Types of surgery

Surgery is performed at different times during treatment. Varying amounts of tumor are removed—from a small biopsy to the whole tumor. This section describes several of the most common surgeries used to treat children with CNS tumors.

## Biopsy

A biopsy involves taking a tiny sample of the tumor through a small incision. Biopsies can help diagnose a child with a CNS tumor that is deep within the brain or brainstem (sometimes even a biopsy is not possible or recommended for a brainstem tumor). A more aggressive surgery in these areas is not possible if the adjacent structures are vital for the body to function. When the pathologist evaluates the tissue removed in a biopsy, she determines if the lesion is a tumor and, if so, what type of tumor it is.

> *Jordan was 3 years old when she was diagnosed with an inoperable pilocytic astrocytoma. Since she was not using her right hand, our*

*pediatrician told me to take her to a pediatric neurologist. But, because of insurance, our first visit was to a local neurologist. Now this doctor was used to seeing adults, so when he saw her MRI, he told us to give her a happy six months. He referred us on to the pediatric doctors at a children's hospital three hours away. They took a biopsy and told us there were treatments available.*

You should have your child's biopsy done at a pediatric center that uses MRI or CT scan to guide the surgeon to the site of the tumor. If the surgeon misses the tumor or the biopsy doesn't obtain adequate tissue, a diagnosis is sometimes not possible. In other cases, the piece of tumor obtained by biopsy is not representative of the whole tumor. Some tumors have areas that are very aggressive ("high grade"); other areas appear "low grade."

Sometimes an area that looks abnormal on an MRI scan is not a tumor. A biopsy to confirm that the lesion is definitely a tumor is usually necessary before major surgery or other treatment begins. However, some tumors that are difficult to biopsy have a typical appearance on MRI, so a biopsy is not done. Examples of this are optic glioma and pontine glioma. In some cases, biopsy is not possible because of tumor location or is not recommended because of the damage the procedure can cause.

## Debulking

Surgical debulking is the partial removal (usually 40 to 75 percent) of the tumor. This type of procedure is done for tumors that are deep within the brain, next to large blood vessels, or growing from the brainstem. In these areas, the risk is too great to allow total removal. The goal of the surgery is to relieve any symptoms caused by the tumor, especially increased intracranial pressure. A debulking procedure is often done prior to giving either radiation or chemotherapy, because these treatments are sometimes more effective on smaller tumors.

A debulking procedure may also slow or stop the growth of a slow-growing tumor for a period of time, thus delaying the need for other treatments.

*Anthony was just over two years old when he was diagnosed with an optic nerve glioma. Radiation was not recommended, because of the risks of serious long-term side effects. We agreed that the pediatric neurosurgeon should debulk as much of the tumor as possible. She removed most of the low-grade tumor that extended into the temporal lobe. Chemotherapy was not needed for several years.*

Delaying treatment if possible may have several advantages. For instance, studies have shown that children who have radiation to the brain at an older age have fewer long-term effects than children who have radiation under the age of five. Slowing tumor growth for several years can also allow time for the discovery of newer and more effective methods of treatment.

> My brain tumor is located in the midbrain, and my neurosurgeon told us at diagnosis that it was inoperable. Since it was diagnosed though, I have had numerous surgeries to shrink it. So, even though they say it is inoperable, they can still go in and reduce its size. My neurosurgeon has always said that the medical field is an ongoing research area. What they couldn't do yesterday, they can do today.

## Surgical resection

The goal of surgery for the majority of CNS tumors is to remove the entire tumor (called maximal surgical resection). It is important to understand what this term means. Unlike a tumor in the intestine, where the surgeon can cut a wide margin on either side of the tumor to ensure that no tumor cells are left behind, CNS tumors can't be removed with large margins because there are vital structures throughout the brain and spinal cord. Surgeons usually remove a CNS tumor by working from the inside of the tumor out, coring out the cavity.

Recent studies have indicated that the best chance for long-term survival and cure occurs with total or near total removal of the tumor. This may not be possible if the tumor is deep within the brain or near a part of the brain responsible for a vital function (for example, near the area that controls breathing). A maximal surgical resection, however, is now possible in many areas within the brain and spinal cord due to new technology in operating equipment and monitoring. The majority of tumors in the frontal, parietal, temporal, and occipital lobes and the cerebellum can be totally or almost totally removed. Similarly, most spinal cord tumors can also have large surgical resections.

> John Michael was 11 years old at the time of surgery. He has a brain tumor located in the thalamus. We were told that it was inoperable by our local neurosurgeon. Then we found a more experienced pediatric neurosurgeon. He did indeed have surgery to remove about 85 percent of his golfball-size tumor, and he has no lasting deficits.

· · · · ·

*Exactly three weeks after being diagnosed with a pilocytic astrocytoma almost the size of an orange in the cerebellum, Christopher went back to school! The tumor was benign and located in the most accessible place possible, so he arrived at school with a full head of hair, no residual effects from surgery, and a bigger smile than he left with three weeks before.*

It is common for children to undergo more than one surgical procedure during the treatment process. Total or near total removal of the tumor is often achieved by operating in more than one stage and/or from different approaches. For example, if an MRI scan after surgery reveals a lump of tumor remaining and the surgeon feels that he can remove it safely, a second surgery is performed. Similarly, a deep tumor may be approached surgically from above and then during a separate operation from the side. Tumors that are very slow growing are debulked and the remaining tumor monitored with MRI scans every three to six months. A second surgery is performed months or years later if the tumor grows.

*About two weeks following surgery, I had to return to the hospital for a post-op check-up and MRI to check the residual tumor. The MRI showed that the pediatric neurosurgeon removed about fifty percent of the tumor, but he informed us that he could see himself going in from another direction to obtain more of the tumor. He said, "Don't be surprised if sometime in the future, I want to go back in just to try and get more of the tumor." We left the office feeling a little peace of mind, because we now knew that the tumor was smaller.*

The results from a number of clinical trials support a second-look operation after a phase of treatment (chemotherapy or radiation) if tumor is still visible on the MRI scan. The second-look surgery is helpful for the pathologist to assess treatment effect on the tumor. Occasionally, on second look an abnormality thought to be tumor on MRI scan turns out to be scar tissue. The results of the second-look surgery provide information to the treating physician that assists him in planning the next step of treatment. In other cases, children have special imaging studies done (i.e., PET) rather than a second-look surgery to evaluate treatment effect.

*Our 10-month-old daughter was diagnosed with medulloblastoma in 1989. Her first surgery took about nine hours to remove the baseball-sized tumor. The pathology showed that it was malignant. She had two and a half years of chemotherapy that she tolerated very well. The first MRI after chemo showed a shadow where the tumor had been. So, they did a second look surgery, which thankfully, only showed scarring. That surgery didn't take as long as the first since they had nothing to remove. After a week in the hospital, we went home. Kristin is now 13 years old, with no late effects from treatment. She is mentally and physically on par with her friends—whom she spends a lot of time talking with on the phone and computer!*

## Intraoperative monitoring

Intraoperative monitoring involves watching the electrical nerve impulses as they travel from an area of the brain to another part of the body, such as the arms, legs, or face and eyes. Electrodes are placed on the scalp and on the extremities (similar to an EEG) to monitor the brain's electrical impulses. By using this technology during an operation, the surgeon can then determine the location of a tumor in relation to important body functions. This helps the surgeon remove the tumor while preserving as much function as possible. Intraoperative monitoring is used for tumors in the frontal and parietal lobes adjacent to the motor strip or the brainstem.

Intraoperative monitoring is also vital for surgery in the spinal cord, because the monitoring allows the surgeon to remove the tumor while observing the nerve activity from the brain, down the spinal cord and out to the arms and legs.

Another type of monitoring uses electrodes to locate seizure activity in the brain. This type of EEG involves placing a grid or strip of electrodes on the surface of the brain after a tumor has been removed. It monitors the tumor cavity and surrounding brain to determine if seizure-generating tissue is still present. If a focus of seizures is not in a vital area, then that seizure-generating tissue is also removed in an attempt to reduce or eliminate the seizures. If the tumor is near the speech center, this procedure is done when the child is awake. By having the person awake, the surgeon can converse with him during the tumor removal, assuring that the speech center remains uninjured. The patient has to be mature enough to cooperate, and this is usually not possible until at least early teen years.

*An attempt to awaken my son Michael during his first awake craniotomy for a mixed tumor of JPA and PNET failed. He was only twelve, but more importantly, I think the person who was talking with him was cold and aloof, as was his surgeon. As he came out of the anesthetic, he tried to move his head while in the cage, was very confused, and they ended up just putting him back to sleep.*

*The second surgery was a whole different story. Now he was fifteen, and we used a major neurosurgery center. Both the pediatric neurosurgeon and his assistant took the time to really talk to Michael, get to know him well and goof around with him (making him feel comfortable with them). When they woke him up, they chatted to him about gymnastics (his first love), his best friend Alex, his desire to be third in his class (to escape having to make a speech at graduation), and so on. The awake surgery was a super success—the surgeon was able to go deeper, get all the tumor, and yet know that Michael's speech would remain intact.*

## Computer-guided surgery

Until recently, neurosurgeons had only an MRI picture to refer to during surgery. Now it is possible to use the MRI along with a computer in the operating room to help the surgeon localize and remove the tumor. Before the surgery, markers (small round stickers) are placed on the patient's forehead. An MRI is performed prior to the surgery. The information from the MRI is transmitted to a computer in the operating room. The surgeon then points with a wand at the stickers on the head of the child and the computer generates a three-dimensional picture of the brain. This allows for localization and removal of the tumor through a much smaller incision.

Surgeons are also working with MRI companies to develop MRI scanners for the operating room. An intraoperative MRI scanner allows the surgeon to obtain an MRI scan during the surgery to update him as to how much tumor is left. This technology should be widely available within the next decade, and it will further improve outcomes of surgeries to remove CNS tumors.

Another new method to help the surgeon to safely remove tumors is intraoperative ultrasonography. Probes that use ultrasound are used to guide the surgical approach. Ultrasonography is also used to examine the ventricles during surgery to look for collections of cerebrospinal fluid (CSF) or cysts.

## Surgical treatment of hydrocephalus

Hydrocephalus is the build up of fluid in the brain caused when a tumor blocks the normal flow of CSF. The surgeon can insert a tube called a drain or ventriculostomy prior to or during the tumor surgery to remove excess CSF. The tube shunts fluid from the brain to a collection bag outside the body. The drain is usually removed a few days following surgery.

> *We were fortunate to be located near one of the most experienced pediatric neurosurgeons in California. They put Megan, who was just 20 months old, in the hospital for two days on Decadron to reduce brain swelling before doing surgery. The tumor, an anaplastic ependymoma, was huge, and they did a gross total resection. They told us ahead of time that she might have language retrieval/word-finding issues and loss of mobility on the right side, but that didn't happen. She did have an external drain after surgery, and they said she might need a permanent shunt because of the tumor's size, but the temporary drain worked well and came out without any fluid buildup, so they didn't need to do that.*

Occasionally, part of the tumor remains or blood from the surgery scars the normal sites of CSF reabsorption, and the hydrocephalus persists after surgery. In this case, a shunt surgery is performed. The shunt functions as a drain inside the body. The tube diverts the excess fluid from the brain into another space in the body—abdomen, chest, or a large vein in the heart. The fluid is then absorbed by the body. If your child has persistent hydrocephalus, an excellent resource is *Hydrocephalus: A Guide for Patients, Families, and Friends* by Chuck Toporek and Kellie Robinson.

> *Tori had a regular ventriculostomy that had a tube that drained out to a bag at the bedside. The reason that they do this is that she had impressive hydrocephalus and they wanted to decrease the pressure during the surgery to resect the medulloblastoma. There was great hope that she might not even need a shunt. They tried for ten days (intermittently clamping the tube) but once they clamped the bag to see if her body could handle the fluid, it started to drain out her incision site. Even if it is only a teaspoon a day that the body cannot handle, the child must have a shunt as it will build up. This was one of the hardest things for me; I really did not want a shunt. It meant to me that she would be a medical device kid her entire life. We could never leave this experience behind. Funny thing—our shunt has been blissfully easy so far. Not a problem at all.*

Like the plumbing in your house, shunts can block and back up. This blockage is called a shunt obstruction or shunt malfunction. Buildup of proteins or debris from surgery that circulates in the CSF can prevent the fluid from draining properly through the shunt. An infection in the shunt can also cause a blockage. Symptoms of a shunt problem are the same as the symptoms of hydrocephalus (headaches, vomiting, double vision). When this happens, the surgeon replaces the entire shunt or repairs the part of the shunt that is obstructed. Rarely, the shunts fracture or become disconnected. Surgical repair is also the treatment for this problem.

*I was 16 when I had my first surgery, when a VP shunt was placed for a large amount of fluid buildup. Then I had a second surgery to remove part of the tumor. About a month later, I started having severe headaches again. This time I could not raise my head up without becoming ill. I was rushed back to the emergency room, and another MRI was done. My neurosurgeon explained that the MRI was showing fluids back in the head again. He said that this was unusual, since I did have the shunt, and the shunt appeared to be working when he completed the last surgery. He performed some tests to see if he could figure out why the fluids were building up in the head. The next day, he told us that he wanted to go back in to check the shunt. He went in and discovered that my shunt had shut down due to a buildup of scar tissue around a valve on the shunt. He replaced the valve so that the shunt began working again. My stay in the hospital this time was about seven days.*

Hydrocephalus caused by a tumor that blocks the flow of CSF is sometimes treated with a procedure called an anterior third ventriculostomy. The surgeon uses an endoscope (a long tube with a camera at the end) to make an opening in the floor of the third ventricle. This new opening is a detour for the fluid around the obstruction caused by the tumor. The opening creates a pathway from inside the brain's fluid spaces to the outside circulation. Here the fluid can be absorbed normally by the subarachnoid space without the need of a shunt tube. For more information, see Chapter 2, *The Brain and Spinal Cord*.

*Although Molly (14 months old) had no outward symptoms of hydrocephalus, the main concern at diagnosis was surgery to relieve the pressure on her brain from the pineoblastoma. We were given the option of either a shunt, or something called a third ventriculostomy. This would create a hardware-free channel for the extra cerebrospinal fluid to leave her brain. This sounded like the best option for Molly, so surgery was scheduled for the next afternoon. Surgery went very well, and she was released the following afternoon. Molly is now three years old, she is followed regularly, but she hasn't had any more problems with pressure in the brain.*

## Palliation

Surgery is sometimes used to improve the quality of life of terminally ill children. Surgery can often relieve pain caused by pressure from tumor growth. Some tumors that do not respond to radiation or chemotherapy can be surgically removed with each

regrowth. This provides a child relief from symptoms and allows the child to participate in normal life activities.

> *Surgery was the only thing that made Laura feel better. She wanted
> to have the tumor operated on each time it came back. Before the last
> operation she spoke to the surgeon and asked him to take it out one more
> time so that she could enjoy her summer.*

## Vascular access

Children with CNS tumors have to endure many months or years of treatment. To
avoid the pain of repeated needle sticks, many children receive a surgically implanted
catheter. Direct access to a blood vessel allows the administration of chemotherapy,
antibiotics, blood products, and hyperalimentation (IV nutrition) and avoids the pain
of repeated needle sticks for the child. For more information, see Chapter 10, *Venous
Catheters*.

## Enteral access

Adequate nutrition plays an important role in children's overall well-being and prognosis. Children who are unable to eat or drink a liquid diet sometimes need enteral
access, a method to deliver nutrients directly to the gastrointestinal tract. Enteral
access can be accomplished in several ways, including the insertion of a nasogastric
tube (a tube passed down the nose to the stomach) or the surgical installation of a
gastrostomy tube (a tube placed through the abdominal wall into the stomach). For
further information, see Chapter 17, *Nutrition*.

# Presurgical evaluation

Soon after a diagnosis of a CNS tumor has been made, parents meet with the pediatric neurosurgeon to discuss the surgery. The consultation is important because it provides the surgeon with background information on your child, including your family
medical history. It is also important for the family because the surgeon will explain
the procedure to you, answer questions, and address any concerns you have. Only an
experienced, pediatric neurosurgeon is equipped to handle the intricacies of treating
a pediatric CNS tumor.

> *My son had several surgeries at different points in his treatment. Each
> time we had a long discussion with his surgeon to review the procedure
> and to talk about the possible complications. It made me feel scared when*

*I thought about my little boy lying on an operating table being cut with a knife. Still, I'm glad that the surgeon was so thorough in explaining everything to us. I think that if I didn't know what was going to happen, my imagination would have really given me a hard time.*

The following is a list of questions that you can ask before signing a consent form for surgery:

- What percentage of your practice is pediatrics?

- How many other children with this type of tumor have you operated on?

- What is the purpose of the surgery? What are the expected findings?

- What are the common and not-so-common deficits that my child might develop after surgery?

- Is this a new procedure? If so, how many other children have had it?

- How much of the tumor do you expect to remove?

- Where will the incision (cut) be?

- How large will the incision be?

- How much hair will be shaved?

- What will cover the incision?

- How long will the operation take?

> *Our son was admitted for surgery to have his tumor resected early on a Monday morning, August 4, 1997. The surgery took five hours. We stuck close by in a waiting room, although the hospital had beepers to call us if we wanted to leave the area. It was an unbearable wait, but we were given updates every hour or so.*

- What are the possible complications of the surgery?

- What types of tubes will my child have after surgery (i.e., number of IV lines, nasogastric (NG) tube, catheter in bladder, drain, or shunt)?

- Will blood transfusions or blood products be required?

- Will my child remain on a ventilator (breathing tube) afterwards? For how long?

> *When my child had surgery, the doctor said that there was a possibility that he would need to stay on the ventilator for a few days. Thankfully, that never happened, and he came from the recovery room breathing completely on his own.*

- How long will my child need to stay in the intensive care unit after the surgery?

- How much pain will my child have after the surgery? How will it be controlled?

- When will my child be able to eat?

- How long will it take my child to recover?

- Will I need to learn how to care for her operation site after she is discharged?

- How long do the stitches or staples stay in?

- What are the possible long-term effects of this procedure?

- Will the scar be very noticeable?

> Our son's surgery was at a major center. I hadn't expected that the incision line that curved along the side of my son's head would at first be raised like a fold, but eventually, the line thinned and flattened then faded to white. It's not indented or jagged-looking, and his hairline hides it pretty well.

Your child may undergo many tests before the operation, depending on the type of surgery and your child's medical condition. This is usually called pre-surgical testing. Some of the tests that are frequently ordered are blood work, urinalysis, x-rays, EKG, echocardiogram, and pulmonary function tests. If computer-assisted surgery is planned, an MRI is done a few hours before the surgery. Your child's surgeon should explain what tests are necessary.

It is important that the pre-operative preparation includes explaining the upcoming surgery to the child. Most large centers have a child psychologist, child life therapist, or a nurse practitioner who can help you prepare your child for surgery. A simple, age-appropriate explanation can be given to the child during the pre-operative testing or, in some cases, just prior to surgery.

The We Can, Pediatric Brain Tumor Network recommends the following explanation prior to surgery for preschoolers: "An operation is where they open the skin to fix something. This time, they will be taking the tumor out. A special doctor will give you medicine that puts you to sleep, but it's really more than sleep; while the medicine is working, you can't feel anything. After the surgery, you'll feel very sleepy. If you have a headache, a nurse will give you medicine to make it go away." Reassure your child that you will stay in the hospital with her. Explain the schedule for each parent. For instance, "Mommy will be here when you wake up, but Daddy will sleep on the couch in the room with you."

The older the child, the more detailed the explanation should be. However, follow your child's lead and give brief but clear answers for each question. Then ask if there is anything else he would like to know. If you don't know the answer, write down the questions and ask the surgeon or nurse practitioner at the next appointment. Make sure you and your child have all of your questions answered prior to the surgery.

# Anesthesia

The anesthesiologist is a key member of the surgical team. It is her responsibility to ensure that the child is properly anesthetized and monitored during the operation. Prior to the surgery, you will have a consultation with the anesthesiologist, during which she will ask you about your child's medical history and any allergies to medications. Take this opportunity to ask the doctor any questions you have or to express concerns. For instance, if your child is very frightened, ask the anesthesiologist if she could prescribe a pre-surgical sedative.

The following is a list of questions you can ask the anesthesiologist before the surgery:

- How will my child be put to sleep (mask or intravenous medication)?

- Will my child be sedated prior to the operation?

- What are some of the common side effects of these drugs?

> Surgery was a scary time for me. My mother and sister don't do very well under anesthesia, and we were afraid that Sean might react badly to it also. Sean did very well and came through the procedure without any complications.

- Will I be able to stay with my child until he is anesthetized?

> For our son's brain surgery, we weren't able to attend the hospital's children's tour for surgery, and he wasn't that well-prepared. But, we had a great experience for his port insertion at our local tertiary care center. We were invited to attend an evening tour of an operating room by Maureen, from Child Life. Our son sat in a circle with other kids while the whole anesthesia process was explained. They all tried on masks and practiced breathing deeply. On the day of surgery, the anesthesiologist spent time talking to our son. My husband, Jim, suited up in scrubs, our son was presedated, and they went off together down the hall to the O.R. chatting with the anesthesiologist.

- Will my child need to remain on a ventilator afterwards? For how long?

You will be asked to sign a consent form prior to the administration of any anesthesia. The anesthesiologist will answer any questions or concerns you might have, and he may include some of the many expected ways children can react when coming out of anesthesia.

> *Anesthesia recovery is horrible for my son. He stands, hits, screams, cries, tries to leave, refuses to leave, you name it. Or rather, I should say his body does these things. The thinking part of him is still anesthetized or dealing with a whopper of a headache. Eventually I get my son back.*

> • • • • •

> *Brendon has been in and out of treatment for the last ten years. He's had numerous surgeries, radiation, and chemo. When he was little he was sedated for all of his scans. I can't count the number of times he's been anesthetized. And he never had a problem. He bounces right back so easily each time. I think that it helps that he is always joking with the staff and thinking up funny pranks.*

## The surgery

The surgical technique used to remove your child's tumor depends on several factors, including the type and location of the tumor, your child's general medical condition, and the type of procedure needed. However, some principles apply to all operations requiring a general anesthetic. Children are usually given anesthesia through a breathing mask, an intravenous injection, or both. A breathing tube is placed in the trachea (windpipe) and connected to a ventilator that will breathe for the child every few seconds. Your child will be anesthetized before the breathing tube is inserted.

During the operation your child will be connected to many different monitors to ensure that there is an adequate supply of oxygen in the blood and that fluids are maintained at proper levels. Blood pressure, heart rate, and other functions are carefully monitored. Your child may also be connected to special monitoring to watch electrical impulses controlling movement of the face, arms, and legs. Brain wave monitoring is sometimes used to detect the presence of seizure activity.

Operating room procedures for neurosurgery are carried out under very sterile conditions. To minimize the risk of infection, parents must put on special gowns to accompany their child into the operating room.

> *The surgery was handled very well. Paige was treated with kindness and prepared, so she wasn't too scared. We were informed of her progress while surgery was taking place, and the surgeon explained the outcome as soon as he could.*

Once the child awakens from the anesthesia, clear liquids are given first and solid foods are offered after the doctor feels that it is safe. Some children are not able to drink and/or eat for several days depending upon the surgery. These children are given nutrition through an intravenous line or through a nasogastric (NG) tube through the nose to the stomach.

> Michelle had a number of major surgeries and more minor ones than I remember. She hated waking up to a liquid diet of Popsicles, Jell-O, and juice. One day she pleaded with the doctor to have something else. The doctor replied, "If you can think of anything else that's clear, you can have it." Michelle thought and thought, and she finally came up with jelly, no seeds. So on her next liquid diet tray were little packets of clear grape jelly.

Most children who have brain surgeries do not experience serious complications. The risk of complications in children is usually lower than in adults, because children recover from postoperative symptoms and weakness at a much faster rate than adults.

> My son was anxious to start moving about a few hours after he had his surgery to remove his tumor. He really amazed me. His mobility was limited for a few days, but he didn't let the operation stop him from trying to do most activities.

A small group of children with CNS tumors experience significant complications from the surgery. These are discussed in the next section.

# Postoperative complications

Postoperative problems are very stressful for the child and family. Symptoms that the child had prior to surgery are usually worse following the operation because of swelling or surgical trauma. This is normal. Less common complications after surgery are:

- Paralysis in arm(s) and/or leg(s)

- Seizures

- Loss of blood supply to an area of the brain (stroke)

- Hydrocephalus that requires another surgery to place a shunt or make a detour via an anterior third ventriculostomy

- Loss of bowel and bladder control

- Leakage of fluid from the incision

- Infection at site of incision

- Memory problems

> *My son Darren is 12, although very mature for 12, and also a whiz at math. Several weeks after surgery when he had recovered enough to talk, we found that his short-term memory had been disrupted. He could not remember all of the letters of the alphabet or what certain numbers were. He also had trouble with word retrieval—he knew what he wanted to say but just couldn't think of the word he wanted to use. For example, he wanted to ask for pain medication, but could only ask us, "Make hurt less." This lasted just over six weeks or so, and I'm happy to say that he is now just as smart as he once was.*

The majority of postoperative complications are not permanent; they can be reversed with additional surgical, medical, or rehabilitative treatment.

> *My son had complications that were worse than the norm. It would have been helpful to me to know that all kids are referred to physical and occupational therapy after brain surgery. Knowing that they expect physical impairment after surgery would have given me some before-surgery perspective.*

Three less common but more serious complications are discussed next.

## Aseptic meningitis

Aseptic meningitis can occur in the first few weeks following surgery, usually when steroids (medications used to decrease swelling and inflammation) are reduced. It is thought that blood and cells from the tumor removal get into the CSF, causing chemical irritation. Symptoms of aseptic meningitis include fever, headache, and stiff neck. If your child has any of these symptoms, the doctor usually asks for a sample of CSF to test for a bacterial infection. This sample is obtained from a spinal tap (see Chapter 4, *Coping with Procedures*) or from fluid near the incision. All cultures (testing for the presence of bacteria) are negative if your child has aseptic meningitis. The symptoms usually improve when the child is given a short course of additional steroids.

## Cranial nerve deficits

Cranial nerves control movement of the eyes, face, and throat. The control center for the cranial nerves is located in the brainstem. Problems with the cranial nerves can be caused by tumors in the brainstem, tumors pressing on the brainstem, or hydrocephalus. Surgery in the posterior fossa (cerebellum or brainstem) can also result in temporary or permanent cranial nerve problems. Some of the deficits that may develop include:

- Double vision
- Bouncing of eyes
- Inability to look up or to one side
- Inability to close eyelid
- Pain in the jaw
- Weakness, droop, or asymmetry of face
- Hoarse or raspy voice
- Difficulty swallowing and coughing
- Respiratory problems, such as difficulty breathing, pneumonias, and frequent respiratory illnesses

If these symptoms are present prior to surgery, they may get worse after surgery. Recovery of cranial nerve function is possible over a long period of time. If eye and facial cranial nerve problems persist, surgery can correct some of them. Children with swallowing problems use a nasogastric or gastrostomy tube. Children with severe respiratory problems have a tube inserted into their throat (tracheostomy) that is connected to a respirator to help the child breathe.

## Posterior fossa syndrome

Posterior fossa syndrome (also called cerebellar mutism) is a complication of posterior fossa (cerebellum or brainstem) surgery. The most common tumors in this area are medulloblastomas, astrocytomas, and ependymomas. Most children wake up from the surgery moving their arms and legs and responding to questions. In some cases, 24 or more hours later the child stops talking, may develop weakness of arms and legs, and cranial nerve deficits appear. Emotionally, the children seem disconnected from their environment and may respond by simply crying.

These symptoms improve over a period of days in the minimally affected child, but improvement may take months in the severely affected child. Physical, occupational, and speech therapy should be started immediately. Children who have severe posterior fossa syndrome require transfer to an inpatient rehabilitation facility to facilitate a quicker recovery.

> Tori developed posterior fossa syndrome and cerebellar mutism after
> surgery. These were slow to improve, but after months in rehab, she was

*eventually able to see and to form short sentences. We have come a long way, and now she is an active five-year-old in regular private kindergarten. She has, however, been basically on a feeding tube for the last ten months since surgery. We occasionally try to have her eat, but usually after a week it needs to go back in because she is getting on the dry side (dehydrated). The tube often is one of the most obvious things that makes her look "sick," so this has had its ups and downs.*

· · · · ·

*Ayla (32 months) was diagnosed with medulloblastoma, a 5×5 cm tumor in the posterior fossa, cerebellarpontine angle, fourth ventricle, and arising from the brainstem. When all of this happens, you are not necessarily in the position or frame of mine to get all opinions. In retrospect, we know we had an excellent pediatric neurosurgeon who removed as much as he felt he could without causing additional deficits. He was very compassionate. When Ayla came out of it after surgery, she said, "I want pasta and salmon with paprika on it." Then she noticed the balloons that we there for her, and she wanted to make sure her sister Jasmine got one. We didn't notice it right away, but she couldn't walk at first and she couldn't drink liquids without choking. All that lasted about a week. They didn't tell us ahead of time about posterior fossa syndrome, though we feel she came out of surgery relatively unscathed.*

A helpful videotape geared for children ages 9 to 13, which describes the experience of brain surgery, is available free from the American Brain Tumor Association. It is called: *Alex's Journey: The Story of a Child with a Brain Tumor.* Contact ABTA at: (800) 886-2282, or go to *http://www.abta.org*.

*Our son had radiation late this summer (23Gr craniospinal and a boost to the tumor bed) and is about to start round two (of eight) of chemotherapy (cisplatin, cytoxan, and vincristine). He was mute for two and a half months post-op, and had a right hemiparesis as well as a gaze palsy. He is back to his hyperactive self in terms of speech, but the physical return has been slower. His vision has improved, but he may still need a surgical correction. However, while he remembers even the worst of his impairments, he has a "today is today" attitude—no complaints, no frustration. He is the youngest of four, and I think the attention he has garnered has made him feel special and loved (he claimed he was "Moses, Prince of Egypt" just two weeks ago). Chemo every three weeks, all the testing, at-home hydration, meds and mouth care, port accessing, GCSF, etc., has just become routine for him. I am trying to catch up to his good spirits.*

# Discharge

When your child is discharged from the hospital after surgery, you are given written instructions on home care. These may include instructions for care of the incision or directions on dressing changes. The most important thing to remember when caring for the operation site is to use proper techniques. Hands should be thoroughly washed with soap and water prior to beginning any dressing changes.

You may also need to ensure that your child complies with daily physical therapy exercises. Before discharge, the physical therapist will discuss this with you, and directions to complete the exercises properly are given in writing. In some cases a physical therapist comes to your home or you take your child for physical therapy several times a week.

> We had some physical therapy as soon as he could tolerate it in the hospital, but the doctor didn't feel he needed it at home. Our child was under three and eligible for early intervention services (which is available to all children younger than school age who have the potential for delayed development) because of his diagnosis, so we asked for and received some physical therapy from them for a period of time.
>
> · · · · ·
>
> Our neurosurgeon told me not to worry about Michael playing soccer (he scored a goal in his first game back—a diving head ball!), that his metal plate was screwed in with titanium screws and wasn't about to move.

At discharge, you will receive a follow-up appointment with your child's surgeon to have any staples or stitches removed. Your surgeon should let you know what the next step in the treatment process is and which member of the multidisciplinary team is in charge of that phase of treatment.

> Chris was born with a condition called gelastic epilepsy, caused by a hypothalamic hamartoma, a rare congenital tumour which can cause intractable seizures, behaviour rages, early puberty, and cognitive decline. Surgery to remove this tumour has had to be the most emotional and most difficult experience of my life. Everything was running through my head, both negative and positive thoughts. Of course it was the overwhelming fear that something might go wrong. I had experienced this in the weeks leading up to surgery, and had tried to prepare myself more for this time, but the

intense feelings were so strong, it is hard to explain. I kept telling myself that we have to go through with it because this was his real chance.

I left Chris asleep in the anaesthetic room. I came out in tears and continued to battle with my emotions. Our neurosurgeon came to see us and assured us that things would be all right, "he was going to take good care of him." I felt a deep inner sense of comfort about this man, that he truly did love and care for all the children he operated on. This helped a lot and we began to settle down a little. The neurosurgeon's associate came up to the ward a few hours later to tell us that he had got the tumour out. We then went down to the parent recovery waiting room and our neurosurgeon came out to talk with us and tell us more about the surgery in detail—the beaming smile on his face said it all.

It was like a dream, there we were, sitting and being told that this terrible thing was no longer inside our son's head. All of a sudden there was this tremendous weight taken off my shoulders and I felt a strange sense of peace within.

Chris slept more or less the whole night and most of the following day. We watched over him as he was constantly checked for responsiveness, blood pressure, signs of seizure, and fluid input and output. That evening he developed a high temperature, we were told to expect this might happen, and it settled down.

Next morning at around 4 A.M., Chris woke up and asked, "Dad, can I have some cola?" You cannot imagine how I felt: I had my son back, he was going to be okay.

# CHAPTER 9

# Clinical Trials

WITHIN DAYS OF ARRIVING at a major pediatric medical center with a child newly diagnosed with a brain or spinal cord tumor, parents are often asked to enroll their child in a clinical trial. A clinical trial is a carefully controlled research study that uses human volunteers to answer specific scientific questions. Pediatric clinical trials are all directed toward improving existing treatments. Clinical trials test approaches that are thought to be promising. They can also fine-tune existing treatments, improve the results or reduce the side effects of known treatments, or develop new ways to assess response to treatments. More than half of all children with CNS tumors in North America are enrolled on a clinical trial at some time during their treatment experience.

Making an informed judgment on whether to participate is crucial, because it will determine what treatment your child will receive in the months to come. This chapter serves as an introduction to clinical trials and protocols and presents information on how different parents made decisions on this important issue.

## Why are children enrolled in clinical trials?

The improvements in treating childhood CNS tumors have been the direct result of clinical trials. In order to accurately evaluate any new treatment, large numbers of patients are needed in each clinical trial.

Because clinical trials offer the most up-to-date treatment available, children who participate in a clinical trial may benefit from the newest research. Many parents derive comfort from knowing that the knowledge gained will make an important contribution to medical science and may help other children with cancer.

## What is standard treatment?

Standard treatment is the best treatment known for a specific type of tumor. As results from ongoing and completed clinical trials are analyzed, more knowledge is accumulated and standard treatments evolve. However, for some types of tumors, no standard treatment exists.

Many clinical trials divide patients into two or more groups (treatment arms). One arm of the trial is the standard-of-care, or best treatment known, and the other arms are the experimental portions, which physicians hope will prove to be more effective or less toxic than the standard treatment. Each arm is based on preliminary, but not conclusive, information that it will be beneficial. Clinical trials are carefully reviewed by experts in the field before implementation.

# What types of clinical trials are there?

There are three main types of clinical trials.

- **Phase I.** These clinical trials are designed to determine the maximum tolerated doses (MTD) of a new drug and to determine the side effects. The dose of a new drug is gradually increased in small groups of children until unacceptable toxicity or side effects are seen. This means that one small group of children gets a low dose. The next small group gets a slightly higher dose, and so on until an unacceptable number of patients experience unacceptable toxicities. The highest dose of a drug that can be safely given to children without unacceptable side effects may then be studied in a Phase II trial.

- **Phase II.** These trials are designed to see if the new drug or treatment is active against specific tumors.

- **Phase III trials.** These clinical trials determine if a new treatment is better than the usual or standard therapy. Some are designed solely to improve survival; others try to maintain survival rates while lowering toxicity of treatment.

The National Cancer Institute, which sponsors COG trials, offers parents several resources to help them understand the clinical trial process. You can call the National Cancer Institute at their local offices at (800) 422-6237. Or you can visit their clinical trials web site online at *http://www.clinicaltrials.gov.*

# What is randomization?

Some scientific studies require a process called randomization. This means that, after parents agree to enroll their child in a clinical trial, a computer will randomly assign the child to one arm of the study. If there are three arms, the parents will not know which of the three (one standard, two experimental) their child will receive until the computer assigns one. The purpose of computer assignment is to assure that patients are evenly assigned to each treatment plan without bias from physicians or families.

One group of patients (the control group) always receives the standard treatment to provide a basis for comparison to the experimental arms.

At the time the clinical trial is designed, there is no conclusive evidence to indicate which arm is superior. It is therefore not possible to predict if your child will benefit from participating in the study. Most arms incorporate standard therapy, and only a small portion of the arm contains the "experimental" therapy. This may consist of new drugs, old drugs used in a new way, duration of treatment that is shorter or longer than standard care, the addition or deletion of certain treatments (such as radiation therapy), or the use of new supportive care interventions, such as preventative antibiotics or new drugs to control nausea.

> We had a hard time deciding whether to go with the standard treatment or to participate in the study. The "B" arm of the study seemed, on intuition, to be too harsh for her because she was so weak at the time. We finally did opt for the study, hoping we wouldn't be randomized to "B." We chose the study basically so that the computer could choose and we wouldn't ever have to think "we should have gone with the study." As it turned out, we were randomized to the standard arm, so we got what we wanted while still participating in the study.

Researchers closely monitor ongoing studies and modify the study if one arm is clearly identified as superior during the course of the trial.

# What about experimental drugs?

Before a promising new drug is used in humans, it undergoes extensive testing in the laboratory. It is then studied in animals to assess its safety and efficacy. In some cases, this may take up to seven years. After pre-clinical testing has been completed, an Investigational New Drug Application (INDA) is filed with the US Food and Drug Administration. The data is analyzed carefully and if results are satisfactory, the drug may be tested in humans. New drugs generally undergo testing in adults before they are used in children, though exceptions do occur.

The first children to receive the drug are usually those who have had their tumors recur multiple times. These first studies are called Phase I studies, and their goal is to identify the maximum tolerated dose (MTD) in humans. The MTD is the dose level below the dose where unacceptable side effects occur. If these studies are successful, Phase II studies begin, which test the drug for activity in a variety of cancers, sometimes including CNS tumors. Most patients enrolled in Phase II studies have also experienced at least one recurrence of their disease. If the drug is effective against one or more types of tumors, it may be incorporated into a Phase III trial to treat newly diagnosed patients. The vast majority of children are treated on Phase III trials to test the new treatment against the standard treatment in large numbers of people. The entire process of drug development takes anywhere from 10 to 15 years.

## Who designs clinical trials?

There were four primary pediatric cancer research groups in North America: Children's Cancer Group (CCG), Pediatric Oncology Group (POG), National Wilms Tumor Study Group (NWTSG), and Intergroup Rhabdomyosarcoma Study Group (IRSG). In July 1998, the four groups decided to form a single pediatric cancer clinical trials organization. The merger is particularly advantageous for children with CNS tumors, because it allows the studies to enroll more patients and facilitates new drug testing in a more timely fashion. The groups officially merged in 2000 under the new name, Children's Oncology Group (COG). New trials developed for children with brain and spinal cord tumors will be offered under the COG name. Trials begun by the previous research groups will continue until they are completed as planned.

More than 350 institutions are members of COG. Researchers from each institution contribute to the design of new clinical trials for children with cancer. The National Cancer Institute and some individual institutions design their own trials for children treated at those institutions.

In 1999, the National Cancer Institute sponsored a new consortium called The Pediatric Brain Tumor Consortium (PBTC). It consists of nine institutions in the US. The purpose of the PBTC is to test new agents and therapies for pediatric brain tumors, and to evaluate cutting edge diagnostic technology. All members of the group have well-established, multi-disciplinary brain tumor programs and are capable of performing technically challenging studies. You can learn more about this group at their website *http://www.pbtc.org.*

## Who supervises clinical trials?

The ethical and legal codes ruling medical practice also apply to clinical trials. In addition, most research is federally funded or regulated, with rules to protect patients (this includes all CCG, POG, NWTSG, and IRSG and, now, COG trials). The research groups also have review boards that meet at prearranged dates for the duration of a clinical trial to ensure that the risks of all parts of the study are acceptable relative to the benefits. If one arm of the trial is causing unexpected or unacceptable side effects, that portion will be stopped, and the children enrolled will be given the other treatment. If one of the arms appears to be significantly less effective than the standard, it will be stopped. Whenever a treatment is proven to be superior, all children have the option to receive it.

All institutions that conduct clinical trials also have an Institutional Review Board (IRB) that reviews and approves the research taking place there. These boards, whose purpose is to protect patients, are made up of scientists, doctors, sometimes clergy, and often citizens from the community. Before patients at an institution are enrolled on a trial, it must be reviewed and approved by the IRB.

# What questions should parents ask about clinical trials?

To fully understand the clinical trial proposed for your child, here are some important questions to ask your treating physician:

- What is the purpose of the study?

- Who is sponsoring the study? Who reviews it? How often is it reviewed? Who monitors patient safety?

- What tests and treatments will be done during the study? How do these differ from standard treatment?

- Why is it thought that the treatment being studied may be better than standard treatment?

- What are the possible benefits?

- What are all possible disadvantages?

- What are the possible side effects or risks of the study? What are the side effects of the study compared to those of standard treatment?

- How will the study affect my child's daily life?

- What are the possible long-term impacts of the study compared to those of the standard treatment?

- How long will the study last? Is this shorter or longer than standard treatment?

- Will the study require more hospitalization than standard treatment?

- Does the study include long-term follow-up care?

- What happens if my child is harmed as a result of the research?

- Compare the study to standard treatment in terms of possible outcomes, side effects, time involved, costs, and quality of life.

- Have insurers been paying for care under this protocol?

When discussing the clinical trial with the physician, you'll need the information to review later. Many parents bring a tape recorder or a friend to take notes. Some parents write down all of the physician's answers for later reference.

> *Our 6-year-old daughter Morgan was diagnosed with a medulloblastoma in her cerebellum when she was two years old. A clinical trial involving very high dose chemotherapy followed by stem cell transplant was proposed. We asked numerous questions, and I wrote down all the answers in my notebook. The two primary questions were: How many kids die during and after this treatment? Are her chances of long-term survival worth the pain we were going to put her through? We struggled with the concept of hurting her if it wasn't going to do any good. We also asked about the specific drugs, their side effects, and what to expect from each treatment. It was a very difficult process and decision.*

# What is informed consent?

Informed consent requires full disclosure and discussion and is usually handled in four stages. First, all the treatments available to the child must be laid on the table and discussed—not just the treatment available at your hospital or through your doctor, but all the treatments that could be beneficial, wherever they are given. Second, the parents and the child should discuss these options and decide whether they want to consider one of them. Next, the option selected is thoroughly discussed, with all its benefits and risks clearly explained. Finally, those aspects of the study that are considered experimental and those that are standard need to be clearly described. A fully informed medical decision weighs the relative merits of a therapy after full disclosure of benefits, risks, and alternatives.

During the discussions between the doctor(s) and family, all questions should be answered in language that is clearly understood by the parents and child, and there should be no pressure to enroll the child in the study. The objective of the informed consent process is to ensure the participants are comfortable with their choice and can comply with it.

> *We had many discussions with the staff prior to signing the informed consent to participate in the clinical trial. We asked innumerable questions, all of which were answered in a frank and honest manner. We felt that participating gave our child the best chance for a cure, and we felt good about increasing the knowledge that would help other children later.*

. . . . .

> *Sean missed the deadline for enrolling in a clinical trial when he was diagnosed. However, when his tumor regrew we did enroll him on a trial. The particular trial he was in was a randomized computer trial that decided if he was getting one or two chemotherapy agents. We felt if we enrolled him in the trial, maybe the results would help other children.*

The form that parents sign has language similar to the following: "The study described above has been explained to me, and I voluntarily agree to have my child participate in this study. I have had all of my questions answered, and understand that all future questions that I have about this research will be answered by the investigators listed above."

By the time a study is published in the literature, doctors on the cutting edge of treatment are two to four years into improving that treatment or learning of its shortcomings. For this reason, it is best to make decisions in partnership with knowledgeable medical caregivers, rather than in isolation.

No matter how comfortable you are with your child's treating physician, it is sometimes helpful to have another medical caregiver help sort out your options. Often, that person will be your pediatrician or family doctor. A list of physicians offering research study treatments for children with brain tumors is available from the American Brain Tumor Association at (800) 886-2282.

> *When my son was diagnosed with an optic glioma, we were told we had two options: a clinical trial or standard treatment. We decided to get a second opinion before making our decision. Our pediatrician, my husband, and I met in the doctor's office for a telephone conference with a pediatric oncologist from a major brain tumor center. We each presented our concerns, including our pediatrician, who thought of some issues we hadn't considered. I think we all came away better informed of our options.*

# What is a protocol?

A protocol is a written plan for treating CNS tumors. Just like a recipe for baking a cake, it has a list of ingredients, the amounts to use, and the order to use them so the recipe has the best chance for success. The protocol document lists the drugs, dosages, and tests for each segment of treatment and follow-up. It usually also contains a diagram (called a roadmap) that shows when each drug and test is given. If your child is enrolled in a clinical trial, the protocol will outline the treatment for each arm.

> The clinical trial that my child was enrolled in had three arms— A, B, and C. He was in the A portion, so we only referred to the A section of the protocol, which clearly outlined each procedure and drug to be given for the duration of the trial. It also listed the follow-up care required by that particular clinical trial.
>
> • • • • •
>
> We referred to the short version of the protocol every week since it provided a chart for the 6-week cycle we were to follow for the entire year-plus on treatment. Our nurse practitioner would respond with a nod and a smile when we came in to clinic saying, "So this week, it's carboplatin only."

A protocol is 5 to 100 pages long, and the family may also be given an abbreviated version (1 to 2 pages) to provide quick and easy reference on a daily basis. Parents and patients should review these documents carefully with the treating physician so that all portions are understood. It will be the parent's responsibility to make the appropriate appointments and give oral medications at the correct times. The protocol also contains specific sections that outline exactly how the therapy is to be given, as well as sections that dictate appropriate modifications in the plan when side effects occur.

Many parents express anguish when their child's protocol changes during treatment. An important point to remember is that the protocol is a guideline that is frequently modified, depending on each child's response to treatment.

> It took me a long time to get over my hang-up that things needed to go exactly as per protocol. Any deviations on dose or days was a major stress for me. It took talking to many parents, as well as doctors and nurses, to realize and feel comfortable with the fact that no one ever goes along perfectly and that the protocol is meant as the broad guideline. There will always be times when your child will be off drugs or on half dose because of illness or low counts or whatever. It took a long time to realize that this

*is not going to ruin the effectiveness, that the child gets what she can*
*handle without causing undue harm.*

. . . . .

*I didn't know what a protocol was when Preston was diagnosed, and I*
*understood from the doctors that this was the "exact" regime which must*
*be followed to cure Preston. It frightened me whenever changes were*
*made in the protocol. After a time, I came to view the protocol as merely*
*a guideline which is individualized for each patient according to his*
*tolerance and reaction to the drugs.*

# Should parents receive the entire trial document?

The clinical trial protocol described earlier is actually a very small portion of an extensive scientific document describing all aspects of the clinical study. The entire document often exceeds 100 pages and covers the following topics: study hypothesis, experimental design, scientific background and rationale with relevant references from the scientific literature, patient eligibility and randomization, therapy for each arm of the study, required observations, pathology guidelines, radiation therapy guidelines (if applicable), supportive care guidelines, specific information about each drug, guidelines for progressive disease, statistical considerations, study committee names and phone numbers, record keeping, reporting of adverse drug reactions, and consent form.

Parents are sometimes not aware that this lengthy document exists. Admittedly, for some parents the full protocol is overwhelming or boring. There are many parents, however, who throw themselves into research to better understand their child's illness. Those parents may benefit from having a copy of the study document for several reasons. First, it provides a description of the clinical trials that preceded the present one and explains the reasons the investigators designed this particular study. Second, it provides detailed descriptions of drug reactions, which may comfort many parents who worry that their child is the only one exhibiting extreme responses to some drugs. Third, motivated parents who have only one protocol to keep track of occasionally prevent errors in treatment. Physicians treat scores of children on dozens of protocols, and sometimes mistakes occur. Finally, for parents who are adrift in the world of cancer treatment, it can provide a bit of control over their child's life. It gives them a sense of control by letting them monitor their child's treatment.

*Since knowledge is comfort for me, I really wanted to have the entire*
*clinical trial document, despite its technical language. Whereas the brief*
*protocol that I had listed day, drug, dose, the expanded version listed the*
*potential side effects for each drug, and what actions should be taken*
*should any occur. I learned the parameters.*

Parents have a right to review all literature and information related to their child's treatment. If you wish to read all of the details of the study, simply ask that a copy be provided to you. Informed consent documents for Children's Oncology Group protocols specifically inform families that they will receive a copy of the full protocol upon request. It may, however, be helpful to schedule an appointment with your physician, nurse practitioner, or research nurse to address any questions or concerns.

# What happens if parents say no?

If the family chooses not to participate in the proposed clinical trial, their child will be given the best-known treatment for his type of tumor (standard care).

*Our son's doctor gave us all the paperwork on the clinical trial and told*
*us that it was our decision. We chose not to join the study, because the*
*second arm of the trial consisted of a combination of four drugs with,*
*we felt, intense side effects. The first arm involved two drugs used as*
*standard treatment and known to be effective in similar cases. We were*
*much more comfortable choosing standard treatment.*

# Can parents remove their child?

Yes. If parents have questions or concerns about any aspect of the trial, they should talk it over with their doctor. If the problem is not resolved, parents have the right to remove their child at any time from a clinical trial. This decision will not be held against the parent, and the child will still receive the best available care for that type of CNS tumor. On the consent form signed by the parent, there will be language similar to this: "You are free to not have your child participate in this research or to withdraw your child at any time without penalty or jeopardizing future care."

*After treatments ended, Jesse was enrolled in a clinical trial to assess*
*long-term consequences of radiation. The testing was free, and we were*
*glad to participate. Unfortunately, the billing department of the hospital*
*continually billed us in error. We tried to correct the problem, but it*
*became such a hassle that we withdrew from the study.*

# Pros and cons of clinical trials

Making the decision whether to have your child participate in a clinical trial is sometimes difficult. The following lists of pros and cons may help you clarify how you feel about this important decision.

Pros of clinical trials are:

- Patients receive either state-of-the-art investigational therapy or the best standard therapy available.

- Clinical trials can provide an opportunity to benefit from a new therapy before it is generally available.

- Information gained from clinical trials will benefit children with CNS tumors in the future.

- Children enrolled in clinical trials may be monitored more frequently throughout treatment.

- The IRB has reviewed the protocol for protection of patient's rights as well as for scientific soundness.

- Review boards of scientists oversee the operation of clinical trials.

- Participating in a clinical trial often makes parents feel that they did everything medically possible for their child.

- Some clinical trials provide all treatment and follow-up care at no cost to the family.

Cons to consider are:

- The experimental arm may not provide treatment as effective as the standard, or it may generate unexpected side effects or risks.

- Not all patients in a study receive the new treatment.

- Some clinical trials require more hospitalizations, treatments, clinic visits, or tests that may be more costly, or more painful, than the standard treatment.

- Some families feel additional stress over which arm is the best treatment for their individual child.

- Participation may generate parental guilt if the child has unacceptable toxicity from the more aggressive experimental arm.

- Insurance may not cover investigational studies. Parents need to carefully explore this issue prior to signing the consent form.

*When we were struggling with the decision of whether to join the study, I asked the oncologist how would we ever know if we made the right decision. He said something very wise. "You will never know and you should never second guess yourself, no matter how the study turns out. Statistics are about large groups of kids, not your child. Your child might respond no matter which arm she is on or she might show no benefit from a treatment arm where most other kids do well. Statistics for you will be either 100 percent or 0 because your child will either live or die. I can't tell you which will be the better treatment, that is why we are conducting the study. But no matter what, we will be doing absolutely the best we can."*

# CHAPTER 10

# Venous Catheters

MANY CHILDREN WITH CANCER require chemotherapy, intravenous (IV) fluids, IV antibiotics, blood and platelet transfusions, frequent blood sampling, and sometimes IV nutrition. The intensity of therapy is determined by the type and stage of disease and by the child's reaction to treatment. Indwelling catheters have proved to be a very effective method for providing entry into the large veins for intensive therapy. They eliminate the difficulty of finding veins for IVs and allow drugs to be put directly into a large vessel of the heart, where they are rapidly diluted and spread throughout the body.

Categories of indwelling catheters include right atrial catheter, implanted catheter, central venous catheter, central line, Hickman, Broviac, Port-a-cath, Medi-port, Infusa-port, or PICC lines.

The two types of indwelling catheters most commonly used in children are the external catheter and the subcutaneous port. PICC lines, or peripherally inserted central catheters, are used less frequently.

## External catheter

The external catheter is a long, flexible tube with one end placed in the right atrium of the heart or the superior vena cava (the large vein leading to the heart) and the other end extending outside the skin of the chest wall. The tube tunnels under the skin of the chest, enters a large vein near the collarbone, and threads inside a big vein leading to the heart (see Figure 10-1). Because chemotherapy drugs, transfusions, and IV fluids are put in the end of the tube hanging outside the body, puncturing the skin is avoided. Blood for complete blood counts (CBC) or other tests is also drawn from the end of the catheter.

The commonly used external catheters are the Hickman or Broviac. With meticulous care, the external catheter can often be left in place for the child's full duration of treatment.

## How it's put in

External catheters are usually put in under general anesthesia. Once the child is anesthetized, the surgeon makes two small incisions. One incision is near the collarbone over the spot where the catheter enters the vein, the other is in the area on the chest where the catheter exits the body. To prevent the catheter from slipping out, it is stitched to the skin where it comes out of the chest. There is a Dacron cuff around the catheter right above the exit site (under the skin), into which body tissue grows. This further anchors the catheter and helps prevent infection.

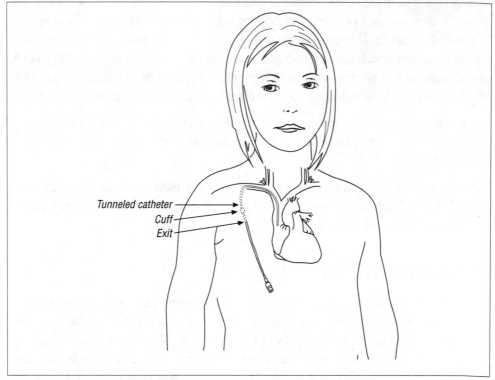

*Figure 10-1. External catheter*

## Daily care

The external catheter requires careful maintenance to try to prevent infection or the formation of clots. The site where the catheter exits the body must be cleaned frequently (schedules range from every other day to weekly) and a fresh, sterile dressing needs to be applied and taped in place. Some pediatric oncology centers also place a small antibiotic-impregnated disk around the catheter at the exit site. The site should be checked for redness, swelling, or drainage. To prevent clots, parents or older patients are taught to flush the line with a heparin solution. Different institutions use different schedules for how often the line should be flushed. During the hospital stay, nurses at the hospital instruct parents in catheter care, and plenty of practice should be provided until both parent and child are comfortable with the entire procedure. At the time of discharge, home nursing visits are sometimes arranged to provide further help.

> We were very grateful for Matthew's Hickman line. Like a lot of children, he was terribly afraid of needles. The maintenance that was necessary to keep his line working properly became second nature to me. After his diagnosis, and again after his relapse, he had a Hickman implanted. In total, he had his external catheter for more than four years.

## Risks

The major complications of using the external catheter are infections—either in the blood or at the insertion site—and the formation of clots in the line. Clots can also form in the blood vessel where the catheter is placed. Rare complications are kinking of the catheter, catheter dislodgement, or breakage of the external segment of the catheter.

### Infections

Even with the best care, infections are common in children with external lines. Children who are immunosuppressed (have low blood counts) for long periods of time are at risk for developing infections. The need for frequent flushing of the external line also increases the chance for bacteria to enter the catheter. Most infections in such patients are caused by the patient's own bacteria that get out of where they belong (skin, mouth, gastrointestinal tract) and enter the bloodstream. The most common organism is a bacterium called staphylococcus epidermidis, which lives on the skin, though a host of other organisms can cause infections in children receiving chemotherapy.

If the child develops a fever over 101°F (38.5°C), redness or swelling at the insertion site, or pain in the catheter area, infection is suspected. To determine if bacteria are present, blood will be drawn from the catheter to culture (grow in a laboratory for 24 to 48 hours). Treatment will start whenever there is a suspected infection and will end if the culture comes back negative. If the culture is positive, treatment usually continues for ten to fourteen days. Treatment with antibiotics is usually effective, though certain organisms are capable of causing a bacterial film to grow on the catheter that is impossible to eradicate, thus necessitating removal of the catheter.

> By November Trevor had completed all his treatments, but his Broviac
> needed to stay in for a few more weeks. However, in December, Trevor
> was admitted back to the hospital when his catheter became infected. The
> doctors treated him with antibiotics and decided to remove it a little early.
> The Broviac prevented a lot of unnecessary pain, and we were grateful that
> he had it.

Some physicians require that the child be hospitalized for antibiotic treatment; others allow the child to go home. If the infection does not respond to treatment, the catheter may have to be removed.

> When my daughter had a line infection, I wanted to use the antibiotic
> pump at home. It was hard, though. It took two hours per dose, three doses
> per day, for fourteen days. I would get up at 5 A.M. to hook her up, so that
> she would sleep through the first dose. The second dose I would give while
> she watched a tape in the early afternoon. Then I would hook her up at
> bedtime so she would sleep through it. I had to wait up to flush and
> disconnect, so I was very tired by the end of the two weeks.

## Clots

Even with excellent daily care, some external catheters develop blockages and/or clots. If the catheter becomes blocked, it will be flushed with a drug capable of dissolving the clot. Examples of such drugs are activase, urokinase, and streptokinase. The agents are given in the clinic or hospital and generally require the child to remain in the area for one to two hours, depending on the institutional protocol. If the catheter is blocked by a drug precipitate, a diluted hydrochloric acid solution may be used to dissolve the blockage. This is a rare occurrence, but may be caused by simultaneous administration of incompatible drugs or long-term administration of intravenous nutrition solutions.

> Two months before the end of Kristin's treatment, her line plugged up. We
> tried several maneuvers at home unsuccessfully. We had to bring her in for
> the IV team to work on it. I think the bumpy ride to the hospital loosened it
> because they were able to dislodge the clot just by flushing it with saline.

## Kinks

Rarely, a kink develops in the catheter due to a sharp angle where the catheter enters the neck vein. In such cases, the fluids may go in the catheter but it is hard to get blood out. Parents and nurses are often able to work around this problem by experimenting with different positions for the child when the blood is drawn. Another method is to teach the child a Valsalva maneuver, such as bearing down as if to have a bowel movement, taking a deep breath, coughing, or laughing.

> My son is 16, and was diagnosed January, 2001, with PNET. His Hickman was giving the nurses problems, so they planned to do a dye study. They didn't even have to inject the dye, the x-ray showed the line had come out and was clear across the opposite side of his chest and kinked! I don't think it had been out long. But it was a little scary to think of that chemo maybe going everywhere. They did a procedure where they go in with a special catheter line and grab the line and pull it back into place. It was still attached to the vein, so the chemo hadn't been going amok. We are all so happy they got it fixed without surgery.

## Catheter Breakage

Breaks in the line do happen, but they are very rare. If the break or rupture of the line occurs when it is not in use, only heparin will leak into surrounding tissues. If the break occurs when corrosive chemotherapy drugs are flowing through the catheter, they may leak and cause damage to surrounding tissue. The risk of an internal line leaking is far lower than the chance of leakage from an IV in a vein of the hand or arm.

Breaks in the external portion of the catheter may also occur. If this occurs, the line should be clamped between the point of breakage and the chest wall covered with a sterile gauze pad, and the physician notified immediately. In most cases, the line can be successfully repaired. Many institutions send a catheter repair kit home with parents.

> I think it is important for parents to obtain clamps from the treating institution to carry on them. The preschool or school the child goes should also have one in case something happens to the external line above the clamps that exist on the catheter. Younger children should wear a snug tank top that helps hold the catheter in place. Pinning it to the shirt is not the best solution for the active or younger kids.

# Other factors to consider

The proper care and maintenance of an external catheter requires motivation and organization. The site needs to be cleaned and dressed frequently, and heparin must be injected using sterile technique. The dressing must be secured to the skin with an adhering dressing. If your child is very tape sensitive (cries whenever tape is removed or skin reddens and breaks out), the external line may not be a the best choice.

Excellent liquid adhesive removers, such as Detachol (Ferndale Laboratories, Ferndale, Mich.), are commercially available that all but eliminate the problem of pain. Additionally, if clear plastic dressings cause skin breakdown, alternate products such as Hypafix, a soft, though adherent, cloth tape that is easy to remove (Smith & Nephew, Inc., Largo, Florida), are sometimes used. More information on dressings and adhesive removers is included at the end of the chapter in the "A word about adhesives" section.

An external catheter may require restrictions regarding swimming, use of hot tubs, and sometimes bathing and showering, though care protocols vary by institution.

> Brendon needed chemo when his astrocytoma came back at age twelve. He was old enough to decide what type of catheter he wanted. I explained about both kinds. We talked about how the port would allow him to swim—he so loves the water. But he hated pokes and he'd need some with the port. We talked about using EMLA for that. On the other hand, he wouldn't need the pokes if he got a broviac. But it would be hanging out of his body. And he was 12. He decided on the port and it worked just fine.
>
> • • • • •
>
> We didn't get a choice when Morgan needed a stem cell transplant. They needed to put in two boviac lines to accommodate all of the meds, fluids, and TPN she needed for the procedure. I remember seeing six bags hanging up at once. I did the dressing changes and we didn't have any trouble with the lines throughout the recuperation.

The external line is a constant reminder of cancer treatment and causes changes in body image. Both parent and child need to be comfortable with the idea of seeing and handling a tube that emerges from the chest. It is noticeable under lightweight clothing and bathing suits, but not heavier clothing like sweaters or coats. If there is a younger sibling who might pull or yank on the catheter, the Hickman or Broviac might not be the appropriate choice.

On the other hand, the reason external lines are chosen so frequently is that there are no needles and no pain. This is a very important consideration for young children or any person who is frightened of needles and/or pain. Some treatment protocols require double lumen access and the external catheter is the only appropriate option. Finally, children who requite long-term continuous venous access or those children in whom a bone marrow transplant is planned require external venous catheters.

> Ben was diagnosed at age 5 with medulloblastoma, had a full resection, low dose radiation to whole brain and spine, and one year of chemo. He

*had a double-lumen Broviac-Hickman, a long tube with two ends that came out of his chest just above his right nipple. When not in use, it was curled and taped against his skin. I hated this thing. It made him Borg-like. I had to clean it every day for more than a year, and flush both ends of the tube. This hated thing, however, was what kept Ben from having to be stuck with needles several times a week. It was direct access to his blood supply, for tests, medication administration and chemotherapy. One day Ben told me he had "made friends with his tubies." They had names, "The red one was Ralph, and the white one was Henry." He liked his tubies, he said, because they kept him from getting "ouchies." I was speechless. His matter-of-fact example showed me that the sooner I made friends with Ralph and Henry, the better off I'd be.*

## Subcutaneous port

Several different types of subcutaneous (under the skin) ports are available by a number of manufacturers. The subcutaneous port differs from the external catheter in that it is completely under the skin. A small metal or plastic chamber (one and a half inches in diameter) with a rubber top is implanted under the skin of the chest wall. A catheter threads from the metal chamber (portal) under the skin to a large vein near the collarbone, then inside the vein to the right atrium of the heart (see Figure 10-2). Whenever the catheter is needed for a blood draw or infusion of drugs or fluid, a special needle is inserted by a nurse through the skin and into the rubber top of the

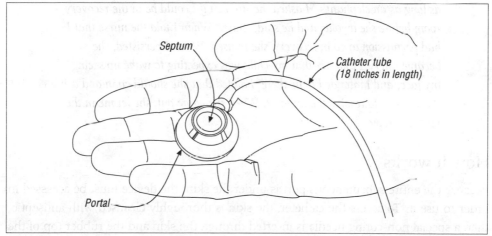

*Figure 10-2. Parts of the Port-a-cath*

portal. Multi-lumen subcutaneous ports are available, but are not appropriate in young children because of the weight of the appliance.

A teddy bear companion equipped with port is available for children via corporate sponsorship by contacting The Kimo Bear Project at *kimo@kimobear.org,* and an interactive web site for kids going through chemotherapy can be found at *http://www. royalmarsden.org.uk/captchemo.*

## How it's put in

The subcutaneous port is implanted under general anesthesia in the operating room in a procedure that generally takes less than an hour. Rarely, local anesthesia is used for older children or teens, though this is not desirable. The surgeon makes two small incisions: one in the chest where the portal will be placed, and the other near the collarbone where the catheter will enter a vein in the lower part of the neck (see Figure 10-3). First, one end of the catheter is placed in the large blood vessel of the neck and threaded into the right atrium of the heart or the superior vena cava. The other end of the catheter is tunneled under the skin, where it is attached to the portal. Fluid is injected into the portal to ensure that the device works properly. The portal is then placed under the skin in the right chest and stitched to the underlying muscle. Both incisions are then closed. The only evidence that a catheter has been implanted is two small scars and a bump under the skin where the portal rests.

> *Christine had her port surgery late at night. The resident gave her some premedication, then the chief resident ordered him to give her more. She felt so silly that she looked at me, giggled, and said, "Mommy has a nose as long as an elephant's." I asked the surgeon if I could be in the recovery room before she awoke, and he said, "Sure." When I told the nurse that I had permission to go in recovery, she refused. When I persisted, she became angry. I told her that my child was expecting to wake up seeing my face, and I intended to be there. I added that she should go in and ask the surgeon to resolve the impasse. When she came out, she let me in the recovery room.*

## How it works

Because the entire subcutaneous port is under the skin, the device must be accessed in order to use it. To access the catheter, the skin is thoroughly cleansed with antiseptic, then a special non-coring needle is inserted through the skin and the rubber top of the portal. The needle is attached to a short length of tubing that hangs down the front of

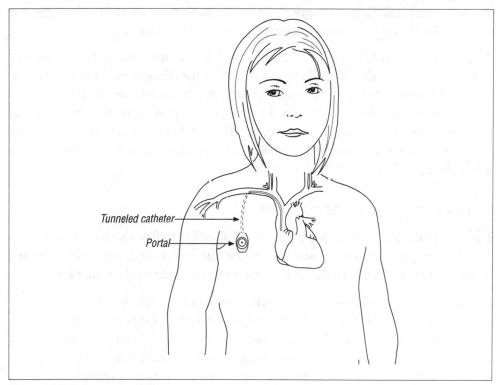

Tunneled catheter
Portal

*Figure 10-3. Subcutaneous port*

the chest. EMLA cream can be applied one hour prior to the needle poke to anesthetize the skin, or ethyl chloride can be sprayed on right before the poke. Subcutaneous
ports have a septum that is self-sealing after needle removal and is designed to withstand years of needle insertions. The non-coring needle is essential because it allows
the rubber septum to self-seal when it is removed. Failure to use this type of needle
will result in leakage of fluid into the tissues.

> Brent (8 years old) has had a Port-a-cath for 33 months with
> absolutely no problems. He uses EMLA to anesthetize it prior to
> accessing. He hates finger pokes so much that he has his port accessed
> every time he needs blood drawn.

If the child is in a part of treatment where the line must be used every day, the nurse
will attach the tubing to IV fluids or will close the end off with a sterile cap after
flushing with saline solution. A transparent dressing will be put over the site where
the needle enters the port. The port can remain accessed in this way for up to seven
days. After that time, to avoid the risk of infection, the needle should be removed and

the port reaccessed when necessary. If the needle and tubing are to be left in place, it is important to tape them securely to the chest to avoid accidents.

If the port is needed only infrequently, this will be the sequence of events: the site will be cleaned, needle put in, line rinsed with saline, drug given or blood drawn, line rinsed with saline, heparin added to line, needle withdrawn, and a Band-Aid placed over the site. In the event that the child may need to be seen at an institution other than the usual cancer treatment center, the family should be given at least one correct size non-coring needle to prevent an inappropriate needle being used to access the port.

## Care of the subcutaneous port

The entire port and catheter are under the skin and therefore require no daily care. The skin over the port can be washed just like the rest of the body. Frequent visual inspections are needed to check for swelling, redness, tenderness, or drainage.

> My 3-year-old was being treated for a low-grade astrocytoma, and had a port inserted for a period of about a year and a half. His port survived all kinds of normal kid wear and tear. I remember that kids with external lines were discouraged from swimming, but with a subcutaneous port, there weren't any restrictions in activity or special precautions, which meant one less thing for us to worry about.

The subcutaneous port must be accessed and flushed with saline and heparin at least once every 30 days, which usually coincides with the monthly clinic visit and blood checks. A nurse or technician does this procedure. The port system requires no maintenance by the parent or patient.

## Risks

The risks for a subcutaneous port are similar to those for the external catheter: infection, clots, and, rarely, kinks or rupture. If the needle is not properly inserted through the rubber septum, fluids can leak into the tissue around the portal.

> Our young son had a Port-a-cath, and never had any line infections, but one time he was so active during an infusion session, the needle pulled out slightly from his port. When the nurse injected a saline flush, it immediately formed a bubble under his skin. It was really uncomfortable and scary for him, but we're glad it didn't happen during his Vincristine injection, which would've burned.

## Infection

Most studies show that the infection rate of subcutaneous ports is lower than that of external catheters. If the subcutaneous port does become infected, it is treated exactly the same as those in external catheters.

> Katy had two infections in her Port-a-cath during treatment. One occurred when the tape loosened during a blood transfusion. She developed a fever the next day and required fourteen days of vancomycin. On another occasion, she became ill in the car on the way home from the clinic. Her skin became white and clammy, and she felt faint and nauseated. She spiked a 102°F temperature which only lasted for two hours. The blood culture both times grew staphylococcus epi.

## Kinks, clots, ruptures

These events rarely occur with the subcutaneous port or the external catheter. If they do occur, they are treated as described earlier in "External catheter."

> When we got to clinic for weekly chemo, no matter what gravity-defying positions we tried (raising arms, lying down, standing up), our nurse couldn't get the line to flush. Adrienne's port was clogged. Luckily, they were able to clear the line with an injection of streptokinase, although it meant entertaining her in clinic for more than an hour while we waited for it to work. They did tell us that if this didn't work we'd have to go in overnight for slow infusion of chemo, but the line cleared, and we did chemo outpatient.

# Peripherally inserted central catheters

A peripherally inserted central catheter is also referred to as a PICC line. This type of catheter is placed in the large antecubital vein (a large vein in the inner elbow area) and threaded into a large vein above the right atrium of the heart (see Figure 10-4). Unlike other catheters, a PICC line can be inserted by an IV nurse, rather than a surgeon.

The PICC line can remain in place for many weeks or months, avoiding the need for a new IV every few days. PICC lines are used to deliver chemotherapy, antibiotics, blood products, other medications, and intravenous nutrition. When the PICC line needs to be accessed, an IV line is connected to the end of the catheter. When it is not in use, the IV is disconnected and the catheter is flushed and capped.

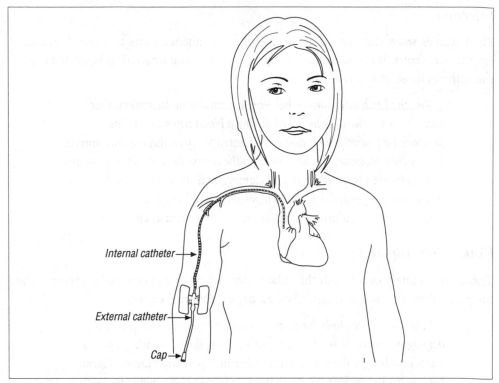

Internal catheter

External catheter

Cap

*Figure 10-4. Peripherally inserted central catheter*

## How it's put in

The peripherally inserted central catheter is inserted in your child's hospital room by an IV nurse or physician. Your child will be positioned on a flat surface, and she will need to keep her arm straight and motionless during the procedure. An injection to numb the area is given to decrease discomfort during insertion. A special needle is used to place the PICC line into the arm vein. The catheter is then threaded through the needle. Once the line is in place, a chest x-ray is taken to ensure that it is positioned properly.

## Care of the peripherally inserted central catheter

The PICC line, like the Hickman catheter, requires meticulous care to prevent problems. You will be taught by the nurses to change the dressing, flush the line, change the injection cap, and inspect the site for possible signs of infection. The dressing covering the exit site is changed on a weekly basis, unless it becomes wet or exposed to the air. The line must be flushed after every use or every day. You should get plenty of practice under the supervision of a nurse until both you and your child are comfortable with caring for the line. The care required for your child's PICC line may be slightly different from what has been described in this section, because institutional preferences vary.

> Kelsey had a PICC line in her right arm, and she would not straighten it out, but kept it a little bent. I definitely think she was protecting it, and also I think when she tried to straighten it, it pulled on the suture and on the dressing in an uncomfortable way that could have been painful, so she just wouldn't try. I had to do a heparin flush every day, and change the dressing twice a week. She could not tolerate Tegaderm so we used another kind of adhesive bandage, and doused it with Detachol, which dissolved the adhesive within a few minutes, allowing us to get the bandage off quite easily. The Detachol was a godsend for her, as removing the adhesive was like pulling teeth and a source of unnecessary pain.

## Risks

The problems associated with a PICC line are similar to those of any external catheter. Veins may become irritated, infection can occur, or the line can be accidentally torn or moved.

### Irritated veins

The vein where the catheter is located may become irritated. This is most likely to occur during the first few days after it has been inserted. Signs of irritation include swelling or pain in the area or the development of small veins near the site. Often, a warm moist cloth or a carefully monitored heating pad placed on the vein will help alleviate discomfort. Elevating the arm on a pillow is also sometimes helpful.

### Infection

Meticulous care using the institution-dictated procedure is very important to reduce the risk of infection. The dressing exit site should be changed every week or if it becomes wet or exposed to the air. Injection caps must also be regularly changed using sterile techniques when the line is not in use, and the line must be flushed on a regular basis. Signs of infection include redness, swelling, pain, drainage, or warmth around the exit site. Fever, chills, tiredness, and dizziness may also indicate that the line has become infected. You should notify the doctor if any of these signs are present or if your child has a fever above 101°F (38.5°C).

### Torn catheter

Accidents sometimes happen, and it is possible that a hole or tear in the line can occur. The only prevention for this is ensuring that care is taken when handling the catheter. You should suspect a torn catheter if fluid leaks out of the line, especially during an injection. If a tear is found, you should find the hole, fold the line above the tear, tape it together and cover it with sterile gauze. You should immediately notify your child's doctor of the problem.

### Displacement of the catheter

Like the external catheters discussed earlier in this chapter, it is important that the PICC line be securely taped to the exit site to prevent movement. Signs of a displaced catheter include chest pain, burning or swelling in the arm above the exit site or in the chest, fluid leaking around the catheter, or pain when fluid is injected into the line. If you suspect that the line has moved, you should tape the catheter in place and immediately notify your child's doctor.

## A word about adhesives

As noted previously, whether your child has a subcutaneous port, an external catheter, or a PICC line, dressing changes will be necessary. Unfortunately, this may become a bone of contention for some children who do not like having the dressing removed. Parents become quite expert in what types of dressings work well for their individual child. Skin type and sensitivity vary from child to child, and you may need to try several skin care regimens before you find the one that works best. The following suggestions from parents may help your child. These can also be used to remove dressings applied to cover EMLA cream.

- Don't use tegaderm if it bothers your child or reddens the skin. Try plastic wrap cut into a square and use paper tape or tape with perforations in it.

- Try Hypafix instead of tegaderm. It's a dressing retention material that looks like gauze with a sticky side. Usually, several sterile 2 × 2 gauze pads are put over the needle entry site, then Hypafix is applied to hold them in place.

- When it's tape removal time, use an effective adhesive remover such as Detachol (an orange colored product). If you douse the paper tape with adhesive dissolver and wait a couple of minutes, it will usually pull right off with no pain.

- Ask for expert advice.

> *Apryl has had skin tears and reactions from the adhesives as a result of using tegaderms and op-sites. We were using Primapore dressings for a while, but after a year she started with the same reaction. When she had her line replaced, I asked for a consultation with the skincare nurse. She recommended All-Dress. It is a waterproof dressing with non-stick gauze in the center surrounded by hypa-fix tape. They are waterproof. Apryl changes hers once every three days, whether it gets wet or not. She also has this pink tape that has zinc oxide in the adhesive to protect the skin. These two have worked out great.*

- Once you have found a routine that works well, negotiate with nursing staff to either do the tape removal yourself or to have them follow your system.

> *I like Hypafix because when it's time to take it off, you can use the adhesive dissolver where it's stuck to the skin, and even without the dissolver, it comes off easier and gentler than Tegaderm. The nurses at our oncology clinic use this all the time. Our local clinic and hospital do not use Hypafix, so I bought a roll and take it with me whenever we go locally for a port access so that we don't have to use Tegaderm.*

· · · · ·

> *Using adhesive dissolver (or peeling off tape or Tegaderm millimeter by millimeter) takes a bit of time—it's not just a swipe and it works. It has to sort of soak in and takes some time to dissolve the sticky stuff. I know the nurses are really busy and under pressure to keep on timelines, so it's probably a conflict for them. I deal with this by always being the one to get the Tegaderm off—took some "muscling in" with nurses who were used to doing it, but it works much better. I try to make a joke of it, "I have a deal with my kid that I'm taking off the Tegaderm. It might take a while and I wouldn't want you to fall asleep waiting on us—how about if I holler out the door when it's off and we're ready?" That way they don't have to stand around and wait, and you don't feel like you need to hurry your child.*

# What about cost?

As noted previously, the external catheter requires supplies for cleaning, dressing, and irrigating the line, but the subcutaneous port does not. The port itself, however, is usually more costly than the external catheter. Both generally require operating room time and the services of a surgeon and an anesthesiologist. The port also requires these services for its eventual removal; the external catheter is removed in the clinic with only intravenous sedation. A good rule of thumb to consider is that, if the lines stay in place at least six months, the overall costs will be almost equal.

Most insurance plans will cover the placement of any central venous catheter and the services of the surgeon, anesthesiologist, and operating room facility. Many plans, however, will not cover the cost of the supplies to maintain the line and this can be an additional financial hardship for families. It is important to consider this when making the final decision about the type of catheter that is best for your child.

## Choosing not to use a catheter

Some physicians do not recommend using implanted catheters in their pediatric patients with specific types of CNS tumors. Ask the physician the reason for this recommendation, and request a second opinion if you think a catheter might be helpful to your child.

> Stephan (6 years old) has no catheter. Sometimes I wish he had one. It seems like it would be easier. We were told he didn't need it. He is running out of usable veins and it is getting harder and harder.
>
> • • • • •
>
> Our physician gave us the option of using a catheter for our six-year-old daughter, but he recommended against it. He said if she could stand the pokes it was better not to use it due to the chance of infections. She had several sessions with the staff psychologist to teach her visualization and imagery which she used successfully to deal with the two years of IVs.
>
> • • • • •
>
> Jordan is four years old and she has had two different ports. She was very protective of them. She would kick and scream and fight being accessed, even with EMLA. In the bath you couldn't touch there, she would wash it very gently. She had port infections so she lost both of them. Now that she receives her chemo through her arm, she doesn't fight that much anymore. I don't know if we will ever put in a new port. She says "No, do it in my arm!!"

To help you make the best decision for your particular situation, the table "Comparison of Catheters" outlines the pros and cons for each catheter. There is no right or wrong choice; different options are available because each child, each parent, each family is unique.

Table 10-1. Comparison of Catheters

| Possible problem | External catheter | Subcutaneous port | Peripherally inserted central catheter (PICC) |
|---|---|---|---|
| Infection rate | Higher | Lower | Higher |
| Maintenance | Daily | Monthly | Daily |
| Body image | Tube outside body | Lump under skin | Tube outside body |
| Pain | Dressing changes | Needle poke to access (use EMLA) | Needle poke to insert the line, dressing changes |
| Anxiety | Low to high | Low to high | Low to high |
| Cost | More because of daily maintenance | Less because of monthly maintenance | More because of daily maintenance |
| Risk of drugs leaking into tissues | Lowest | Low | Low |

# The decision: which catheter for your child?

After reviewing the information presented and the comparison chart, discuss the merits of each catheter with your child's doctor. Involve your child in the decision at a developmentally appropriate level. Then make the rounds of the cancer ward, asking both parents and children which type of catheter they chose and why. You will probably hear many strong opinions on the benefits and drawbacks for each catheter.

> When we asked one of the young children on the ward which catheter she had, she pulled up her shirt with a big grin to show us her Hickman. She had a coil of white tubing neatly taped to her chest. My husband's face turned as white as her tubing.

· · · · ·

> My 4-year-old daughter loved ballet and was extremely interested in her appearance. Her younger sister was very physical, and we were worried that if we chose the Hickman she would grab and pull on the tubing. We chose the port so that she could wear her tutus without reminders of cancer and so that the children could play together without mishap.

The nurses in the clinic and on the ward are another source of valuable information. They will have seen dozens (or hundreds) of children with catheters and will be able to give excellent advice, given your family situation. There is no right or wrong choice, just different options for each unique child.

Removal of indwelling catheters is explained in Chapter 21, *End of Treatment*.

*When Scott (age 3) was diagnosed, his doctor gave us a choice of which central line we could use. He showed us a mannequin with a Broviac and a Port-a-cath. He also told us the pros and cons of each type, then asked us to decide. We chose the Broviac, and feel it was the best decision for Scott. The day it was installed was the end of a lot of unnecessary pain (from needle sticks) for Scott.*

*Scott finished all his treatments three months ago, and yesterday he had his Broviac removed. It went extremely smoothly. He had only one cuff and it was halfway out already. And to think, I fretted and worried about the removal all week!*

# CHAPTER 11

# Radiation Therapy

RADIATION IS A LIFE-SAVING THERAPY that has dramatically improved survival rates for some childhood tumors. Radiation can shrink small tumors and help decrease pain. However, radiation therapy can cause acute short-term side effects and sometimes permanent damage that may not be evident until months or years after treatment. The benefits and risks of treatment with radiation must be carefully weighed by both doctors and parents.

This chapter explains what radiation is, when and how it is used, and its potential side effects. It clearly explains what the parent and child can expect from radiation treatment.

## Types of radiation therapy

Radiation treatment, also called radiotherapy, directs high-energy x-rays at targeted areas of the body to destroy tumor cells. Radiation can be given internally or externally. Several different types of radiation are used to treat children with CNS tumors.

### External radiation

External radiation uses high-energy x-rays to kill tumor cells. A large machine called a linear accelerator directs x-rays to the precise portion of the brain or spinal cord where the tumor is located. The treatment is usually given in small doses measured in units called centigrays (cGy).

Radiation is usually given every day for a specific number of days, excluding weekends. This is called standard or conventional fractionation. Radiation given more than once a day is called accelerated fractionation, or hyperfractionation. It uses smaller amounts of radiation for each treatment. Hyperfractionation theoretically reduces long-term side effects, but short-term side effects are sometimes more pronounced.

Specific types of external radiation therapy include:

- **3D conformal radiation therapy.** This type of therapy delivers high-dose radiation tailored to the precise area of the tumor, while delivering a lower dose to the normal tissue surrounding the tumor. Recent advances in MRI and CT technology coupled with the availability of sophisticated computer systems have facilitated the development of this form of radiation therapy. This type of radiation is particularly beneficial for children, whose brains are still developing. Available at most large treatment centers, it is expected to replace the conventional two-dimensional systems within the next few years.

- **Intensity modulated radiation therapy (IMRT).** This is a type of 3D conformal therapy that modifies the radiation beam based on the shape of the target to be treated. IMRT can spare adjacent critical structures by varying the intensity of one beam (field) of irradiation. It is a sophisticated conformal treatment. Like 3D conformal, it is a new but important type of radiation delivery that is increasingly available to children with CNS tumors when appropriate.

- **Stereotactic radiosurgery.** This is a sophisticated 3D technique that directs radiation to a small, precisely defined target. This type of radiation is delivered by multiple independent beams directed to a single target. Stereotactic radiosurgery can be delivered as a single treatment (radiosurgery) or as fractionated treatment (stereotactic radiotherapy). This innovative treatment requires precise planning and the combined efforts of multiple specialties. Use for childhood brain tumors is limited as yet, although consideration is reasonable after some types of relapse.

  > *My daughter Stacia's inoperable tumor (a GBM) located in the basal*
  > *ganglia was treated with stereotactic radiosurgery by way of focused*
  > *radiation beams. She had to put on the bird cage, she thought the screws*
  > *in her head were annoying, and the anesthetic shots in the scalp were a*
  > *nuisance, but otherwise she was fine. Two months after this treatment, her*
  > *basal ganglia tumor was completely dark, and she clinically was terrific.*
  > *Two months after that, recurrence, on the edges of the cavity had begun.*
  > *But in my opinion this treatment was effective in increasing both the*
  > *quantity and quality of her life. This treatment was a good one for Stacia.*

- **Proton beam radiation.** This uses large, positively charged particles having a larger mass than standard proton-beam radiation. This type of radiation provides excellent beam definition. Proton beam therapy is available at only a few specialized centers.

*In 1991, our daughter Megan (age 8) was we believe the first pediatric optic glioma patient to receive proton beam therapy at a major California radiation facility. Megan laid on a table where they placed pliable plastic mesh over her face first to get a mold, then the mask was bolted to a board during treatment. She was so full of spunk she would run down the hall with her pink blanket dragging behind her and jump on the table. The radiation took about a minute per location, and there were three locations. She had this treatment for six weeks, there was no sickness, no skin burning. After proton treatment, the tumor stopped growing for about seven years.*

Children do not become radioactive from external treatments, and no specific precautions or activity restrictions are necessary.

*I was very proud of my 6-year-old son for handling his radiation treatments so well. In total, he had ten days of external radiation. He never required sedation and was always cooperative. I'm convinced that it was partly because of his personality, and partly because of how the staff treated him. Every day that he received radiation, his favorite stuffed toy, Mr. Bear, was radiated, too.*

For further information on radiation therapy, contact the Radiation Therapy Oncology Group at *http://www.rtog.org.* For a listing of facilities that offer specific kinds of radiation treatment, contact the American Brain Tumor Association, listed in Appendix B, *Resources.*

## Internal radiation

Internal radiation—also called brachytherapy, implant therapy, or interstitial therapy—is less commonly used than external radiation to treat childhood CNS tumors. Brachytherapy uses radioactive materials (called seeds or implants) placed directly at the tumor site. Radioactive material can be placed directly into tissue (interstitial implants) or applied to the surface of tumor sites (plaques). Brachytherapy may be useful in treating CNS tumors because it delivers high-dose radiation directly to the tumor site, while sparing surrounding, healthy tissue. It differs from external radiation because it provides a continuous low dose of radiation to the tumor, rather than intermittent bursts one or two times per day. The disadvantage of implants is that one dose may not penetrate deeply enough.

Internal radiation is delivered through a catheter that is placed surgically with CT scan guidance. The catheter remains in place for a specific number of days (usually two to five days), until the required amount of radiation has been given, and it is then removed.

Your child will become radioactive from internal radiation. He will need to stay in a special isolation room with a private bath during treatment. The room has plastic covers on all permanent fixtures, and disposable serving plates and utensils are used. Parents are allowed to spend a limited amount of time with their child, typically several hours a day. You are usually able to sit outside your child's room throughout the day and talk or read to him. Children and pregnant women cannot visit as long as the child remains radioactive.

Although experience with internal radiation in children is limited, efforts are ongoing to evaluate various methods of internal radiation in children with recurrent CNS tumors.

> Megan had an anaplastic ependymoma in the left occipital/parietal region of her brain. She had a gross total resection of the tumor. This was followed by chemo under CCG-9921. While all of her MRIs were clear following the initial surgery, we all know that you can't get every cell in surgery and we don't know how well chemo works on these brain tumors. So, we went with the aggressive approach and (two and a half years ago now) Megan had a second surgery to implant brachytherapy seeds.
>
> The doctor had 150 seeds ready to be implanted in the tumor bed. Our doctor called us from the operating room, happy and amazed that there were no visible traces of tumor. Five biopsies were done while Megan was in surgery, only one showed traces of tumor. The doctor then removed some tissue in the area where the traces of tumor were and then did five more biopsies in that area. Those five biopsies came back clear. As there was only one are that had any active tumor cells, that is the only area where the seeds were implanted and they only used 34 seeds.
>
> Megan had no side effects, either at the time of surgery or since, from this type of radiation. Her MRIs are still clear and do not show any signs of radiation damage to the area where the seeds were implanted. We do know that some of the seeds have since "fallen" out of place and rest at the bottom of her spine. The doctors aren't concerned about this and they don't affect her.

## Experimental treatments used with radiation

Two other treatments are used in conjunction with radiation in some clinical trials to treat children with CNS tumors. They are radioimmunotherapy and chemical modifiers.

Radioimmunotherapy uses radiolabeled antibodies to act as radiation carriers. The antibodies are attached (labeled) to a radioactive material and then injected into the body through a venous catheter or IV. Once injected, the antibodies begin a "seek and destroy" mission, searching for specific tumor cells. Radiolabeled antibodies lessen the chance of radiation damage to normal cells. Experience with this method of radiation in children is limited.

Chemical modifiers are compounds used at the same time as radiation therapy. Two classes of compounds are currently under study in children: Radiation sensitizers and radioprotectors. Radiation sensitizers increase delivery of oxygen to tumor cells, thereby rendering them more sensitive to the effects of radiation. Radioprotectors are designed to shield normal cells from radiation damage by using substances absorbed by healthy normal cells but not by tumor cells. Numerous studies using these compounds are ongoing or under development in the Children's Oncology Group and may provide important new avenues of treatment for children with CNS tumors.

# Who needs radiation treatment?

Your child's physician will recommend radiation treatment based on your child's type and location of CNS tumor. Some CNS tumors do not respond to radiation; others are especially sensitive to it. Childhood CNS tumors that usually respond to radiation include high-grade gliomas, medulloblastomas, ependymomas, germinomas, and some low-grade astrocytomas. Although radiation to the brain or spinal cord can cause long-term complications, it is still considered the gold standard and is an important part of successful treatment of many types of CNS tumors.

> *My daughter Ayla had maximum craniospinal radiation the day after she turned three. Prior to that she had a 50% resection of a brainstem PNET and the highest dose chemo. While taking chemo her cancer spread to several locations throughout her midbrain. We were told that she had a 10% chance to live. We chose radiation as a last recourse and it is my belief that this was what "zapped" that cancer! She is doing great now and even attended school full time a few weeks after completing the radiation.*

*I know that every kid is different but there are many successes from radiation, so it should not be discounted. I also know that in the future she may have some cognitive problems, but at least we have her.*

# When is radiation treatment given?

Radiotherapy is given according to the schedule outlined in your child's treatment protocol or as planned by the radiation oncologist. Radiation lasts for days or weeks, depending on your child's situation. For example, standard radiation treatments for many CNS tumors usually last five to seven weeks. It is sometimes used to shrink the tumor prior to surgery or to prevent the spread of disease after surgery. In very young children, radiation therapy is usually delayed until after several months of chemotherapy, in an effort to allow your child's brain to develop more fully.

In rare situations, radiation is given to children during life-threatening emergencies. If disease or pressure from a tumor causes spinal cord compression, radiation may be used.

# Questions to ask about radiation treatment

If radiation has been recommended as a treatment for your child, you should ask the oncologist the following questions:

- Why does my child need radiation?

- What type of radiation does she need?

- What type of radiation treatments do other facilities offer?

- What part of his brain or spinal cord will be treated with radiation?

- What is the total dose of radiation that she will receive?

- How many treatments of radiation will he get?

- How much experience does this institution have in administering this type of radiation to children?

- How will she be positioned on the table?

- Will any restraints be used?

- Will anesthesia or sedation be needed?

- How long will each treatment take?

- What are the possible short-term and long-term side effects?

- Could this type and dosage of radiation cause cancer later?

- What are the alternatives to radiation?

- Are there any precautionary procedures to be done prior to spinal radiation therapy (such as moving the ovaries or sperm banking)?

> *My daughter Rachel (age 14) had medulloblastoma. She had one of her ovaries moved to protect it from the field of spinal radiation. It's not a guarantee, but it does seem to be the standard procedure.*

# Where should your child go for radiation treatment?

To have optimal treatment, children should receive radiation therapy only at major medical centers with experience in treating children with CNS tumors. Physicians who are experienced in pediatric radiation oncology should supervise all treatments. State-of-the-art equipment, expert personnel, and vast experience with many types of childhood tumors are what you should look for when choosing a center. Pediatric anesthesiologists should administer sedation or general anesthesia during radiation.

# Radiation oncologist

A radiation oncologist is a medical doctor with years of specialized training in using radiation to treat disease. In partnership with the other members of the treatment team, the radiation oncologist develops a treatment plan tailored specifically for each individual child.

The radiation oncologist will explain to both child and parents what radiation is, how it is administered, and any possible side effects and will answer all questions regarding the proposed treatment. Parents will be given a consent form to review prior to signing (ask to take it home if you need more time to read it over). Parents should not sign the consent form until they thoroughly understand all benefits, risks, and possible side effects of the radiation. The radiation oncologist should meet at least weekly with child and parents to discuss how the treatment is going and to address concerns or answer questions.

# Radiation therapist

The radiation therapist is a specially trained technologist who operates the machine that delivers the dose of radiation prescribed by the radiation oncologist. This member of the medical team will give your child a tour of the radiation room, explain about the equipment, and position the child for treatment. The technologist will operate the x-ray machine and will monitor the child via closed-circuit TV and a two-way intercom.

> When 3-year-old Katy was being given the tour of the radiation room by her technologist, Brian, he was just wonderful with her. He gave her a white, stuffed bear that he used to demonstrate the machine. He immobilized the bear on the table using Katy's mask (device to hold the head still during treatment), then moved the machine all around it so that she could hear the sounds made by the equipment. He then took a Polaroid picture of the bear on the table, in the mask, for Katy to take home with her.

# Immobilization devices

Different institutions use a variety of devices to immobilize children (and adults) to ensure that the radiation beam is directed with precision. Some of the products used are custom-made plaster of paris casts, thermal plastic devices, vacuum-molded thermoplastics, polyurethane foam forms, and sandbags. Custom fitting the forms on a child who has already undergone numerous painful procedures requires skill and patience. This is especially true for children being fitted for a mask in preparation for radiation to the head or spine. Great care should be taken to ensure that making the mask is not traumatic. This can often be accomplished by utilizing play therapy to demonstrate the procedure.

Masks are made from a lightweight, porous mesh material. First, the technologist should explain and demonstrate the entire mask-making process to the child. The child then lies down on a table. The technologist places a sheet of the mask material in warm water to soften it. This warm mesh sheet is placed over the child's face and quickly molded to his features. The child can breathe the entire time through the mesh material, but must hold still for several minutes as the mask hardens. The mask is lifted off the child's face, and the technologist cuts holes in it for the eyes, nostrils, and mouth.

*My 4-year-old son needed six weeks of radiation scheduled to begin just weeks after his stem cell transplant. His immune system was still so low, although he was starting to recover from the month-long ordeal. The technicians thought he would lay face down quietly in a tub of warm plaster so that they could make his mold. I don't think so! He was scared, and kicked and screamed so we went home. We came back the next day, they sedated him with propofol, and then it took just a few minutes to make the mold and prepare him for radiation.*

• • • • •

*The cancer center staff had scheduled two hours for mask making for my three-year-old daughter. I asked them to very quietly explain every step in the process. I told her that I would be holding her hand, and I promised that it would not hurt, but it would feel warm. I asked her to choose a story for me to recite as they molded the warm material to her face to make the time go faster. She picked "Curious George Goes to the Hospital." She held perfectly still; I recited the story; the staff were gentle and quick; and the entire procedure took less than twenty minutes.*

For children having radiation to areas other than the head, immobilization devices can be as simple as Velcro straps to hold the body in place. Some children will have special foam or plaster molds made to allow greater accuracy when directing the radiation.

Immobilization devices can be fitted on well-prepared, calm children or sedated children. The following are parent suggestions for preparing a child for the fitting of her immobilization device and for radiation treatment:

• Give the child a tour of the room where the fitting and treatment will take place and introduce her to the staff.

• Explain in clear language each step in the process.

• Be honest in describing any discomfort the child may experience.

• For small children, fit the device onto a mannequin or stuffed animal to demonstrate the process.

• For older children or teenagers, show a video or read a booklet describing the procedure.

The more time spent on preparation, the less time generally is needed to fit a device. If the fitting goes well, it establishes trust and good feelings that will help make the actual radiation treatments proceed smoothly.

# Sedation

All infants, most preschoolers, and some school-age children require sedation or anesthesia to ensure that they will remain perfectly still during radiation therapy. Most radiation facilities use a combination of anesthetics that are effective, yet allow the child to recover quickly.

The radiation facility should give parents written instructions concerning pediatric anesthesia, including guidelines for when to stop eating and drinking before sedation or anesthesia. Children can eat and drink after treatment, as soon as they are alert enough to swallow.

> About one month after he was diagnosed with ependymoma, Sam started a course of 30 daily radiation treatments. In some ways, this was the easiest part. Each day we woke up at the same time we always had, got dressed and went directly to the hospital. Because of Sam's young age, he received anesthesia so that he would lie still for the radiation session. He had a Hickman catheter in his chest, so that made getting the anesthesia into him a quick process. The anesthesia acted very quickly, and the technicians and nurse would place him in position and the treatment would start. Each session lasted about fifteen minutes. He'd then be moved into a recovery area where I'd wait while he awoke. He usually came out of it happy, but hungry. I learned to pack lots of easy snacks, like cheerios, crackers, and juice boxes. Once he was fully awake, I'd wheel him to the car in the baby stroller. Most days we were home by 9:30 A.M. One of the blessings of daily radiation is seeing nurses and technicians every day. I was very touched by the caring and comfort of the staff in the radiation department. Another benefit of the daily radiation was being able to change the dressing on Sam's Hickman while he was under anesthesia.

Anesthesia is given through a mask or through the child's catheter or IV, sometimes while the parent is holding or comforting him. The parent must leave the room while the radiation treatment takes place. Once the child is easily aroused and can swallow, the child and parents can go home. The entire procedure generally takes from 30 to 90 minutes. Nausea and vomiting are occasional side effects of anesthesia, but are well-controlled by antinausea drugs such as ondansetron (Zofran).

> Gilbert was three when he started spinal radiation for medulloblastoma. First, we were highly motivated not to do sedation

because the ones with anesthesia were scheduled first thing in the morning and we were commuting 45 miles. Traffic was a killer that time of morning, and if Gilbert had to remain NPO during that drive, it was a nightmare. We explained that he could eat if he did treatment while awake, and that there also wouldn't be any "pokes" if he did it awake. He hated having his port accessed, so that helped. We would sing a silly song "No pokes today" over and over on the way to the hospital. We also stressed that he could do it sleeping if he really wanted. At the hospital, the technicians let him move the machines around a little, and when he was getting marker put on, they talked about drawing road maps on his back.

The mask was tough, but they called it a spiderman mask, and we brought a little hand mirror so that he could see himself in it, and use it to laugh afterwards at the funny imprints on his face. I was in the room touching and stroking him while they positioned the machines, and during the shots (we called them "jumpouts") we could talk to him over an intercom. It also helped for him to ask the technicians each time how many jumpouts there would be. We brought a birthday cake to the dungeon where they do the radiation therapy as an extension of the feeling that these were our friends. I can't overemphasize how much easier our lives were during that seven weeks without the anesthesia. We could follow our routine, play on the escalators, ride our riding toy, peek in at the cafeteria eaters from the window above. I think he looked forward to it because so much play was involved! An added benefit was he did all his MRIs unsedated too.

During a course of radiotherapy, the dose, drugs, and methods to sedate or anesthetize the child may need to be changed because some children develop a tolerance to certain drugs. Good communication between parent and members of the treatment team should prevent unnecessary anxiety about increased dosages or the use of a different drug. In some cases, less anesthesia is needed if the child is gently coached on ways to hold still.

Each time my young son came in for radiation, part of the routine was to place the hard plastic mesh mask over his face while he was awake, just for an instant, to get him used to the idea of trying to wear it for treatments without sedation. No pressure was ever put on him about it, it was just mentioned as a possibility of something he could try, something *that would let him keep eating and drinking all through the day, instead of having to fast for a few hours before each sedation, which was very hard for such a small boy who was getting sedation twice a day.*

*They left the mask on him for a tiny bit longer each time, until he was tolerating it for several seconds, and by the end of the third week, close to a minute. His fifth birthday was at the exact middle of treatment, and he decided that since he was such a big boy now, he would try to do it without sedation. I know he was trying to please and impress all these kind people. He worked it out quietly with a favorite technician, asked the "sleepy medicine doctor" to wait outside the treatment room, let them screw the mask down to the table and did the whole thing awake.*

*I've never been more proud in my life. Everyone cheered and hugged him. He finished the last three weeks of treatments without sedation, sometimes eating and drinking on his way in the door just to show off that he could!*

# What is a radiation treatment like?

Radiation treatments can be very stressful for both children and parents. Knowledge and preparation, however, can make the entire process much easier. This section describes radiation simulation and the various types of radiation therapy.

## Radiation simulation

Prior to receiving any external radiation therapy, measurements and technical x-rays are taken to map the precise area to be treated. This preparation for therapy is called the "simulation." The simulation will take longer than any other appointment, from 30 minutes to 2 hours. Because simulation does not involve any high-energy radiation, parents may be allowed to remain in the treatment room to help and comfort their child. As discussed previously, some children will require sedation for the simulation.

During simulation, the radiation oncologist and technologist use a specialized x-ray machine or a CT scanner to outline the treatment area. They will adjust the table that the child lies on, the angle of the machine, and the width of the x-ray beam needed to give the exact dosage in the proper place. In addition, the radiation oncologist or technologist will put small ink marks on the skin to pinpoint the area to be treated. These marks should not be scrubbed in the bath or shower. They do fade with time, so the technologist may need to add more ink at some point in the child's treatment.

Children who wear masks during treatment will have these ink marks put on the mask, not their skin. At some institutions, children who require spinal radiation may have tiny black dots permanently tattooed on their skin. These tattoos are made by putting a drop of India ink on the skin, then pricking with a pin. They look like tiny black freckles.

After the simulation is completed, the child can leave while the radiation oncologist carefully evaluates the developed x-ray film and measurements to design the treatment field.

## External radiation treatment

To receive external radiation, children are given appointments to visit the radiation clinic for a specific number of days, usually the same time each day. They usually have the weekends off. At some institutions and for some protocols, children go more than once a day to receive hyperfractionated dosing. When the parent and child arrive, they must check in at the front desk. The technologist or nurse comes out to take the child into the treatment room. Often, parents accompany young children into the room. If the child requires anesthesia, it is usually given in the treatment room.

The technologist will secure conscious children or teens in place with an immobilization device. Measurements are taken to verify that the child's body is perfectly positioned. Frequently, the technologist will shine a light on the area to be irradiated to ensure that the machine is properly aligned. The technologist and parents leave the room, closing the door behind them.

At some institutions, parents are allowed to stay and watch the TV monitor and talk to their child via the speaker system. If this is the case, the parent should be careful not to distract the technologist as he administers the radiation. At other institutions, parents are asked to wait in the waiting room. It's important that parents understand the department's policies; they should ask the therapist if anything is unclear.

The treatment takes only a few minutes and is stopped at any time if the child experiences any difficulty. When the treatment is finished, the technologist turns off the machine, removes the immobilization device, and parents and child can go home. There is no pain at all when receiving x-ray treatment.

> I desperately wanted my 3-year-old to be able to receive the radiation without anesthesia. I asked the center staff what I could do to make her comfortable. They said, "Anything, as long as you leave the room during the treatment." So I explained to my daughter that we had to find ways for

*her to hold very still for a short time. I said, "It's such a short time, that if*
*I played your Snow White tape, the treatment would be over before Snow*
*White met the dwarves." Katy agreed that was a short time, and asked*
*that I bring the tape for her to listen to. She also wanted a sticker (a*
*different one every day) stuck on the machine for her to look at. I brought*
*her pink blanket to wrap her in because the table was hard and the room*
*cold. Each day, she chose a different comfort animal or doll to hold during*
*treatment. So we'd arrive every day with tapes, blanket, stickers, and*
*animals. She felt safe, and all treatments went extremely well.*

· · · · ·

*There was something about the radiation or the anesthesia that*
*frightened Shawn terribly. He would scream in the car all the way to the*
*hospital. It was a scream as if he was in pain. He had nightmares while*
*he was undergoing radiation and every night after it was over. We decided*
*a month after radiation ended to bring a box of candy to the staff who*
*had been so nice. Shawn asked, "Do I have to go in that room?" When*
*I explained that it was over and he didn't need to go in the room anymore,*
*he asked if he could go in to look at it once more. He stood for a long time*
*and just looked and looked at the equipment. Somehow he made his peace*
*with it, because he never had any more nightmares.*

## Internal radiation treatment

Children are admitted to the hospital to receive internal radiation. A hospital room is specially designed for patients undergoing this type of treatment. The walls may contain lead, and often items such as sheets and eating utensils are disposable. This is because the child and everything he touches will become radioactive during therapy.

Internal radiation may be given in the child's hospital room after catheters have been placed in the radiology department or in the operating room. The child is then transported to the special room, where he will remain until he is no longer radioactive. The brachytherapy or interstitial plaques will generally remain in place for several days. Once they are removed, your child may resume normal activity and will no longer require isolation. When a child receives internal radiation, he poses a radiation risk to others. Children and pregnant women should not visit while the child is receiving internal radiation. Parents and nursing staff can spend a limited amount of time in the child's room. This may be distressing for very small children, who are unable to understand why people must maintain a safe distance. It may be possible to keep the door to the child's hospital room open. In these instances, parents can sit in the hall and talk to their child to help alleviate any fears or feelings of boredom. Parents should talk with the nursing staff and the play therapist and ask if they have suggestions on how to make the child as comfortable as possible.

> *Our son was 5 years old when he was admitted for his internal radiation. The biggest issue we had to deal with was boredom. It was hard for him to understand that I wasn't allowed to spend all my time at his bedside. The door to his room was open at all times, so I moved a reclining chair into the hall, and that was where I stayed for four days. I would read him stories, stopping from time to time to hold up the book so he could see the pictures. He had a Nintendo machine and a VCR in his room, and that helped to keep him entertained. The nurses even thought of clever games to play. They would inflate rubber gloves and bat them into his room as they passed by his door. After a while they became more and more creative, taking time to draw faces and hair onto the rubber gloves.*

# Possible short-term side effects

Generally, radiation therapy given to children with CNS tumors takes place over four to six weeks. When side effects occur, it is often hard to differentiate those caused by radiation from those caused by the high-dose chemotherapy that is sometimes given at the same time. The severity of the side effects depends upon the sensitivity and the size of the area being radiated. The radiation oncologist is familiar with these possible side effects and is responsible for their treatment.

> *The side effects Sam experienced from the radiation were typical: hair loss, sunburned skin in the radiated area, irritability, and headaches. Eventually, he started on Decadron to reduce the internal brain swelling. The side effects of this were markedly increased appetite, mood swings, and irritability. A 3-year-old on Decadron is no picnic! There were many days that all I did was prepare and serve food! On those days I was too worn out to worry.*

Possible short-term side effects follow:

* Loss of appetite

> *Calories are most important, nutrition can come after treatment. We use whole milk, and put butter on everything. Ethan would eat any time, any thing. When Ethan completely lost his appetite during radiation, we used megase. It has fairly few side effects and did seem to work for him.*

- Nausea and vomiting

    *About a month after radiation was over for my residual pilocytic astrocytoma, I started experiencing all my side effects. I started having problems with my stomach, and was vomiting every morning. I also had balance problems, headaches, cold chills, and had problems with my shunt. I am still experiencing side effects six months later. Radiation did stop the growth of my brain tumor.*

- Ear, nose, or throat problems
- Mouth and throat sores

    *There are several concoctions that radiation oncologists prescribe, sometimes called "Miracle Mouthwash," that often work wonders.*

- Fatigue
- Reddened, itchy, or peeling skin

    *Where the beams entered at two places, his scalp was burned like a sunburn, and aloe vera gel helped to keep that soft.*

    · · · · ·

    *During radiation I was told to use baby shampoo, not to use a hair dryer, and was given samples of a cream for my scalp called Aquaphor.*

- Hair loss (sometimes permanent)

    *My son, Dan, experienced really no side effects for the first three weeks of radiation to treat anaplastic astrocytoma. Then, at the beginning of the fourth week, his hair began to fall out in quite big clumps. By the end of radiation, he had no hair on his head except for a small ball-shaped spot on top, and a sharp line between his ears and below to his neck. Now, 14 months later, he has all of his hair back except in two places, the two spots where the beams entered his head. The exit spots have all filled in nicely, just the two entrance spots remain. One is very bald while the other has a thin fine film of hair. The rest is long and black and curly again. The docs have told Dan that if the hair hasn't come back by now, it probably won't. But Dan is handling it. Hats are still cool. And he doesn't really care what people think.*

- Low blood counts
- Changes in taste and smell (sometimes occurring during treatment sessions)
- Increased or decreased saliva or dry mouth (ask your physician about saliva substitutes such as Moi-Stir or Salivant)

*My daughter Mandy (age 4) had a problem with thick saliva while she was being treated. We started to give her about 200 ml of extra water each day through her G-tube. This seemed to help although she would still have the problem some days, just not as much.*

Additional methods of coping with most of the above side effects are contained in Chapter 13, *Common Side Effects of Chemotherapy.*

Somnolence syndrome is uniquely associated with cranial radiation and is characterized by drowsiness, prolonged periods of sleep (up to twenty hours a day), low-grade fever, headaches, nausea, vomiting, irritability, difficulty swallowing, and difficulty speaking. It may occur during radiation or as late as twelve weeks after radiation treatment ends; it can last from a few days to several weeks.

*Nine weeks after ending her cranial radiation, my daughter started complaining of severe headaches. She would hold her head and just sob with pain. She also vomited several times. Then she became very sleepy, and dozed on the couch most of the day. She developed a low fever and choked when she tried to swallow liquids or solid food. This lasted for about a week, and I was worried sick. I called her oncologist, her radiation oncologist, and her pediatrician, and they all said they didn't think that it was related to the radiation or chemotherapy. I went to the medical library and discovered somnolence syndrome.*

• • • • •

*Stephan (8 years old) had no side effects from the cranial and spinal radiation other than sleepiness, but he was very affected by it. First, he just started taking naps and generally slowing down. Then the naps got longer, and he was awake less. Finally, he only woke up to eat. Luckily, that part coincided with Christmas vacation so he didn't miss much school. Altogether, it lasted about six weeks.*

# Possible long-term side effects

Many children and teens with CNS tumors receive 2,400 cGy to the whole brain, with a boost up to 5,400 cGy to the tumor bed (place of origin of the tumor). Others receive high-dose radiation to the tumor itself. In certain tumors, such as medulloblastoma, where spread of the tumor to the spinal cord is possible or has already occurred, radiation is delivered to the spine as well. Specific disabilities depend on the age of the child, the dose of radiation, and the location of the radiation.

Although short-term effects appear and subside, long-term side effects may not become apparent for months or years after treatment ends. The effects of radiation on cognitive functioning, bone growth, soft tissue growth, teeth and sinuses, puberty, and fertility, range from no late effects to severe, life-long impacts. Brain tumor survivors can develop seizure disorders, gait and balance problems, hand/eye coordination problems, personality changes, as well as learning disabilities. Vision problems and cataracts can also develop after radiation. Second tumors in the radiation field are also a possible long-term side effect. Detailed information about possible late effects are described in *Childhood Cancer Survivors: A Practical Guide to Your Future* by Nancy Keene, Wendy Hobbie, and Kathy Ruccione.

## Cognitive problems

Injury to the central nervous system can result from a multitude of factors, including tumor extension, surgical procedures, radiation, and chemotherapy. Children with CNS tumors develop learning disabilities that can start immediately or develop later. Typically, poor performance is noted in mathematics, spatial relationships, problem solving, attention span, visual disturbances, and concentration skills.

> In 1991, Megan's tumor was growing and even after chemo the tumor was getting bigger. Our consultants gave us no other options for treatment, so we sought out proton beam radiation treatment ourselves. Because proton radiation was so new, we were not given any information beforehand about long- or short-term effects. Being that Megan has neurofibromatosis (NF1) and optic glioma and that NF is associated with learning disabilities, slow motor skills, and processing problems, it would be very difficult to determine which may be the cause anyway. Megan has an IEP and resource special education (RSP) teachers and classes, and is a solid 3.5 (B+/A−) student going into the twelfth grade.

It is important to remember that doctors cannot predict which children will develop cognitive problems. Children at greatest risk for cognitive problems are those treated with irradiation to large portions of the brain when less than 5 years of age, with those under 2 years of age at the highest risk. Chapter 20, *School,* discusses in great detail the types of educational problems some children face and how to deal with them.

## Growth

The brain contains the hypothalamus and the pituitary gland, which control many body processes, including growth and reproduction. Effects on growth usually begin to be seen in those children receiving 2,400 cGy or more. Studies are under way, however, to evaluate the effectiveness of decreased doses of radiation to the spine in young children. If your child receives radiation therapy for treatment of a CNS tumor to the brain and/or spine, growth can be slowed or stopped. Your child's growth will require close observation, and he should be measured (sitting and standing) at every follow-up visit. Your child's growth chart should be kept up-to-date so that it will be easier to quickly observe subtle changes that may indicate early plateauing of your child's growth.

If your child is one of the rare individuals who experience premature puberty (before the age of 8 for girls and 10 for boys), growth may also be affected. An early growth spurt with early sexual maturation results in short stature because the bones stop growing when sexual maturity is reached. When this happens at a young age, the child loses two or three years of additional growth. After completion of treatment for a CNS tumor, growth hormone injections are sometimes given to support your child's growth until he reaches his final height.

Adrenal and thyroid function need monitoring after spinal radiation.

> Mandy (age 16) is a tad short-waisted, but grew seven inches on growth hormone treatment! The doctors closely monitor wingspan (that is, outstretched arms fingertip to fingertip), to make sure it correlates to height. Otherwise they may have longer arms and be out of balance. The growth hormone adds energy and good spirits as well.

## Early or delayed puberty

Some young children who receive radiation to the brain do not experience puberty at the appropriate age. A very small percentage of children develop precocious puberty, which means that puberty begins several years earlier than normal. This is most common in children who also have impaired growth. Conversely, puberty is significantly delayed in some children who have received cranial radiation. Children or teens who receive radiation to the area of the hypothalamus and pituitary may develop a variety of hormonal abnormalities. They are at risk for growth hormone deficiency and deficiencies in the production of other important hormones, such as follicle stimulating hormone (FSH), luteinizing hormone (LH), adrenal corticotrophic hormone (ACTH), and thyroid stimulating hormone (TSH). They may also produce too much prolactin.

These problems may develop years after treatment, so long-term follow-up is essential. A pediatric endocrinologist should evaluate teenage girls who do not show signs of puberty—pubic and underarm hair, breast development. Similarly, teenage boys who show no signs of puberty—growth of body hair, deepening voice—should also consult an endocrinologist.

## Endocrine function

The hypothalamus and pituitary (endocrine glands in the brain) can be damaged by radiation, the tumor itself, or surgery. Several rare problems that can occur are listed below:

- Surgery for a CNS tumor in the vicinity of the pituitary can damage specific functions regulated in the area of surgery. These surgeries typically don't cause short stature because they don't result in an overall pituitary malfunction.

- Hyperprolactinemia (excess prolactin production) can occur in children who receive more than 3,000 cGy to the area of the hypothalamus and pituitary. In females, prolactin is involved in breast development when there is adequate estrogen, progesterone, and growth hormone. Teens or women with too much prolactin stop having menstrual periods. Sexual potency can be reduced in men who produce too much prolactin.

- Pan hypopituitary axis dysfunction is a rare complication in children with CNS tumors who receive more than 5,500 cGy to the area. In these cases, the production and secretion of all the substances produced by the hypothalamus and pituitary ceases. In such cases, long-term hormonal supplementation and close observation and supervision by an endocrinologist are important.

## Vision

Problems with vision may occur as a result of tumor location, tumor spread, surgery, or radiation therapy. If such problems are present, the early involvement of a pediatric ophthalmologist and serial evaluations are important. Subtle changes may indicate tumor growth in a sensitive area. Your child may need special glasses, selective seating in the classroom, or a reading machine. If your child has significant visual impairment or is considered legally blind, he is probably eligible for a variety of services, including Talking Books. It is important that you keep a copy of all reports of your child's vision testing for your records. Such reports are very useful in dealings with your child's teachers and school administrators.

## Teeth

Early cranial radiation may result in disrupted tooth development and in the blunting of roots of your child's permanent teeth. This can result in your child's missing certain permanent teeth or in early tooth loss because of shortened roots. The involvement of a pedodontist (children's dentist) is important. Panorex x-rays of your child's jaw are routinely done as part of comprehensive dental care and will assist your child's dentist in making an appropriate plan if there has been radiation damage to permanent teeth.

Any child who has received cranial or spinal radiation is at additional risk for dental decay because of diminished function of the salivary glands. Appropriate dental evaluations and treatment with fluoride preparations may be necessary.

> Mandy is eight years out from having had radiation for medulloblastoma, and has had NO teeth problems at all. She's had more radiation than most kids on present protocol. A few weeks ago she had her wisdom teeth removed due to impaction and they were even normal (she is 16). We were told that her rear teeth may be affected by the radiation scatter but so far not. She also has no hearing issues related to the radiation. I still wonder if the area of posterior boost that was radiated (tumor bed) is a potential culprit for some of these issues. Most children have the area from ear to ear behind the head done. Like the bottom part of a bowl haircut only in the back. The amount of radiation back there is over 5200 Gy. This is close to the ears, and teeth and the amount of scatter is much higher. Mandy only had a 2 × 4 inch area around her incision done in the occipital area. Of course she had 3600 Gy to her whole head and spine done too.

## Secondary cancers

Children who receive cranial radiation have an increased risk of developing another tumor years after treatment. The risk is reported to range from 1 to 5 percent.

> Our only son Clint was diagnosed with a low-grade astrocytoma in 1976. At the time, treatment called for whole brain cobalt radiation, which left him with the cognitive ability of a 4-year-old. In 1997, I heard about a sheltered workshop for people with disabilities that made fishing tackle. The people who opened the place were wonderful. Clint (age 24) went there for awhile, but then he started showing signs of a secondary meningioma. He needed surgery for this second brain tumor, and after that, he never went back. In July, 2001, an MRI showed recurrent tumor growth, and Clint is scheduled for gamma knife surgery in September.

Radiation therapy remains an important treatment for children with CNS tumors. Although it is very effective in eradicating tumor cells, this treatment is not without its share of short- and long-term complications.

*As I carried my unconscious son back to the waiting room after radiation treatment, a woman there stared intently. On impulse, I took the seat next to her. As I arranged Ben into a bear hug with my arms wrapped around him, she whispered to me, "I'm so jealous." I was taken aback by the heat in her voice. She told me she was making these daily treks with her son, too. Only, he was 21 years old, and wouldn't let her hold him or hug him. It broke her heart to see Ben and I wrapped up in ourselves in that unique mom-child world of clinging hugs, multiple kisses, and rubby-faces. Her son was brave, a valiant independent young man, and she was proud of him. But what she really wanted to do was wrap herself around him, tuck his head under her chin, and make everything all better like she used to.*

# CHAPTER 12

# Chemotherapy

THE WORD CHEMOTHERAPY is derived from words meaning "chemical" and "treatment." When used in reference to oncology, it means using drugs, singly or in combination, to destroy or disrupt the growth of tumor cells without permanently damaging normal cells.

This chapter describes the most common drugs that are used to treat CNS tumors, as well as drugs that prevent nausea, stimulate bone marrow recovery, and treat pain. Numerous stories are included that show the range of responses to different chemotherapy drugs.

Reading about potential side effects of chemotherapy can be disturbing. However, it is important to be aware of the possibilities in order to recognize symptoms early and report them to the doctor so that swift action can be taken to make your child more comfortable. On rare occasions, side effects may be life-threatening, and some can persist throughout life. Most are merely unpleasant and subside soon after treatment ends. Remember that your child or teen may experience several, a few, or none of the side effects discussed here.

## How chemotherapy drugs kill tumor cells

Normal, healthy cells divide and grow in a well-established pattern. When normal cells divide, an identical copy is produced. The body makes only the number of normal cells that it needs at any given time. As each normal cell matures, it loses its ability to reproduce and it is also pre-programmed to die at a specific time.

Tumor cells, on the other hand, reproduce uncontrollably and grow in an unpredictable way. There are several groups of chemotherapy drugs that act on cancer cells in very different ways:

- Alkylating agents. All cells use building blocks (DNA and RNA) to make exact copies of themselves. Alkylating agents poison cancer cells by interacting with DNA to prevent cell reproduction.

- Antimetabolites. These drugs starve cancer cells by replacing essential cell nutrients that are necessary during the synthesis (growth in preparation for cell division) phase of the cell cycle.

- Antibiotics. This type of drug prevents cell growth by blocking reproduction, weakening the membrane of the cell (outer wall), or interfering with certain cell enzymes.

- Alkaloids. These drugs, derived from plants, interrupt cell division through a variety of mechanisms, including interfering with the synthesis of DNA, specific enzyme activities, and actual cell division and, also, disrupting the membrane (outer wall) of the cell to cause cell damage or cell death.

- Hormones. These drugs create a hostile environment that slows cell growth.

- Enzymes. These drugs interfere with tumor cells' ability to reproduce by depriving the cell of specific proteins necessary for cell growth and division.

- Anti-angiogenesis agents. Drugs in this category have the ability to disrupt the blood supply to the tumor, depriving it of nutrients necessary for growth.

# How chemotherapy drugs are given

The most common ways drugs are given during treatment for CNS tumors are:

- Intravenous (IV). Medicine is delivered directly into the bloodstream via a right atrial catheter or IV needle in the arm or hand. These may be administered as a slow IV push or an infusion over a number of hours.

- Oral (PO). Drugs taken by mouth in liquid, capsule, or tablet form are absorbed into the blood through the lining of the stomach and intestines.

- Intramuscular (IM). Drugs that need to seep slowly into the bloodstream are injected into a large muscle, such as the thigh, buttocks, or upper arm.

- Intrathecal (IT). Doctors perform a spinal tap and inject the drug directly into the cerebrospinal fluid (the fluid surrounding the brain and spinal cord), circumventing the barrier between the blood and brain.

- Intracavitary/Interstitial/Implanted. Drugs are delivered directly into a body cavity through a catheter or placed in a tumor bed in the form of a product that will slowly dissolve.

- Subcutaneous (Sub-Q). Drugs that need to enter the bloodstream at a moderately rapid rate are injected into the soft tissues under the skin of the upper arm, thigh, or abdomen.

# Dosages

Dosages vary among protocols; however, most are based on your child's weight or body surface area (BSA). BSA is calculated from your child's weight and height and is measured in meters squared ($m^2$). Doses of medications your child is scheduled to receive should be recalculated at the beginning of each new phase of treatment. Recalculating doses more frequently is necessary if your child has experienced significant weight gain or loss (more than 10 percent of initial weight).

> My son's protocol required that his height and weight be measured each time chemotherapy was to start. When we would arrive in clinic, the nurses would take his measurements, then calculate his body surface area using those figures. His weight fluctuated considerably over the course of his treatment, so the actual dosage of the drugs that he received was never quite the same.

# Chemotherapy drugs and their possible side effects

The following drug information contains not only common and infrequent side effects, but also parent and survivor experiences and suggestions. You may be overwhelmed after reading the potential side effects of each drug. Please remember that each child is unique and will handle most drugs with few problems. Most side effects are unpleasant, not serious, and subside when the medication stops. Parent experiences are included to alert new parents to possibilities and provide comfort and suggestions should their child have an unusual side effect. Consult your child's pediatrician, oncologist, or nurse practitioner should any concerns arise after reading the following information. Remember to keep all chemotherapy drugs at home in a locked cabinet away from children and pets. Please refer to Chapter 13, *Common Side Effects of Chemotherapy*, for additional family stories.

> The chemotherapy made Rachel's tastes change, so we adapted to what she liked or would eat. She lived on bland or very salty foods, like pickles and bacon. Basically, we gave her whatever she wanted, whenever she wanted.
>
> • • • • •
>
> Kristin was only 10 months old when she began two and a half years of chemo for medulloblastoma. I think being a baby helped so much. She mostly slept through it. She had nausea and lost her hair, but she has no memory of it. She recovered quickly and is now a wonderful 13-year-old.

## Questions to ask the doctor

Prior to giving your child any drug treatment for his CNS tumor, you should be given basic information about the drugs:

- What is the dosage? How many times a day should it be given?

- What are the common, as well as the rare but serious, side effects?

- What should I do if my child experiences any of the side effects?

- Will the drug interact with any over-the-counter drugs (e.g., Tylenol) or vitamins?

- Will my teen be given detailed counseling on avoiding risks, such as drinking alcohol, smoking cigarettes or marijuana, and pregnancy?

- What should I do if I forget to give my child a dose?

- What are both the trade and generic names of the drug?

- Should I buy the generic version?

## Guidelines for calling the doctor

Sometimes parents are reluctant to call their child's physician or nurse with questions or concerns. Here are general guidelines for when calling is necessary:

- Temperature above 101°F (38.5°C)

- Shaking or chills

- Shortness of breath

- Severe nausea or vomiting

- Unusual bleeding, bruising, or cuts that won't heal

- Pain or swelling at chemotherapy injection site

- Exposure to chicken pox or measles

- Severe headache or blurred vision

- Constipation lasting more than two days

- Severe diarrhea

- Painful urination or bowel movements

- Blood in urine

- Severe headache

- Worsening of neurological symptoms

- Whenever child appears sick and parent is concerned

# Chemotherapy drug list

Drugs used for chemotherapy are known by a variety of names. You may hear the same drug referred to by its generic name, its abbreviation, or one of several brand names, depending on which doctor, nurse, or pharmacist you are talking to. Chemotherapy drugs are covered in detail in this chapter and are listed alphabetically. The list below gives various names of chemotherapy drugs and what name to look under in this chapter:

| Name | Look under | Name | Look under |
|---|---|---|---|
| ARA-C | Cytarabine | Lomustine | Lomustine |
| BCNU | Carmustine | Methotrex | Methotrexate |
| Blenoxane | Bleomycin | Methotrexate | Methotrexate |
| Busulfan | Busulfan | MTX | Methotrexate |
| Camptosar | Irinotecan | Myleran | Busulfan |
| Carboplatin | Carboplatin | Oncovin | Vincristine |
| Carmustine | Carmustine | Paraplatin | Carboplatin |
| CCNU | Lomustine | Platinol | Cisplatin |
| Cyclophosphamide | Cyclophosphamide | Procarbazine | Procarbazine |
| Cytarabine | Cytarabine | Temodar | Temozolamide |
| Cytoxan | Cyclophosphamide | Temozolamide | Temozolamide |
| Cytosar | Cytarabine | Thalidomide | Thalidomide |
| Cytosine arabinoside | Cytarabine | Thalomid | Thalidomide |
| DTIC-Dome | Dacarbazine | Thiotepa | Thiotepa |
| Droxia | Hydroxyurea | Topotecan | Topotecan |
| Etoposide | Etoposide | Velban | Vinblastine |
| Hycamtin | Topotecan | VePesid | Etoposide |
| Hydroxyurea | Hydroxyurea | VCR | Vincristine |
| Idarnycin | Idarubicin | Vinblastine | Vinblastine |
| Ifex | Ifosfamide | Vincristine | Vincristine |
| Ifosfamide | Ifosfamide | VP-16 | Etoposide |

# Bleomycin (Blee-oh-MY-sin)

*Also called:* Blenoxane, BLM

*How given:* Intramuscular (IM), subcutaneous (SQ), intravenous (IV), intracavitary

*How it works:* Bleomycin binds with DNA in order to stop cell growth.

*Precautions:* A small percentage of children are allergic to this drug. Lung function tests are used to detect possible lung toxicity.

*Common side effects:*

- Hair loss (alopecia), generally not permanent
- Mouth sores (stomatitis)
- Nausea, vomiting
- Weight loss and loss of appetite (anorexia)
- Darkening of the skin
- Thickening of skin on palms, fingers, soles of feet
- Fever, with or without chills

*Infrequent side effects:*

- Lung toxicity (potentially permanent)
- Allergic reactions
- Joint swelling

*Hints for Parents:* Plan on staying with your child during the short time that the drug is given, in case an allergic reaction occurs. Report any shortness of breath, cough, or other breathing difficulties to your nurse or physician promptly. Your child can take ibuprofen or Tylenol for joint discomfort.

---

## Busulfan (Byoo-SUL-fan)

*Also called:* Myleran, busulphan

*How given:* Pills by mouth (PO)

*How it works:* Busulfan is an alkylating agent that interferes with DNA to prevent cell division.

*Precautions:* The child should have lung function tests for early detection of possible toxicities.

*Common side effects:*

- Low blood counts (myelosuppression)
- Patchy darkening of the skin (hyperpigmentation)

- Nausea, vomiting, and diarrhea (usually mild)
- Fever
- Loss of appetite (anorexia)
- Mouth sores (stomatitis)
- Dry mouth
- Elevated liver function tests (temporary)

*Infrequent side effects:*
- Lung toxicity (potentially permanent)
- Cataracts (with long-term use)
- Blurred vision
- Mental confusion
- Seizures

*Hints for Parents:* Giving your child the medicine at bedtime often decreases nausea and vomiting. Report any respiratory, visual, or neurological symptoms to your physician or nurse promptly. Schedule your child's pulmonary function tests the week prior to starting a new cycle of therapy, so that test results will be available for your physician to review.

# Carmustine (CAR-mus-teen)

*Also called:* BCNU, BiCNU, bis-chloronitrosurea

*How given:* Intraveneous (IV)

*How it works:* Carmustine is an alkylating agent that disrupts DNA and RNA replication, resulting in cell death.

*Precautions:* Give through right central venous catheter or newly placed peripheral IV. Baseline pulmonary function tests are necessary.

*Common side effects:*
- Low blood cell counts with delayed nadir (lowest point)
- Nausea and vomiting
- Hair loss that is not permanent (alopecia)

- Patchy brown discoloration of the skin

- Low blood pressure if rapidly infused

- Irritation along the vein if given through a peripheral IV

*Infrequent side effects:*
- Diarrhea

- Inflammation of the esophagus

- Clots in blood vessels in the liver (veno-occlusive disease)

- Permanent lung damage

- Permanent kidney damage

- Second malignancies (cancer occurring as a result of treatment)

- Facial flushing and dizziness

*Hints for parents:* The serious side effects of this drug are generally only seen at the high doses used as part of a bone marrow or stem cell transplant. Report any shortness of breath or dry, non-productive cough to your child's physician promptly. Your child should have pulmonary function tests performed prior to starting therapy with this drug and at specified intervals thereafter. The drug is reconstituted in alcohol, and some children act intoxicated after high-dose therapy is infused.

> My daughter, Jennifer, had the gliadel wafers implanted during her surgery. Gliadel wafers are BCNU chemo wafers and they provide chemo directly to the tumor. The neurosurgeon put about eight disks in the tumor bed. The wafers were about the size of a dime. Gliadel wafers are a great way to dispense chemo. They are biodegradable so there's no surgery to remove them. Some of the side effects of gliadel wafers can be seizures, brain edema (swelling), and slow healing of the incision site. Some people develop cerebrospinal fluid leaks.

## Carboplatin (CAR-bo-plat-un)

*Also called:* Paraplatin

*How given:* Intravenous (IV)

*How it works:* Carboplatin is a platinating agent that inhibits DNA replication, RNA transcription, and protein synthesis.

*Precautions:* The child may be given extra fluids to prevent possible kidney toxicity. Mannitol, a diuretic medication, is sometimes given with this drug to promote a good urine output.

*Common side effects:*

• Low blood counts (myelosuppression)

• Nausea and vomiting

• Loss of appetite (anorexia)

• Altered taste

*Infrequent side effects:*

• Ringing in the ears (tinnitus)

• Hearing loss

• Loss of appetite (anorexia)

• Numbness or tingling in fingers and toes (peripheral neuropathy)

• Kidney damage

*Hints for parents:* Make sure that you have adequate antinausea medication at home after your child receives this drug. Taste distortion may alter your child's food preferences. Report any hearing problems, such as ringing in the ears, problems hearing in the classroom, or background noise interference, promptly. Report any fine motor coordination problems, such as difficulty buttoning clothes, writing, or picking up small objects.

> *Our son did experience ringing in his ears and had some questionable hearing tests during treatment with carboplatin, but a recent thorough hearing test after we finished showed his hearing is near perfect.*

## Cisplatin (sis-PLAT-un)

*Also called:* CDDP, cisplatinum, Platinol

*How given:* Intravenous (IV)

*How it works:* Cisplatin is a platinating agent that inhibits DNA replication, RNA transcription, and protein synthesis.

*Precautions:* The child should be given large amounts of IV fluids while receiving cisplatin to prevent damage to the kidneys. A diuretic drug, called Mannitol, may also given to decrease the risk of kidney damage. All urine output should be measured during the infusion. The child should be monitored for possible hearing loss.

*Common side effects:*

- Nausea and vomiting
- Low blood counts (myelosuppression)
- Loss of appetite (anorexia)
- Taste distortion
- Hearing loss
- Ringing in the ears (tinnitus)
- Abnormalities of sodium, potassium, calcium, and magnesium
- Kidney damage
- Tingling and weakness in the hands and feet (peripheral neuropathy)
- Hair loss that is not permanent (alopecia)

*Infrequent side effects:*

- Low blood pressure (hypotension)
- Allergic reactions
- Rapid or slow heart rate (tachycardia/bradycardia)
- Damage to the liver
- Dizziness, agitation, paranoia
- Temporary blindness, color blindness, or blurred vision

> *Missy's protocol required her to have both cisplatin as well as carboplatin (for her stem cell transplant). Both of these drugs, over the course of her treatment, damaged her high-pitch frequency hearing so much that her speech development took a turn for the worse. She needed hearing aids to help correct the problem.*
>
> · · · · ·
>
> *Molly had a pineoblastoma, had surgery, then was placed on a clinical trial for infants with medulloblastoma. She was too young for radiation. She had vincristine and cisplatin, cytoxan, thiotepa, carboplatin, and a few others. She had a good bit of muscle wasting from the vincristine, but*

*did really well with the "platins" with no hearing loss. Molly is 3 years old now, and is doing physical therapy twice a week just for muscle strength issues from the vincristine and being in the hospital for so long.*

*Hints for parents:* Home IV fluids for several days after receiving cisplatin can help eliminate the drug from your child's system. Because elimination of this drug is much slower than many other agents, make sure that you have adequate antinausea medication on hand at home. Report any hearing or neurologic symptoms promptly to your physician or nurse.

## Cyclophosphamide (Sye-kloe-FOSS-fa-mide)

*Also called:* Cytoxan

*How given:* Pills by mouth (PO), intravenous (IV)

*How it works:* Cyclophosphamide is an alkylating agent that disrupts DNA in cancer cells, preventing reproduction.

*Precautions:* The child should drink lots of water or be given large amounts of IV fluids while taking cyclophosphamide to prevent damage to the bladder. Mesna is often given as a precaution to prevent bladder irritation. Antinausea drugs should be given before and for several hours after this drug is administered.

*Common side effects:*
- Low blood counts (myelosuppression)
- Nausea, vomiting, and diarrhea
- Loss of appetite (anorexia)
- Hair loss that is not permanent (alopecia)
- Mouth sores (stomatitis)

*Infrequent side effects:*
- Bleeding from the bladder (hemorrhagic cystitis)
- Cough or shortness of breath (dyspnea)
- Skin rash, dryness, and darkening of the skin (hyperpigmentation)
- Metallic taste during injection of the drug
- Blurred vision

- Irregular or absent menstrual periods in girls
- Permanent sterility in post-pubertal boys

> Christine breezed through the Cytoxan infusions. She would go to the children's hospital in the afternoon, they would give her lots of IV fluids, and then ondansetron (Zofran) a half hour before the Cytoxan. She would sleep through the night with absolutely no nausea because they were so good about giving her the ondansetron all night and the next morning. It was harder on me because I had to wake up every two hours to change her diaper so that the nurse could weigh it to make sure she was passing enough urine.

*Hints for parents:* Have your child drink plenty of fluids prior to going for treatment; this will help get the therapy started earlier in the day. Your child must urinate every one to two hours during treatment, because emptying the bladder will help prevent cystitis (bleeding from the bladder). Make sure you have plenty of antinausea medication at home after the treatment. Menstrual irregularities do not mean your child is infertile. Pre-therapy sperm storage should be considered in adolescent or young adult males.

## Cytarabine (Sye-TARE-a-been)

*Also called:* ARA-C, Cytosar, cytosine arabinoside

*How given:* Intravenous (IV), intrathecal (IT), subcutaneous (SQ)

*How it works:* Cytarabine kills cancer cells by disrupting DNA.

*Common side effects:*
- Low blood counts (myelosuppression)
- Nausea, vomiting, and diarrhea
- Loss of appetite (anorexia)
- Hair loss that is not permanent (alopecia)
- Mouth sores (stomatitis)
- Redness and irritation of the eyes (conjunctivitis)

*Infrequent side effects:*
- Fever with or without chills

- Yellow skin or eyes (jaundice)

- Lethargy and excessive sleepiness (somnolence)

- Flu-like symptoms, including bone and joint pain

- Seizures

- Headache

- Numbness or tingling of fingers and toes (peripheral neuropathy)

*Hints for parents:* This drug is generally given over a period of several days, and your child's nausea and vomiting may be cumulative. Make sure you have an adequate supply of antinausea medication at home. If possible, give the medication at bedtime, rather than early in the day; your child may sleep through some of the nausea. Ask if prophylactic eye drops are appropriate for your child to prevent eye irritation. Give your child ibuprofen or Tylenol for flu-like symptoms.

> *I told my daughter's oncologist how happy I was that she had not had any severe nausea after her first few doses of ARA-C. His only reply was, "It's cumulative." Within an hour, on the long drive home, she was vomiting constantly. We became ensnared in a two-hour traffic jam. She ran out of clean clothes, so for two hours, I repeatedly carried her to the side of the road, a naked, bald, 25-lb. 4-year-old with tubing hanging from her chest, and supported her as she dry-heaved. The people in the cars around us were in tears, and kept asking if there was anything they could do to help. I just focused on comforting her, and getting her home to that vial of ondansetron in our fridge.*

## Dacarbazine (Da-KAR-ba-zeen)

*Also called:* DTIC-Dome

*How given:* Intravenous (IV)

*How it works:* Dacarbazine is an alkylating agent that prevents cancer cell reproduction.

*Precautions:* The child should be given an antinausea drug prior to infusion. Dacarbazine causes severe skin reactions if it leaks outside the IV.

*Common side effects:*

- Low blood counts (myelosuppression)
- Nausea, vomiting, and diarrhea
- Hair loss that is not permanent (alopecia)
- Sun sensitivity
- Loss of appetite (anorexia)
- Mouth sores (stomatitis)
- Flu-like symptoms, including low fever and body aches

*Infrequent side effects:*

- Pain on injection if the drug is given through a peripheral vein
- Clotting in blood vessels in the liver
- Allergic reactions
- Confusion, blurred vision, and seizures

*Hints for parents:* Make sure to have an adequate supply of antinausea medication at home during treatment with this drug. Ibuprofen or Tylenol will help relieve flu-like symptoms if your child develops these. Report any neurological or visual symptoms promptly. Avoid prolonged sun exposure and use SPF 30 sunscreen liberally when your child is outside.

---

## Etoposide (E-TOE-poe-side)

*Also called:* VP-16, VePesid, Etopophos, Toposar

*How given:* Intravenous (IV), pills by mouth (PO)

*How it works:* Etoposide prevents DNA from reproducing and also causes death of dividing cells.

*Common side effects:*

- Low blood counts (myelosuppression)
- Loss of appetite (anorexia)
- Nausea and vomiting
- Hair loss that is not permanent (alopecia)

*Infrequent side effects:*

- Low blood pressure (hypotension)

- Shortness of breath (dyspnea)

- Numbing of fingers and toes (peripheral neuropathy)

- Fever with or without chills

- Secondary cancers (new cancers that occur years after initial treatment)

*Hints for parents:* If your child takes this drug orally, give the dose at bedtime to decrease nausea. Allergic reactions and low blood pressure are rare, but may occur if the drug is administered too rapidly (less than one hour). Ask your child's physician what total dose of the drug is planned for your child's treatment.

> *Derick is 12 years old and he has an anaplastic astrocytoma grade 3 in his left frontal lobe. After surgery, his first round of chemo was carboplatin and VP-16. He handled it very well. He then followed with four of five scheduled rounds of BCNU, VP-16, cisplatin, and procarbazine. He was unable to do the last round because of toxicity which left him unable to eat and resulted in what we came to call "food in a bag" for about a month. So far the only problems he has are language related (aphasia), right-sided weakness and memory problems. He is currently on his third cycle of maintenance chemo which is a protocol consisting of Temodar and Celebrex with his Tegretol for seizure control. We are now in the wait and see mode with scans every three months.*

## Hydroxyurea (Hi-DROX-ee-yoo-REE-ah)

*Also called:* Droxia

*How given:* Pills by mouth (PO)

*How it works:* Hydroxyurea has an action that is not well understood, but it is thought to work by stopping DNA production.

*Common side effects:*

- Low blood counts (myelosuppression)

- Skin rash, itching, darkening of the skin (hyperpigmentation)

- Redness of the skin in areas of prior radiation ("radiation recall")

*Infrequent side effects:*

- Nausea, vomiting, and diarrhea
- Loss of appetite (anorexia)
- Fever, chills, and flu-like symptoms
- Headache, drowsiness, dizziness
- Disorientation, hallucinations
- Seizures

*Hints for parents:* Give pills at bedtime to decrease nausea and vomiting. Over-the-counter steroid cream may be helpful if your child develops a dry skin rash. Ibuprofen or Tylenol will relieve flu-like symptoms if your child develops these. Report any redness or skin blistering to your physician or nurse; special skin care measures may be needed. Report any neurological symptoms, such as hallucinations or seizures, promptly.

## Idarubicin (Eye-dah-ROO-bah-sin)

*Also called:* Idamycin

*How given:* Intravenous (IV)

*How it works:* Idarubicin is an anthracycline that works to destroy cancer cells by changing the shape of their DNA.

*Precautions:* The child should have her heart tested (echocardiogram and EKG) prior to starting this drug and at specified intervals thereafter.

*Common side effects:*

- Low blood cell counts (myelosupression)
- Nausea, vomiting, and diarrhea
- Hair loss that is not permanent (alopecia)
- Abdominal pain
- Mouth sores (stomatitis)

*Infrequent side effects:*

- Heart damage

- Pain and burning to the tissues if the drug leaks out of the vein during administration

*Hints for parents:* Make sure that you have adequate nausea medicine at home for your child after he receives this drug; nausea and vomiting are usually gone within 24 hours. The drug will turn the urine red to orange for a period of time, and this is normal. Mouth sores can be painful and often require medication for your child to be comfortable.

## Ifosfamide (Eye FOSS-fah-mide)

*Also called:* Ifex, IFF

*How given:* Intravenous (IV)

*How it works:* Ifosfamide is an alkylating agent that disrupts DNA in cancer cells, preventing reproduction.

*Precautions:* The child should be given extra fluids by mouth or intravenously during infusion. Mesna, a drug that protects the bladder, should also be given. Your child must urinate every one to two hours during the treatment, and her urine will be tested for blood.

*Common side effects:*
- Hair loss that is not permanent (alopecia)
- Low blood cell counts (myelosuppression)
- Nausea and vomiting
- Dizziness
- Excessive sleepiness and mental confusion

*Infrequent side effects:*
- Kidney damage that may be permanent
- Bladder irritation and bleeding (hemorrhagic cystitis)
- Liver damage
- Irritation to veins used for administration

*Hints for parents:* Have your child drink plenty of fluid if possible prior to coming for treatment. Your child must urinate every one to two hours during the treatment, and his urine will be tested for blood. This drug is usually given over three to five consecutive days, so make sure you have an adequate supply of nausea medicine at home for your child. This drug may cause the kidneys to lose important substances, such as calcium and phosphorus, and it may be necessary for your child to take oral supplements.

## Irinotecan (Eye-rin-oh-TEE-can)

*Also called:* Camptosar, CPT-11

*How given:* Intravenous (IV)

*How it works:* Irinotecan is a plant alkaloid that disrupts the structure of DNA, preventing cell reproduction.

*Common side effects:*

- Loss of appetite (anorexia)
- Low blood cell counts (myelosuppression)
- Nausea and vomiting
- Abdominal cramping and diarrhea
- Excessive sweating, salivation, and facial flushing during administration
- Hair loss that is not permanent (alopecia)
- Fatigue

*Infrequent side effects:*
- Mouth sores (stomatitis)
- Muscle cramps
- Temporary damage to the liver
- Skin rash
- Sugar in the urine
- Dizziness
- Numbness and tingling of hands and feet

*Hints for parents:* Many of the side effects that occur while or immediately after your child receives this drug may be controlled by the administration of a drug called atropine.

> *The big side effect that comes along with CPT-11 like a shadow is diarrhea. There are two forms: early and late. Early diarrhea could happen even during the infusion (we had this problem during the second dose). Late diarrhea is every bit as much CPT-11's fault but might not be so obvious, because it can take 4 to 11 days post infusion to show up. I guess I should say that there are really two other forms: the kind you can tolerate as a mild inconvenience and the more potent kind. Most doctors suggest that Imodium A-D (over the counter) be given per label instructions, and if that doesn't control the diarrhea, you should call them for something more. Our second-line drug was Lomotril by prescription (we gave that AND Imodium and still had no luck). Use commonsense with any diarrhea. Call in if it seems out of line, and hydrate, hydrate, hydrate to replace the fluids.*

Seizure medications may affect the metabolism of irinotecan, and families should check with their medical team about interaction of seizure medications with other chemotherapy drugs as well. One oncologist states:

> *Dilantin and certain other seizure medications (Tegretol, phenobarbital) cause the body to metabolize CPT-11 much faster. Clinical trials in progress use a much higher dose of CPT-11 to compensate for the faster metabolism.*

---

## Lomustine (Low-MUS-teen)

*Also called:* CCNU, CeeNu

*How given:* Capsules by mouth (PO)

*How it works:* Lomustine is an alkylating agent that interferes with DNA and RNA replication, resulting in cell death.

*Precautions:* Baseline pulmonary function tests are necessary if prolonged therapy is planned.

*Common side effects:*

- Low blood cell counts (myelosuppression)

- Nausea and vomiting

- Loss of appetite (anorexia)

- Hair loss that is not permanent (alopecia)

*Infrequent side effects:*

- Mouth sores (mucositis)

- Kidney damage

- Permanent lung damage

- Disorientation and confusion

- Menstrual cycle irregularities

- Second new cancers that occur years after treatment (secondary cancers)

*Hints for parents:* Give your child her dose of this drug at bedtime to decrease the possibility of nausea and vomiting. Report any shortness of breath or dry, non-productive cough to your child's physician promptly. Your child will probably have baseline pulmonary function tests performed, and these will be repeated at specified intervals throughout treatment with this drug.

## Methotrexate (Meth-o-TREX-ate)

*Also called:* Methotrex, MTX

*How given:* Pills by mouth (PO), intravenous (IV), intrathecal (IT)

*How it works:* Methotrexate is an antimetabolite that replaces nutrients in the cancer cell, causing cell death.

*Precautions:* Children should not be given extra folic acid in vitamins, or the methotrexate will not be effective.

*Common side effects:*

- Low blood cell counts (myelosuppression)

- Extreme sun sensitivity (photosensitivity)

- Diarrhea
- Fatigue
- Skin rashes
- Headache, tingling pain down legs, and spinal irritation (when given intrathecally)

*Infrequent side effects:*
- Mouth sores (stomatitis)
- Hair loss that is not permanent (alopecia)
- Nausea and vomiting
- Loss of appetite (anorexia)
- Fever with or without chills
- Temporary liver damage
- Temporary kidney damage
- Shortness of breath and dry cough
- Temporary or permanent nervous system damage

*Hints for parents:* Most of the common side effects of this drug are temporary and reversible. Mouth sores can be quite painful, and your child may not eat or drink well at this time. Always remember to have your child use sunscreen when he plays outside (SPF 30 or higher). Minor skin rashes can be effectively treated with over-the-counter cortisone cream. When given as "high-dose" therapy, this drug requires administration of a reversing (antidote) agent called leucovorin. It is critical that your child begin this drug at the correct time to prevent serious, possibly irreversible, side effects.

> *My son developed learning disabilities from his high-dose methotrexate protocol. He received tutoring through high school and is doing extremely well in college.*
>
> • • • • •
>
> *My daughter had serious problems with rashes during treatment with methotrexate. The doctors thought that she had developed an allergy. She often would be covered with rashes that looked like small, red circles with tan, flaky skin inside. They were extremely itchy.*

## Prednisone (PRED-ni-sone) and Dexamethasone (Dex-a-METH-a-sone)

These two steroids are grouped together because they are closely related chemically and have similar action and side effects. Dexamethasone is given in high doses as a chemotherapy drug and in low doses to prevent nausea. To see the side effects of dexamethasone when it is used as an antinausea drug, look under "Drugs Given to Prevent Nausea."

*Also called:* Dexamethasone is also called Decadron.

*How given:* Pills by mouth, liquid by mouth, IV.

*How they work:* These drugs are hormones that kill lymphocytes.

*Precautions:* Every parent interviewed described problems that their children had while on prednisone. The side effects ranged from very mild to severe, but were universal. At high doses, prednisone creates major behavioral problems in children, which gradually subside after the drug is stopped.

*Common side effects:*

- Mood changes
- Increased appetite
- Food obsessions
- Increased thirst
- Indigestion
- Weight gain
- Fluid retention
- Round face and protruding belly
- Sleeplessness
- Nightmares
- Nervous, restless, hyperactive
- Loss of potassium
- Hypersensitive to lights, sound, motion
- Extreme irritability

*Infrequent side effects:*

- Decreased or blurred vision
- Seeing halos around lights
- Increased sweating
- Weakness with loss of muscle mass
- Muscle cramps or pain
- Swelling of feet or lower legs
- High blood pressure
- High blood sugar
- Hallucinations
- Aseptic necrosis (destruction of blood supply to bones)

*When Jennifer first came home from the hospital (first week on Decadron), I didn't think I would ever get any sleep. She would come in and talk to me at all times of the night. I thought she was scared but it ended up being the Decadron. Once we knew the insomnia was from Decadron, we started adjusting it so she took it long before bedtime. And I prayed that the Dilantin would make her feel tired so I could get some sleep. Now she takes all of the Decadron in the morning and the Dilantin right before going to bed.*

• • • • •

*Oh that Decadron. The medicine we both love and hate. However, I must come to the defense of Decadron. It has given Jennifer the quality of life to enable her to return to the third semester of college since her diagnosis. Jennifer has never been able to get rid of the swelling in the left temporal and parietal lobes but she is able to do everything a young woman normally does. Yes, Jennifer has had the weight gain, developed the moon face, developed some arm weakness, but she is still with me, attending college, and driving herself back and forth from school. Although it is the goal of most doctors and patients to come off of Decadron as soon as possible, there are times when a person can never come off of it. I don't look for Jennifer to ever separate from Decadron. I do caution people of the weaning of this drug. Jennifer was on Decadron in the hospital, she came home on a Monday and ended up back in the hospital on a Wednesday. We didn't think she was going to make it. The cause: complete withdrawal from Decadron. No one had ensured that Jennifer was given a prescription for Decadron upon discharge. Take the time when weaning off this medication, especially those who have been on it for a long time. Don't get discouraged if it takes someone longer to be weaned off. Some people have more brain swelling than others. Some people lose the swelling, and some people don't. Opt for the quality of life that Decadron gives.*

## Procarbazine (pro-KAR-ba-zeen)

*Also called:* Matulane, Natulanar, N-methylhydrazine

*How given:* Pills by mouth (PO)

*How it works:* Procarbazine is an alkylating agent that prevents cancer cell reproduction.

*Precautions:* Drug is best taken at bedtime, and it is often helpful to take antinausea medicine 30 minutes before taking the drug. Adverse effects, such as headache, tremor, excitation, heart arrhythmias, and visual problems, may occur if the drug is taken with foods rich in tyramine (red wine, imported beers, fermented cheese), chocolate, and fava beans.

*Common side effects:*
- Low blood counts (myelosuppression) 2 to 3 weeks after taking the drug
- Nausea, vomiting, and diarrhea
- Mouth sores (stomatitits)
- Skin rash and itching
- Sun sensitivity
- Light sensitivity, double vision
- Low blood pressure
- Rapid heart rate
- Flu-like symptoms, including low fever and body aches
- Tingling and weakness in hands and feet, dizziness, lethargy, nightmares, hallucinations, seizures

*Infrequent side effects:*

- Urinary frequency

- Blood in the urine

- Drug interactions with alcohol, ephedrine, epinephrine, tricyclic antidepressants, certain narcotic drugs (Demerol), antihistamines, barbiturates, and certain high blood pressure medications.

- Increased side effects if the drug is taken with tyramine-rich foods, such as those listed above.

*Hints for parents:* Make sure to have an adequate supply of antinausea medication at home during treatment with this drug. Give your child the antinausea medication about 30 minutes before giving this drug, and give both before bedtime. Ibuprofen or Tylenol will help relieve flu-like symptoms if your child develops these. Report any neurological or visual symptoms promptly. Avoid prolonged sun exposure, and use SPF 30 sunscreen liberally if your child is outside. Be sure to tell your physician if your child is taking any drugs that can enhance the side effects of this drug. Avoid tyramine-rich foods, chocolate, and fava beans during the times your child is taking this drug.

## Temozolamide (Tem-oh-zo-LA-mide)

*Also called:* Temodar, Temodal

*How given:* Capsules by mouth (PO)

*How it works:* Temozolamide works as an alkylating agent to interfere with DNA replication, causing cell death.

*Precautions:* Capsules should not be broken open. If this inadvertently occurs, avoid inhaling the powder or directly touching it.

*Common side effects:*

- Low blood cell counts (myelosuppression)

- Hair loss that is not permanent (alopecia)

- Nausea and vomiting

- Headache

- Constipation
- Fatigue

*Infrequent side effects:*
- Seizures
- Dizziness
- Poor coordination
- Weakness on one side of the body (hemiparesis)
- Infertility
- Second cancers (cancer that occurs as a result of treatment)

*Hints for parents:* Give your child this medication at bedtime to decrease nausea. Capsules should be swallowed whole and not chewed. The manufacturer states that mixing with applesauce or apple juice is acceptable for children who cannot swallow capsules.

> *I gave Nikki her Zofran and Temodar every night for 42 nights on and 28 off. I let her eat dinner and dessert and do a time check. One hour after her last bite, she would take 4 mg Zofran and one hour following that, I'd give her the Temodar.*

## Thalidomide (Tha-li-DO-mide)

*Also called:* Thalomid

*How given:* Capsules by mouth (PO)

*How it works:* Thalidomide is an anti-angiogenesis agent that may disrupt the blood supply to the tumor, resulting in death of tumor cells.

*Precautions:* Girls of childbearing age must not become pregnant while taking this drug, because it can cause serious birth defects.

*Common side effects:*
- Drowsiness and excessive sleeping
- Tingling and weakness of the hand and feet (peripheral neuropathy)
- Constipation

- Dizziness and low blood pressure on sitting up or arising
- Low blood cell counts (myelosuppression)

*Infrequent side effects:*
- Slow heart rate
- Allergic reactions
- Severe skin reactions (Stevens-Johnson syndrome)
- Severe birth defects

*Hints for parents:* Your child should take this drug at bedtime. Your child should take a stool softener during therapy with this drug to prevent constipation.

---

# Thiotepa (Thigh-oh-TEE-pah)

*Also called:* Thioplex

*How given:* Intramuscular (IM), intrathecal (IT), intravenous (IV)

*How it works:* Thiotepa is an alkylating agent that disrupts DNA and inhibits protein synthesis.

*Precautions:* A small percentage of children have an allergic reaction to this drug.

*Common side effects:*
- Low blood cell counts (myelosuppression)
- Nausea and vomiting
- Loss of appetite (anorexia)
- Headache and dizziness
- Weakness of the legs and tingling after intrathecal injection

*Infrequent side effects:*
- Hair loss that is not permanent (alopecia)
- Allergic reactions
- Severe mouth sores (bone marrow transplant doses)
- Bronzing, redness, peeling skin (bone marrow transplant doses)
- Confusion, cognitive impairment (bone marrow transplant doses)

- Impaired fertility (bone marrow transplant doses)

- Second cancers (cancers occurring as a result of treatment)

*Hints for parents:* The serious side effects that your child may develop occur in conjunction with bone marrow transplant doses. Two to three showers per day are necessary under these circumstances to reduce the possibility of serious skin reactions. When skin peeling occurs, keeping the skin clean and dry is very important. Your child may become very confused for several days after receiving this drug and, depending on her age and developmental level, may require much patience and comforting on your part.

## Topotecan (Toe-poe-TEE-can)

*Also called:* Hycamtin

*How given:* Intravenous (IV)

*How it works:* Topotecan is a derivative of a plant alkaloid and interferes with an enzyme involved in maintaining the structure of DNA.

*Precautions:* Dose may need to be adjusted for children with kidney damage.

*Common side effects:*
- Low blood cell counts (myelosuppression)

- Nausea, vomiting, and diarrhea

- Loss of appetite (anorexia)

- Hair loss that is not permanent (alopecia)

- Headache during the infusion

- Dizziness and light-headedness during the infusion

- Fever

- Fatigue

*Infrequent side effects:*
- Mouth sores (mucositis)

- Skin rashes

- Kidney damage

- Elevated blood pressure and fast heart rate

- Blood in the urine (hematuria)

*Hints for parents:* Your child may have diarrhea starting during treatment and persisting for several days after therapy is completed.

> *Matthew tolerated the topotecan very well. He had the usual nausea and vomiting that he experienced with other chemotherapy drugs, though. He wouldn't eat much during the treatments, but within a day or two he was usually back to his old self again.*

## Vinblastine (vin-BLAS-teen)

*Also called:* VLB, Velban

*How given:* Intravenous (IV)

*How it works:* Vinblastine is an alkaloid derived from the periwinkle plant that causes cells to stop dividing.

*Precautions:* Care should be taken to prevent leakage of vinblastine from the IV site. The child may need to start on a program to prevent constipation.

*Common side effects:*
- Low blood cell counts (myelosuppression)

- Nausea and vomiting, usually mild

- Constipation

- Pain and a burn if the medicine leaks into the tissues

*Infrequent side effects:*
- Hair loss that is not permanent (alopecia)

- Mouth sores (stomatitis)

- Headache

- Numbness or tingling in fingers and toes (peripheral neuropathy)

*Hints for parents:* This drug is often given weekly for a number of weeks. Start a mild stool softener when your child begins treatment with this drug. If your child develops a "burn" from the medication, notify your physician or nurse promptly.

## Vincristine (Vin-CRIS-teen)

*Also called:* Oncovin, VCR

*How given:* Intravenous (IV)

*How it works:* Vincristine is an alkaloid derived from the periwinkle plant that causes cells to stop dividing.

*Precautions:* Care should be taken to prevent leakage of vincristine from the IV site. The child may need to be started on a program to prevent constipation.

*Common side effects:*

- Constipation, progressing to a mechanical bowel obstruction
- Jaw pain (may be severe)
- Progressive weakness and tingling of arms, fingers, legs, toes (peripheral neuropathy)
- Loss of reflexes in the lower extremities (foot drop)
- Loss of muscle mass and extreme weakness
- Drooping eyelids (ptosis)
- Hair loss that is not permanent (alopecia)
- Pain, blisters, and skin loss if the drug leaks into the tissues

*Infrequent side effects:*

- Headaches
- Dizziness and light-headedness
- Seizures
- Inappropriate production of anti-diuretic hormone
- Paralysis

*Hints for parents:* This drug is given weekly for a number of weeks. Start a stool softener when your child begins treatment with this drug and give it consistently. Jaw pain is an early and temporary side effect, but is often severe enough to warrant an oral narcotic. Watch your child's gait and strength, especially going up and down stairs and performing fine-motor activities, such as coloring, writing, or buttoning clothes. Report problems in these areas to your physician promptly so that appropriate dose modifications may be made and/or physical therapy started.

*Erica (diagnosed at 1 year old) once had a vincristine burn on her arm at the IV site. It was red when we went home from the clinic, but by the second day it was badly burned. She developed a blister as big as a half dollar, which left a bad scar. It hurt and was sensitive for a long time. She also developed severe foot drop (she could not lift up the front part of her foot) and fell a lot. This went away when treatment ended.*

· · · · ·

*Stephan is a very tough boy who rarely complains, but he cries when he gets the vincristine because it gives him severe bone pain. I insisted that he get a strong pain killer, and we give him Tylenol with codeine when the pain starts. It usually only lasts a few days.*

# Colony-stimulating factors

Colony-stimulating factors play an important role in cancer therapy. High-dose chemotherapy reduces the number of white blood cells used by the body to fight infections. The administration of colony-stimulating factors, such as granulocyte colony-stimulating factor (G-CSF) and granulocyte-macrophage colony-stimulating factor (GM-CSF), can reduce the severity and duration of low white blood counts, reducing the chance of infection. G-CSF may be administered IV or by subcutaneous injection. GM-CSF must be administered as a subcutaneous injection.

*Kenny was only 2 years old when he was receiving G-CSF, so he was too young to understand why he needed the shots. He would cry and beg us not to hurt him, that he was sorry. My heart would break, but I would have to stick him. We finally developed a really good system. Right before being discharged after a round of chemo, we would put EMLA on Kenny's arm and then have the nurse place an insulflon. It was a small catheter that Kenny didn't even notice was in his arm. It was good for seven to ten days, which was the duration of his G-CSF for the entire month. We would draw up the amount needed for injection, then place it in the insulflon and inject very slowly. Kenny never felt it and no longer begged us not to do the G-CSF. Oh, how I wished we had done this from the beginning! Kenny's counts would usually start to decline about four days after his chemo. At about day ten the G-CSF would kick in and his counts would skyrocket.*

Erythropoietin (Epogen and Procrit are the brand names) is a protein normally produced by the kidneys that stimulates red blood cell production. It is manufactured using recombinant DNA technology and is sometimes used in chemotherapy patients to reduce anemia and, hence, the need for blood transfusions. It is given as an injection, either IV or subcutaneously, usually three times a week. Once a week dosing is also possible.

Oprelvekin (Neumega is the brand name) is a copy of a protein called IL-11, which stimulates the formation of platelets. It is manufactured using recombinant DNA technology. It is used to lessen the degree of thrombocytopenia (low platelets) associated with chemotherapy. It is given as a daily subcutaneous injection, usually starting after chemotherapy is complete and continuing until the platelet count recovers.

All these drugs are very costly and generally pre-approval by your insurance company is required. In some cases, your child must demonstrate the problem (i.e., low white blood count, anemia requiring a transfusion, etc.) before the drug will be approved. If you do not have third-party coverage, most pharmaceutical companies that manufacture these drugs have drug programs available that will provide the drug to your child at no cost.

# Antinausea drugs used during chemotherapy

Antinausea drugs, also referred to as antiemetics, make chemotherapy treatments more bearable, but can potentially cause side effects. The following section lists some commonly used antinausea drugs.

## Antinausea drug list

As with chemotherapy drugs, several different names are used to refer to each of the antinausea medications. You may hear the same drug referred to by its generic name, abbreviation, or one of several brand names, depending on which doctor, nurse, or pharmacist you are talking to. The list below gives various names of antinausea drugs and what name to look under in this chapter:

| Name | Look under | | Name | Look under |
|------|-----------|--|------|-----------|
| Ativan | Lorazepam | | Kytril | Granisetron |
| Benadryl | Diphenhydramine | | Lorazepam | Lorazepam |
| Compazine | Prochlorperazine | | Ondansetron | Ondansetron |
| Decadron | Dexamethasone | | Phenergan | Promethazine |
| Dexamethasone | Dexamethasone | | Prochlorperazine | Prochlorperazine |
| Hexadrol | Dexamethasone | | Zofran | Ondansetron |

## Dexamethasone (dex-a-METH-a-sown)

*Also called:* Decadron, Hexadrol

*How given:* Intravenous (IV), usually given in combination with other antinausea drugs at the beginning of treatment. May also be given by mouth (PO).

*Common side effects:*

- Euphoria, confusion
- Stinging sensation in perineal area if injected rapidly

Side effects are different from those experienced when it is given in high doses for long periods of time.

## Diphenhydramine (Die-fen-HIGH-dra-meen)

*Also called:* Benadryl

*How given:* Liquid, pills, or caplets by mouth (PO), intravenous (IV)

*When given:* Diphenhydramine is usually given every six to eight hours.

*Common side effects:*

- Drowsiness
- Dizziness
- Impaired coordination
- Dry mouth
- May cause excitation in young children.

## Granisetron (Gra-NI-se-tron)

*Also called:* Kytril

*How given:* Intravenous (IV), pills by mouth (PO)

*When given:* Kytril is usually given prior to the start of chemotherapy infusion. Doses may be repeated every 12 to 24 hours.

*Common side effects:*

- Headache

*Infrequent side effects:*

- Diarrhea

- Constipation

> *Kytril is an antinausea pill. It is incredibly expensive but brilliant in treating chemo-related sickness. It sometimes takes a bit of juggling to get the timing right; Michael used to take it an hour before taking the CCNU, which he then took at bedtime and slept right through with no ill effects. None of the other antiemetics worked for him nearly as well.*

## Lorazepam (lor-AZ-a-pam)

*Also called:* Ativan

*How given:* Pills by mouth (PO), intravenous (IV), or intramuscular (IM)

*When given:* This is a tranquilizer and is generally given in combination with other antinausea drugs. It is useful for "breakthrough" nausea.

*Common side effects:*

- Drowsiness and sleepiness

- Poor short-term memory

- Impaired coordination

- Low blood pressure (hypotension)

- May cause excitation in young children.

## Ondansetron (on-DAN-se-tron)

*Also called:* Zofran

*How given:* Intravenous (IV), liquid or pills by mouth (PO)

*When given:* Ondansetron is usually given 30 minutes prior to chemotherapy drugs and every four to eight hours until nausea ends, or in a higher dose once a day.

*Common side effects:*

• Headache with rapid IV administration

*Infrequent side effects:*

• Constipation

> *The absolute best for me were the Zofran lozenges, simply dissolve on or under the tongue for instant relief. The prescription must state lozenges. You'll love those "melty pills."*

· · · · ·

> *Ondansetron works great for Ethan, he does have late nausea after chemo, so he takes it once a day for 10 days afterwards, and hasn't vomited or felt nauseated.*

## Prochlorperazine (pro-chlor-PAIR-a-zeen)

*Also called:* Compazine

*How given:* Pills or long-acting capsule by mouth (PO), rectal suppository, intramuscular (IM), or intravenous (IV)

*When given:* Prochlorperazine is used alone if only mild nausea is expected.

*Common side effects:*

• Drowsiness

• Low blood pressure (hypotension)

• Nervousness and restlessness

• Uncontrollable muscle spasms, especially of jaw, face, hands (dystonic reaction)

If your child takes this medication, keep diphenhydramine on hand to "reverse" this reaction if it occurs. It can be frightening if it occurs unexpectedly and may mimic a seizure.

> *Compazine is an older antinausea drug that many (not very current) oncologists prescribe for brain tumor patients, and people invariably have breakthrough nausea. We had nine rounds with Temodar (and Zofran an hour beforehand) and he never got sick once.*

## Promethazine (Pro-METH-ah-zeen)

*Also called:* Phenergan

*How given:* Pills by mouth (PO), rectal suppository, intramuscular (IM), or intravenous (IV)

*When given:* Promethazine is usually given every four to six hours.

*Common side effects:*

- Drowsiness
- Dizziness
- Impaired coordination
- Blurred vision
- Insomnia
- Euphoria

# Drugs used to relieve pain

As with other drugs, medications used for pain relief can be given by various methods and can cause side effects. The following section lists some of the commonly used drugs to relieve pain.

## Pain medication list

Several different names can be used to refer to each of the pain medications. You may hear the same drug referred to by its generic name or one of several brand names, depending on which doctor, nurse, or pharmacist you are talking to. The list below gives various names of pain medications and what name to look under in this chapter:

| Name | Look under | | Name | Look under |
|------|-----------|---|------|-----------|
| Codeine | Codeine | | Meperidine | Meperidine |
| Demerol | Meperidine | | Methadone | Methadone |
| Dilaudid | Hydromorphone | | Morphine | Morphine |
| EMLA cream | EMLA cream | | Numby Stuff | Numby Stuff |
| Fentanyl | Fentanyl | | Percocet | Oxycodone |

## Codeine

*How given:* Intramuscular (IM), pills or liquid by mouth (PO)

*How it works:* Codeine is an alkaloid obtained from opium.

*Common side effects:*
- Light-headedness
- Dizziness
- Sedation
- Euphoria
- Constipation

*Infrequent side effects:*
- Nausea
- Vomiting

## Meperidine

*Also called:* Demerol

*How given:* Intravenous (IV), liquid or pill by mouth (PO)

*How it works:* Meperidine is a narcotic similar to morphine. Oral absorption is poor.

*Common side effects:*
- Sedation
- Constipation

*Infrequent side effects:*
- Dizziness
- Nausea and vomiting
- Flushing and excessive sweating
- Respiratory depression
- Decreased blood pressure (hypotension)

- Seizures
- Headache
- Visual disturbances

## EMLA cream

*How given:* Applied to the skin and covered with an airtight dressing one to two hours before such procedures as spinal taps, bone marrow aspirations, or injections.

*How it works:* EMLA cream is an emulsion that contains two anesthetics, lidocaine and prilocaine. It may take longer than an hour to achieve effective anesthesia in dark-skinned individuals.

> We use EMLA for everything: finger pokes, accessing port, shots, spinal taps, and bone marrows. I even let her sister use it for shots because it lets her get a bit of attention, too. Both of my children have sensitive skin which turns red when they pull off tape, so I cover the EMLA with saran wrap held in place with paper tape. I also fold back the edge of each piece of tape to make a pull tab so the kids don't have to peel each edge back from their skin.

## Hydromorphone

*Also called:* Dilaudid

*How given:* Intravenous (IV), pill by mouth (PO), rectal suppository

*How it works:* Hydromorphone is a narcotic pain reliever.

*Common side effects:*
- Dizziness and light-headedness
- Sedation
- Nausea and vomiting
- Excessive sweating
- Euphoria and other mood alterations
- Headache
- Constipation

- Respiratory depression

*Infrequent side effects:*
- Hallucination and disorientation
- Respiratory arrest
- Diminished circulation
- Shock
- Cardiac arrest

## Methadone

*Also called:* Dolophine

*How given:* Intravenous (IV), pill or liquid by mouth (PO)

*How it works:* Methadone is a narcotic pain reliever.

*Common side effects:*
- Light-headedness and dizziness
- Sedation
- Nausea and vomiting
- Excessive sweating
- Loss of appetite (anorexia)
- Constipation
- Euphoria

*Infrequent side effects:*
- Respiratory depression
- Decreased circulation
- Shock

## Morphine

*How given:* Intravenous (IV), pill or liquid by mouth (PO)

*How it works:* Morphine is a narcotic derived from the opium plant.

*Common side effects:*

- Euphoria
- Nausea and vomiting
- Drowsiness
- Constipation

*Infrequent side effects:*

- Reduction in body temperature
- Itching
- Respiratory depression
- Allergic reactions
- Seizures

> *Zachary's first surgery was fairly easy to recover from. His second, however, had a horrible three-week recovery period, involving painful bladder spasms, extreme diarrhea, an infection in his Hickman line, and massive weight loss. It took a lot of morphine to help him feel comfortable.*

## Numby stuff

*How given:* Numby Stuff provides a needle-free method of delivering pain medication through the use of low-level electric currents applied to the skin.

*How it works:* Numby Stuff is an emulsion that contains two anesthetics, lidocaine and prilocaine. It anesthetizes skin and tissue in ten to fifteen minutes. Some children and teens do not like the electrical sensation that goes from the site to the battery pack.

## Oxycodone

*Also called:* Percocet, oxycotin

*How it works:* Oxycodone is a narcotic derived from opium.

*Common side effects:*

- Light-headedness
- Dizziness

- Sedation
- Constipation
- Nausea and vomiting

*Infrequent side effects:*
- Repiratory depression
- Skin rash

# Adjunctive treatments

In recent years there has been increasing research on mind-body medicine and its effect on coping with the side effects of illness. Adjunctive therapies are those that can be expected to add something beneficial to the ongoing treatment program. For example, imagery and hypnosis are widely used in established treatment programs to help children and teens prepare for or cope with medical procedures. Other helpful adjunctive therapies are relaxation, biofeedback, massage, visualization, acupuncture, meditation, aromatherapy, and prayer. Chapter 4, *Coping with Procedures,* discusses adjunctive therapies and how to obtain information about them.

# Alternative treatments

Alternative treatments can be defined as those that are used in place of conventional medical treatment or, if used in addition to treatment, may have unknown or adverse effects. Sometimes these therapies are illegal or unavailable in the United States or Canada, and patients travel to other countries to obtain them.

Alternative treatments are usually based on word-of-mouth endorsements, called anecdotal evidence. Medical therapy is based on scientific studies using large groups of patients. In treating cancer, these large clinical trials have resulted in increases in survival rates in the past three decades.

Many alternative treatments can help parents and children feel that they are aiding the healing process. Even with a good prognosis for your child, it is difficult to ignore the advice of friends and relatives extolling the virtues of various alternative treatments. Parents just want to help their children in every way possible; they often feel helpless, and they agonize over the pain and misery that their child endures for many months while on conventional therapy. Conventional treatment can be brutal, but it is effective in many cases.

It is extremely important that any therapy that involves ingestion or injection into the body (herbs, vitamins, special diets, enemas) only be given with the oncologist's knowledge. The involvement of the physician is necessary to prevent giving something to your child that could lessen the effectiveness of the conventional chemotherapy or could cause harm. For instance, folic acid (a B vitamin) replaces methotrexate in cells and reduces or eliminates methotrexate's effectiveness, allowing cancer cells to flourish. The oncologist will be much more knowledgeable about these potential conflicts than a parent, herbalist, or health food store salesperson.

Despite the effectiveness of childhood CNS tumor treatment, you may wish to research one or more alternatives. Parents of children who have had their tumors come back one or more times often are drawn to exploring alternative treatments. To help you evaluate claims made about alternative treatments, here are several ways to collect enough information to make an educated judgment:

- Go to or call your local American Cancer Society or Canadian Cancer Society's division office and ask for their information on the therapy you are considering. They have compiled information on many therapies describing the treatment, its known risks, side effects, opinion of the medical establishment, and any lawsuits that have been filed. The American Cancer Society has an online database at *http://www.cancer.org* with information about many alternative treatments.

- Check the National Institutes of Health's National Center for Complementary and Alternative Medicine to see if any scientific evidence exists on the treatment that interests you. The office can be reached at (888) 644-6226 or online at *http://nccam.nih.gov.*

- Ask specifically what this treatment is expected to do for your child; ask what is in it; ask what tests will be done to ascertain whether your child needs it and whether your child is benefiting from it.

- Collect and study all available objective literature on the treatment. Ask the alternative treatment providers if they have treated other children who have cancer, what results have been achieved, how these results have been documented, and where they have reported their results. Ask for the reports so that your doctor can review them.

- Talk with other people who have gone through the treatment. Inquire about the training and experience of the person administering the treatment. Be sure to find out how much the therapy costs, because your insurance company may not pay for alternative treatments.

- Beware of any practitioner who will give your child the alternative therapy only if you stop taking the child in for conventional treatments.

Take all the information you have gathered to your child's oncologist to discuss any positive or negative impact that it may have on your child's current medical treatment. Do not give any alternative treatment or over-the-counter drugs to your child in secret. Some treatments negate the effectiveness of chemotherapy; other substances, such as those containing aspirin or related compounds, can cause uncontrollable bleeding in children with low platelet counts.

> At one point, we decided to try some alternative therapies with our son. Our plan was to use it in conjunction with his conventional treatment. I scheduled a meeting with his oncologist and discussed the alternatives with him. I wouldn't dare attempt to start anything, not even vitamin supplements, without first talking it over with the doctor, because I was scared that I would cause him more harm than good. I was grateful that he was willing to listen to what I had to say and offer his opinion.
>
> We both agreed that the alternative therapy we had in mind wouldn't do any damage or interfere with the chemotherapy he was receiving. Two months later, we decided that it was doing absolutely nothing for him, so we stopped. I figured the money would be better spent at the toy store than on a useless alternative therapy. I learned a valuable lesson from that experience. I'm much more skeptical now than I used to be. My new motto is "show me the proof."

· · · · ·

> I gave my son echinacea when he received chemotherapy. I checked with his doctor first. He didn't think it would hurt, but didn't think it would help, either. Still, all the nurses in emergency swore by the stuff. We got good results, too. We started the echinacea after lots of treatment, and it was the first time that he didn't have to be readmitted three days after chemo for febrile neutropenia. I'm convinced that it helped him during the recovery period when his counts would bottom out.

If, after thorough investigation, you feel strongly in favor of using an alternative treatment in addition to conventional treatment and your child's oncologist adamantly opposes it, listen to his reasoning. If you disagree, go get a second opinion. Remember, the child is the most important person here. Don't give the treatment in secret or your child may be the loser.

Treatment of your child's CNS tumor requires that you gain a good understanding of the drugs used to treat the tumor and to minimize the side effects she experiences. Such knowledge will help you function in a collaborative role with your child's treatment team and may avert major problems and lessen discomfort your child may experience.

*When Zack (age 6) was treated, he always developed a fever after chemotherapy. I could tell when his counts were dropping because the fever would start off low and go up to around 102°. When his fever went over 101°, the doctor would put him on IV antibiotics and draw blood cultures every day. His fevers usually started about seven days after the first day of chemo. His counts would drop real fast. For us, it became normal. He'd always need platelet and red blood cell transfusions after chemotherapy, also. It was a scary time but we became used to it.*

*I thank God daily for sustaining Zack this long. Yesterday was just a horrible day. But today I arose with positive thoughts. I will take care of my son and live life for we have been blessed to be his parents.*

# CHAPTER 13

# Common Side Effects of Chemotherapy

CHEMOTHERAPY DRUGS interfere with tumor cells' ability to grow or reproduce. Because rapidly dividing cells are more susceptible to chemotherapy drugs, tumor cells may be severely affected. Unfortunately, healthy cells that multiply rapidly can be damaged as well. These normal cells include those of the bone marrow, mouth, stomach, intestines, hair follicles, and skin.

This chapter explains the most common side effects of chemotherapy drugs and explores ways to effectively deal with them. Chemotherapy side effects that prevent good nutrition are discussed in Chapter 17, *Nutrition*.

## Hair loss

Chemotherapy drugs destroy not only cancer cells, but also normal cells that are produced at a rapid rate. Because hair follicle cells reproduce quickly, chemotherapy causes some or all body hair to fall out. The hair on the scalp, eyebrows, eyelashes, underarms, and pubic area may slowly thin out or may fall out in big clumps.

Hair regrowth usually starts one to three months after intensive chemotherapy ends. The color and texture may be different from the original hair. Straight hair may grow back curly; blond hair may be brown. If your child receives cranial radiation for treatment of a CNS tumor, some or all of the hair follicles may be permanently damaged, and your child may only experience partial or patchy regrowth in the area that was irradiated.

Parents suggest the following ways to deal with hair loss:

- When hair is thin or breaking, use a brush with very soft bristles.
- Avoid bleaches, permanents, curlers, blow dryers, or hair spray, as these may cause additional damage.

- If hair is thin, use a mild shampoo specifically designed for overtreated or damaged hair.

- A flannel receiving blanket placed on the pillow at night will help collect hair that is falling out.

- Recognize that hair loss is traumatic for all but the youngest children. It is especially hard on teenagers.

- Emphasize to your child that the hair loss is temporary and that, in many cases, it will grow back.

> During the first year after Belle was diagnosed (and lost her hair), her brother and I found some Barbie hats/bandanas with wigs attached at the local dollar store. So the Barbies whose heads were shaved had something to wear while their hair grew out! Belle also made numerous outfits for "chemo Barbie" out of supplies at the hospital: napkins, masks, various kinds of tape. She even made furniture out of straws and stuff!

- Try to have your child meet other children who have undergone similar treatment, especially if that treatment included cranial radiation therapy.

- Allow your child or teen to choose a collection of hats, scarves, or cotton turbans to wear. These are tax-deductible medical expenses that may be covered by insurance.

- If your child expresses an interest in wearing a wig, take pictures of her hairstyle prior to hair loss. Also cut snippets of hair to take in to allow a good match of original color and texture. The cost of the wig may be covered by insurance if the doctor writes a prescription for a "wig prosthesis." This should include the medical reason for the wig, such as "Alopecia due to cancer chemotherapy." To find a wig retailer, look in the yellow pages of your phone book under "Hair Replacements, Goods, and Supplies." The American Cancer Society, (800) ACS-2345; the Canadian Cancer Society, (888) 939-3333; and some local cancer service organizations offer free wigs in some areas.

- Advocate that school-age children be permitted to wear hats or other head coverings to school.

- Separate your feelings about baldness from your child's feelings. Many parents rush out to buy wigs and hats without discussing with their child how she wants to deal with her baldness. An oncologist comments:

> Consider whether hair loss bothers your child. If it bothers him, then you should pursue things to hide or resolve the problem. If it bothers you but not

*him, then focus your efforts on trying to deal with your concern and anxiety. Think of this as an opportunity to teach him that it is what is on the inside that counts. In today's culture that places so much emphasis on outward appearance and conformity, this is a valuable lesson. It has been my experience that kids who have visible late effects after cancer treatment can adjust quite well to external differences if they are given a lot of support at home. As a parent, if you let him know he is a great kid, he will believe it.*

- Allow your child to choose whether to wear head coverings or not. Let it be okay to be bald.

Hair loss is quite variable for children being treated for cancer. Some only lose part of their hair, some have hair that thins out, and some quickly lose every hair on their body.

*Preston never completely lost his hair, but it became extremely thin and wispy. When he was first diagnosed, a friend bought him a fly-fishing tying kit, and he became very good at tying flies. He even began selling them at a local fishing shop. When his hair began to fall out, we would gather it up and put it in a plastic bag. He started tying flies out of his hair, and they were displayed in the shop window as "Preston's Human Hair Flies." He was only eleven, but the shop owner hired him to help around the shop. He became very popular with the clientele, because everyone wanted to meet the boy who tied flies from his own hair. He really turned losing his hair into something positive.*

· · · · ·

*My daughter, Katie (age 11), cut and dyed her hair bright fuchsia as soon as she realized she had cancer. It made her hair seem less hers than something to play with. Then, when she started receiving chemo, she asked that it be cut and shaved really short like some of her boy friends in her class. Our local coach came over and shaved it for her. It was only about ¼ inch long at that point. Then when it fell out a week later, it was no big deal for her, because she had already taken it off. That was her way of controlling the situation.*

*Now we celebrate her baldness by painting henna designs on her head and using face paints to paint fancy designs whenever we go somewhere special, or visit the hospital. On July Fourth, we painted stars and rockets in red, white, and blue. On our last visit to the hospital, we painted a floral vine with flowers and lightning bolts above her ears to show she's hot stuff. She even had her sisters add two eyes at the back of her head ... to watch the doctors and nurses when her back is turned. Everyone loves to check out her head when she comes in the hospital and she receives tons of attention as a result of it. Also now she's beginning to play with the rub-on tattoos and is placing them where the doctors like to inspect, just to surprise them when they pull up her shirt.*

*She also loves to dress up her head with funny wigs and masks. Last week she was dancing in the front yard with a black/blue fright wig, monster ears, a Grateful Deadhead shirt and black platform heels. She literally stopped traffic! It was a riot. She absolutely refuses to talk to most of her doctors and nurses, and is extremely shy, but this is her silly way of poking fun at them and the whole situation with her cancer.*

# Nausea and vomiting

The effects of anticancer drugs vary from person to person and dose to dose. A drug that makes one child violently ill may have no effect on other children. Some drugs produce no nausea until several doses have been given; others cause nausea after a single dose. Because the effects of chemotherapy are so wildly variable, each child's treatment must be tailored to his individual needs. There is no relationship between the amount of nausea and the effectiveness of the medicine.

The following is a list of suggestions for helping children and teenagers cope with nausea and vomiting:

- Give your child antinausea medications as prescribed. Do not skip any doses.

- Ask your doctor to prescribe a drug that blocks gastric secretions, such as Pepcid or Zantac, to go along with the antinausea medication (note that these medications might need to be given well before or after other meds).

- Your child should wear loose clothing because it is both more comfortable and easier to remove if soiled.

- Parents should always have at least one change of clothes for their child in the car.

- Carry a bucket, towels, and baby wipes in the car in case of vomiting.

- Large zip lock plastic bags provide an easily used container if your child gets sick in the car. They can be sealed and disposed of quickly and neatly, ridding the car of unpleasant odors that could make your child's nausea worse.

- Keep your child in a quiet, well-ventilated room after chemotherapy.

- Smells can trigger nausea. Try not to cook in the house when your child feels ill. If possible, open windows to provide plenty of fresh air.

- If your child is nauseated by smells, use a covered cup with a straw for liquids.

- Do not serve hot foods, as the odor can aggravate nausea.

- Serve dry foods, such as toast, pretzels, or crackers, in the morning or whenever the child is feeling nauseated.

- Serve several small meals rather than three large ones.

- Have the child keep her head elevated after eating. Lying flat can induce nausea.

- Serve plenty of clear liquids, such as water, juice, Gatorade, or ginger ale.

- Avoid serving sweet, fried, or very spicy food. Instead, serve bland foods, such as potatoes, cottage cheese, soup, or toast.

- Watch for any signs of dehydration. These include dry skin and mouth, sunken eyes, dizziness, and decreased urination. Call the physician if your child appears dehydrated.

- Use distractions such as TV, videos, music, games, or reading aloud to divert attention from nausea.

- After the child vomits, rinse his mouth with water or a mixture of water and lemon juice to remove the taste.

- If your child develops a metallic taste in his mouth, chewing gum, sucking on Popsicles, or hard candy may help.

- Acupuncture, aromatherapy, meditation, or yoga may also help to alleviate symptoms.

> A friend whose wife had undergone radiation for breast cancer recommended acupuncture to us as being good for energy and mood and lessening of nausea. We were certainly worried about his regimen, which for medulloblastoma is thirteen sessions to the full cranium and spine and then eighteen sessions to the tumor bed, that's an awful lot of radiation. So, Ezra went to the acupuncturist every week while he did radiation and certainly the doctors were impressed with his energy level. The fact that he managed to pull off his bar mitzvah on the last day of six weeks of radiation speaks well of his stamina.

*Another reason we liked the acupuncture was this: because cancer treatment is so grueling, it seems everything we do for the kids harms them in some overt way. They never saw the cancer, and in our case, did not experience any significant harm prior to diagnosis, but since then Ezra's life has been a series of painful, damaging, exhausting, and nauseating treatments. Acupuncture was something that was only there to make him feel better, no bad effects. He likes the warm room, the soft table, the soothing music, there is a trickling fountain in the room which he loves. Because it's hard to fit this treatment into a school week, he didn't go to the acupuncturist during the six week rest period or the first six week round of chemotherapy, but at that point he was so miserable, had been vomiting every morning and basically had no good days for six weeks, we sent him back to the acupuncturist and he went weekly during the second six week round. Maybe it was a coincidence, but his mood has been wonderful and the nausea almost nonexistent over this period. He likes and looks forward to his sessions.*

If the various antinausea medications do not work well for your child, you may want to investigate the FDA-approved Relief Band. This wristband gives an electrical stimulation (too faint to feel) to an acupuncture point in the wrist that affects the portion of the brain that controls nausea. Information about the band is available at (888) 297-9728 and online at *http://www.reliefband.com.*

*Kytril is an antinausea pill. It is incredibly expensive but brilliant in treating chemo-related sickness. It sometimes takes a bit of juggling to get the timing right; Michael used to take it an hour before taking the CCNU, which he then took at bedtime and slept right through with no ill effects. None of the other antiemetics worked for him nearly as well.*

• • • • •

*Liquid Phenergan worked fine for controlling nausea, but James' preschool teacher mentioned how drowsy he was at school, so we asked for something else.*

• • • • •

*During Megan's treatment for anaplastic ependymoma, nausea at first was a big problem. I made a point to work with the staff to address this, and this is the plan we came up with: Megan would be given the maximum tolerated dose of Zofran the first time chemo was administered, then four hours later she'd get the regular dose, then we would give the regular dose every six hours.*

# Low blood counts

Bone marrow, the spongy material that fills the inside of the bones, produces red cells, white cells, and platelets. Chemotherapy drugs destroy the cells inside the bone marrow and dramatically lower the number of cells circulating in the blood. Frequent blood tests are crucial in determining whether the child needs transfusions. Many children treated for CNS tumors require transfusions of red cells and platelets to treat anemia and prevent bleeding. When the number of infection-fighting white cells is low, the child is in danger of developing serious infections.

## What is an ANC? (also called AGC)

The activities of families of children receiving chemotherapy for treatment of a CNS tumor revolve around the sick child's white count, specifically the absolute neutrophil count (ANC). This is sometimes called an absolute granulocyte count (AGC). The ANC (or AGC) provides an indication of the child's ability to fight infection.

When a child has blood drawn for a complete blood count (CBC), one section of the lab report will state the total white blood cell (WBC) count and a "differential," in which each type of white blood cell is listed as a percentage of the total. To perform a WBC differential, a laboratory technologist examines a slide of your child's blood and counts 100 white blood cells, assigning them by subtype (i.e., segs, bands, lymphs, etc.). For example, if the total WBC count is 1,500 mm3, the differential might appear as in the following table:

| White blood cell type | Percentage of total WBCs |
| --- | --- |
| Segmented neutrophils (also called polys or segs) | 49% |
| Band neutrophils (also called bands or stabs) | 1% |
| Basophils (also called basos) | 1% |
| Eosinophils (also called eos) | 1% |
| Lymphocytes (also called lymphs) | 38% |
| Monocytes (also called monos) | 10% |

To calculate the ANC, add the percentages of neutrophils and bands, and multiply by the total WBC. Using the example above, the ANC is 49% + 1% = 50%. 50% of 1500 (.50 × 1500) = 750. The ANC is 750.

> Erica ran a fever whenever her counts were low, but nothing ever grew in her cultures. They would hospitalize her for 48 hours as a precaution. She was never on a full dose of medicine because of her chronically low counts. She's five years off treatment now and doing great.

## How to protect the child with a low ANC

Generally, an ANC between 500 and 1,000 provides the child enough protective neutrophils to fight off exposure to infection caused by bacteria and fungi. With an ANC this high, you can allow your child to attend all normal functions, such as school, athletics, and parties. However, it is wise to keep close track of the pattern of the rise and fall of your child's ANC. If you know that the ANC is 1,000, but is on the way down, it should affect your decision on what activities are appropriate. Each hospital has different guidelines concerning appropriate activities for children with low ANCs.

The following are parents' suggestions for detecting and preventing infections:

• Insist on frequent, thorough hand washing for every member of the family. Use antibacterial hand soap and warm water, lather well, and rub all portions of the hands. Children and parents need to wash before preparing meals, before eating, after playing outdoors, and before and after using the bathroom.

> We always had antibacterial baby wipes in our car. We washed Justin's hands, and our own, after going to any public places such as parks, museums, or restaurants. They can also be used to wipe off tables or high chairs at restaurants. We even asked family members to follow the same steps when they were in contact with him.

• Make sure that all medical personnel at the hospital or doctor's office wash their hands before touching your child.

• Keep your child's diaper area and skin creases clean and dry.

• When your child's ANC is low, make arrangements with your pediatrician to use a back entrance to the office to avoid exposure to sick kids in the waiting room. It sometimes helps to make all appointments for early morning so that your child can be seen in a room that hasn't had several sick children in it.

• Whenever your child needs a needle stick, make sure that the technician cleans your child's skin thoroughly with both betadine and alcohol.

• Protect your child if he has a low ANC.

> When my son's ANC was low, we took extra care to avoid situations that increased his risk of infection. We kept him home from school and restricted the number of visitors to our home. Little things that many people take for granted were dependent upon whether his ANC was high enough. For example, we wouldn't take him to see a movie if his ANC was low. Sitting in an enclosed theater with so many people would have definitely been a bad idea without enough neutrophils.

- If your child gets a small cut, wash it with soap and water, rinse with hydrogen peroxide, and cover with a clean Band-Aid.

- When your child is ill, take her temperature every two to three hours.

- Do not allow anyone to take your child's temperature rectally (in the anus) or use rectal suppositories, as this may cause anal tears and increase the risk of infection and bleeding.

    *Believe it or not, we once stopped the nursing assistant from doing a rectal temp during an inpatient admission. When we had a room on the pedi oncology side, this never happened, but those rooms were full and we were on the other side of the floor for that admission.*

- Do not use a humidifier, because the stagnant water can become a reservoir for bacterial or fungal contamination.

- Apply sunscreen whenever your child plays outdoors. Children taking certain chemotherapy drugs, such as methotrexate, or who have received recent cranial radiation therapy, are sun sensitive, and a bad sunburn can easily become a site for infection.

- Your child should not receive routine immunizations while on chemotherapy. Your physician or nurse can prepare medical exemption cards for your child's school.

- Siblings should not be vaccinated with live polio virus (OPV). They should get the killed polio virus (IPV). Verify that your pediatrician is using the appropriate vaccine for the siblings.

    *Katy was diagnosed just a week after her younger sister Alison had been given the live polio vaccine. Because there was a small risk that Alison could infect any immunosuppressed child with polio, we were not allowed to stay on the cancer floor of the hospital.*

- If your child's ANC is low, an infected site may not become red or painful.

    *My daughter kept getting ear infections while on chemo. They would find them during routine exams. I felt guilty because she never told me her ears were hurting. I told her doctor that I was worried because she didn't complain of pain, and he reassured me by telling me that she probably felt no pain because she didn't have enough white cells to cause swelling inside her ear.*

- Never give aspirin for fever. Aspirin or aspirin-containing drugs interfere with blood clotting. Ibuprofen may be given if approved by your child's oncologist. If your child has a fever, call the doctor before giving any medication.

- Ask your child's oncologist about using a stool softener if he has problems with constipation. Stool softeners can help prevent anal tears.

- Call the doctor if any of the following symptoms appear: fever above 101°F (38.5°C), chills, cough, shortness of breath, sore throat, severe diarrhea, bloody urine or stool, or pain and burning while urinating.

> Some people choose to keep their kids away from everything and everyone during treatment, while others restrict their activities when they're neutropenic or receiving a particularly heavy dose of chemo. You will learn how to trust your instincts and your doctor's advice, and also learn how to take your cues from your child. For us, we try to walk a fine line between keeping Hunter's life as normal and stimulating as possible, while not taking any foolish risks with his health. When he's neutropenic (ANC below 500) or when he's in a particularly heavy round of chemo, or when there's chicken pox going around we keep him at home. When he's doing well then we take him out a bit more, but sensibly: no shopping malls on Saturdays, no contact with anyone who's sick, and limited contact with other kids. During the week, I will take him with me to the grocery store, or to see his grandparents or cousins providing everyone is healthy. When he's feeling well we also go to the park, ride our bikes and do normal kid stuff. I carry around anti-bacterial hand wipes with me so I can keep him clean after playgrounds.

Two serious infections that plague children during treatment for cancer are pneumonia and chicken pox.

## Pneumonia

Pneumonia is inflammation of the lungs caused primarily by bacteria, viruses, or other organisms. The symptoms of pneumonia are rapid breathing, chills, fever, chest pain, cough, and bloody sputum. Children with low blood counts can rapidly develop a fatal infection and must be treated quickly and aggressively. Most cancer centers recommend an annual influenza shot to help prevent this cause of pneumonia.

> My son received chemotherapy just days before he was scheduled to go to the American Cancer Society's camp. His ANC was 1,200 and he looked so sick, but he begged to go and I let him. It was early in his treatment and I didn't realize the pattern of his blood counts. They called me from camp on Friday to say he had a temperature of 103°F (39.5°C) and needed to go to the hospital. He was very weak and feverish; his WBC was 140, and his

*ANC was 0. Both lungs were full of pneumonia. I was furious at the doctor for giving him permission to go to camp and at myself for not paying closer attention to how quickly his counts dropped. I'm sure he had the pneumonia before he even went to camp. They started him on five different antibiotics, and his fever went up to 106°F (41.1°C) that night. We didn't know if he would live or die. He started to gradually improve the next morning and was completely recovered in a week.*

If your child has received carmustine (BCNU), lomustine (CCNU), or bleomycin, she may be at greater risk for respiratory infections as a result of lung damage from these drugs. Children taking steroids (prednisone, dexamethasone, hydrocortisone) are often immunosuppressed and are at increased risk to contract serious and potentially life-threatening lung infections from an organism called Pneumocystis carinii. In most cases, the infection can be completely prevented by taking trimethoprim-sulfamethoxazole (septra, bactrim) two or three consecutive days per week.

## Chicken pox

Chicken pox is a common childhood disease caused by a virus called varicella zoster. Its symptoms are headache, fever, and malaise, rapidly followed by eruptions of pimple-like red bumps. The bumps typically start on the stomach, chest, or back. They rapidly develop into blister-like sores that break open, then scab over in three to five days. Any contact with the sores can spread the disease, and children are contagious up to 48 hours prior to breaking out.

Chicken pox can be a fatal disease for immunosuppressed children, so extreme care must be taken to prevent exposure. It will be necessary to educate all teachers and friends to be vigilant in reporting any outbreaks. Your child can be kept home from school or preschool until the outbreak is over.

Chicken pox can be transmitted through the air or by touch. Exposure is considered to have occurred if a child is in direct contact or in a room for as little as ten minutes with an infected person. If your child has never had chicken pox, it is better to take him to beaches or parks rather than indoor play areas, especially in the spring or fall when the outbreaks of the disease peak.

Untreated chicken pox or shingles can result in life-threatening complications, including pneumonia, hepatitis, and encephalitis. Parents must make every effort to prevent exposure and be vigilant in watching for signs of the diseases while their child is on treatment.

Your child should be tested for antibody of varicella virus (varicella IgG) soon after diagnosis and prior to beginning treatment. If your child has evidence of immunity to varicella, either through prior infection or immunization, prophylaxis is generally not necessary if your child is exposed, but you should still notify your physician or nurse practitioner.

If your child has no antibodies, she will need to receive prophylactic treatment and you should call the doctor immediately if exposed. If the doctor is able to administer a shot called VZIG (Varicella Zoster Immune Globin) within 72 hours of exposure, it may prevent the disease from occurring or minimize its effects.

> We knew when Jeremy was exposed, so he was able to get VZIG. He
> did get chicken pox, but only developed a few spots. He didn't get sick;
> he got bored. He spent two weeks in the hospital in isolation. We asked
> for a pass, and we were able to go outside for some fresh air each day.

If a child develops chicken pox while on chemotherapy, the current treatment is hospitalization or, if possible, home therapy for IV administration of acyclovir, a potent antiviral medication. This drug has dramatically lowered the complication rate of chicken pox.

> Kristin broke out with chicken pox on the Fourth of July weekend. Our
> hospital room was the best seat in the house for watching the city fireworks.
> She did get covered with pox, though, from the soles of her feet to the very
> top of her scalp. We'd just give her gauze pads soaked in calamine lotion
> and let her hermetically seal herself. They kept her in the hospital for six
> days of IV acyclovir, then she was at home on the pump (a small
> computerized machine that administers the drug in small amounts for
> several hours) for four more days of acyclovir. She had no complications.

A child who has already had chicken pox may develop herpes zoster (shingles). If your child develops eruptions of vesicles similar to chicken pox that are in lines (along nerves), call the doctor. The treatment for shingles is identical to that of chicken pox.

> Kristin also got a herpes zoster infection, this time on Thanksgiving.
> It looked like a mild case of chicken pox, limited to her upper right arm,
> her upper right chest, and her right leg. They kept her overnight on IV
> acyclovir and then let her go home for nine more days on the pump.

An immunization for chicken pox has been developed and is likely to be given to children with cancer in the future. Currently, there is insufficient data to indicate its usefulness or safety in these children.

## Can pets transmit diseases?

It is very unlikely that your child will be harmed from living with a household pet, but several common sense precautions are needed to protect a child with a low ANC from disease, worms, or infection.

- Make sure that the animal is vaccinated against all possible diseases.

- Have pets checked for worms as soon as possible after your child is diagnosed, and then every year thereafter (more often for puppies).

- Do not let pets eat off plates or lick your child's face.

- Keep children away from the cat litter box and any animal feces outdoors.

- Have children wash hands after playing with the pet.

- Make sure that your pet has no ticks or fleas.

- If you have a pet that bites or scratches, consider finding another home for it. On the other hand, if you have a gentle, well-loved pet, do not give it up.

> *I think parents should know that you should not automatically get rid of your dog because your child has a low ANC. We went through a small crisis trying to decide whether to give away our large but beloved mongrel. The doctors wouldn't really give us a straight answer, but a parent in the support group said, "DO NOT get rid of your dog. Your son will need that dog's love and company in the years ahead." She was right. The dog was a tremendous comfort to our son.*

If your child wants to buy a pet while undergoing treatment for cancer, here are some suggestions:

- Do not get a puppy. All puppies bite while teething, increasing the chance that your child may contract an infection.

- Do not get a parrot or parakeet, unless it has been tested for psittacosis.

- Do not get a turtle or other reptile (snake, iguana) as they sometimes carry salmonella.

- Avoid buying any animal that is likely to bite or scratch.

If you have any concerns or questions about pets you already own or are thinking of purchasing, ask your oncologist for advice.

> *We had an odd situation when Christopher (age 3) was diagnosed. Our oncologist told us about not letting Christopher around any birds or animals*

*with a lot of fur. The problem was I am a farmer. Not just cattle, but I also raise turkeys. When the houses are full, we hold about 60,000 at a time.*

*Even before Christopher could walk he would go to work with me. He especially enjoyed helping me feed baby birds. Christopher had a huge plastic dump truck he would put feed in and push around while I fed with a wheelbarrow. We would take our shirts off and be silly together—a very special time. When Christopher was diagnosed, I told the doctors I had no problem selling or shutting the farm down if it gave Christopher a better chance of surviving or would reduce the chance of infection. They told us to keep Christopher away from the animals and especially the turkeys and to keep him inside when his ANC was low, which we did. Every time I got baby turkeys in, I would move his truck to that house. Sometimes I would cry, sometimes I wouldn't. But I absolutely hated taking care of the little birds.*

*In late June when Christopher was declared in remission, again we happened to get a house full of baby turkeys in. This time, Christopher didn't want his truck, but he pushed my wheelbarrow and we got silly again. I really missed that.*

# Diarrhea

Chemotherapy destroys cancer cells, as well as any cells that are produced at a rapid rate—such as those that line the mouth, stomach, and intestines. This damage can cause diarrhea, ranging from mild (frequent, soft stools) to severe (copious quantities of liquid stool). Diarrhea during chemotherapy can also be caused by some antinausea drugs, antibiotics, or intestinal infections. After chemotherapy ends and immune function returns to normal, the lining of the digestive tract heals and the diarrhea ends.

The following suggestions for coping with diarrhea come from parents:

- Do not give any over-the-counter drug to your child without approval from the doctor. He may want to test your child's stool for infection prior to treating the diarrhea. Frequently recommended drugs for diarrhea are Kaopectate, Lomotil, or Immodium.

- It is very important that your child drink plenty of liquids. This will not increase the diarrhea, but will replace the fluids lost.

  *My 3-year-old had stopped drinking from bottles months before her diagnosis. When she first began her intensive chemotherapy, she had uncontrollable, frequent diarrhea. Liquid would just gush out without warning. It was hard for her to drink from a cup, so one night she said in a small voice, "Mommy, would it be okay if I drank from a bottle again?" I said, "Of course, honey." It was a great comfort to her, and she took in a lot more fluids that way.*

• Hot or cold liquids can increase intestinal contractions, so serve plenty of room-temperature clear liquids or mild juices, such as water, Gatorade, ginger ale, peach juice, or apricot juice.

• Diarrhea depletes the body's supply of potassium. Provide foods high in potassium, such as bananas, oranges, baked or mashed potatoes without the skin, broccoli, halibut, mushrooms, asparagus, tomato juice, and milk (if tolerated).

• Low potassium can cause irregular heartbeats and leg cramps. If these occur, call the doctor.

• Do not serve greasy, fatty, spicy, or sweet foods.

• Do not serve roughage, such as bran, fruits (dried or fresh), nuts, beans, or raw vegetables.

• Do serve bland, low-fiber foods, such as bananas, white rice, noodles, applesauce, unbuttered white toast, creamed cereals, cottage cheese, fish, and chicken or turkey without the skin.

*In the middle of treatment, my son had severe diarrhea for a week. He had large amounts of liquid stools twenty times a day. I felt so sorry for him. The doctor cultured a stool specimen, but they never identified a cause. It cleared up after a week of the BRAT diet (bananas, rice, applesauce, toast). He had a problem with diarrhea almost weekly throughout his treatment.*

• Keep a record of the number of bowel movements and their volume to keep the doctor informed. Call the doctor if you notice any blood or mucous in the stool or if your child has any signs of dehydration, such as dry skin, dry mouth, sunken eyes, decreased urination, or dizziness.

• Keep the area around the anus clean and dry. Wash with warm water and mild soap after every bowel movement. Pat dry gently.

• If the anus is sore, check with the doctor before using any nonprescription medicine. She may recommend using Desitin, A&D ointment, or Bag Balm after each bowel movement.

*While taking ARA-C my daughter had a terribly sore rectum, which was a big problem. It hurt to have bowel movements—she'd cry and have*

*to squeeze our hands to go, then the urine would run back and burn. She*
*was very itchy. We carried around bags with Q-tips and every known*
*brand of rectal ointment—A&D, Preparation H, Desitin, Benadryl.*

- Call the doctor if your child has significant pain with bowel movements, especially if your child has low blood counts.

# Constipation

Constipation means a decrease in the normal number of bowel movements. There are many reasons that constipation occurs on chemotherapy. Some drugs, such as vincristine, slow the movement of the stool through the intestines, resulting in constipation. Pain medication, decreased activity, decreased eating and drinking, and vomiting can all affect the normal rhythm of the intestine. When movement through the intestine slows, stools become hard and dry.

The following are parents' suggestions for preventing and helping constipation:

- Encourage your child to be as physically active as possible.

- Encourage your child to drink lots of liquids every day. Prune juice is especially helpful.

- Serve high-fiber foods, such as raw vegetables, beans, bran, whole wheat breads, whole grain cereals, dried fruits (especially prunes, dates, and raisins), graham crackers, and nuts.

- Check with the doctor prior to using any medications for constipation. He may recommend a stool softener like colace. If the doctor suggests liquid ducosate, be aware that many kids don't like the taste. Senokot, another frequently prescribed stool softener, comes in a tablet, liquid (chocolate flavored), and granules (also chocolate flavored) that can be mixed in yogurt or ice cream. Metamucil or Citrucel increase the volume of the stool, which stimulates the intestine. Milk of magnesia, magnesium citrate, or a new product called Miralax help the stool to retain fluid and remain soft.

- Do not give enemas or rectal suppositories. These can cause anal tears, which can be dangerous for a child with a weakened immune system.

- When your child feels the need to have a bowel movement, sipping a warm drink can help.

# Fatigue and weakness

Fatigue—a feeling of weariness—is an almost universal side effect of treatment for CNS tumors. General weakness, although different from fatigue, is caused by many of the same things and is treated the same way. Fatigue and weakness may be constant throughout therapy or intermittent. They can be minor annoyances or totally debilitating. Many parents worry that if fatigue is present, so is the cancer, but this is not the case. Fatigue and weakness can be caused by one, or a combination, of the following things:

- Your child's body working overtime to heal tissues damaged by treatment and rid itself of dead and dying cancer cells

- Medications to treat nausea or pain

- Mineral imbalances caused by chemotherapy, diarrhea, or vomiting

- Infection

- Emotional factors, such as anxiety, fear, sadness, depression, or frustration

- Malnutrition caused by vomiting, loss of appetite, or taste aversions

- Anemia (low red cell count)

- Disruption of normal sleep patterns (common when hospitalized or when taking certain drugs, such as prednisone)

- Cranial radiation therapy

The following suggestions come from parents:

- Make sure that your child gets plenty of rest. Naps or quiet times spaced throughout the day help.

    *Erica took a two-and-a-half hour nap every afternoon throughout therapy. She's 4 now and off treatment, but her endurance is low and she still tires easily.*

- Limit visitors if your child is weak or fatigued.

    *While in the hospital, my daughter was very weak. She had too many visitors, yet didn't want to hurt anyone's feelings. We worked out a signal that solved the problem. When she was too tired to continue a visit, she would place a damp washcloth on her forehead. I would then politely end the visit.*

- Serve your child well-balanced meals and snacks, but don't get upset if she doesn't eat them (see the next point).

- Parents and children should try to avoid physical or emotional stress.

- Encourage your child to pursue hobbies or interests if he is able. For example, if your child is too weak to play on his athletic team, let him go to cheer the team or help keep score.

> My eighth-grade daughter was a fabulous athlete prior to her cancer diagnosis. When she went back to school after missing a year, she wasn't very competitive, but she managed the softball team and dressed for basketball. So she was still part of the social scene and was able to do things with the teams.

- Help your child make a prioritized list of what she wants to accomplish. If she feels strongly that she wants to attend a certain activity and you think she may run out of energy, throw a wheelchair or stroller into the car and go.

- Encourage your child to attend a kid's support group, and go to the parent group yourself. Seeing that others have the same problems and talking about how you are feeling can lighten the load.

- Plan more strenuous activities earlier in the day when your child will have more energy.

Many children complete their chemotherapy protocols without fatigue or weakness; other children are not so lucky.

> Before Brent was diagnosed at age 6, he was exceptionally well coordinated and a very fast runner. During treatment, he slowed down to about average. He played soccer and T-ball throughout, and was very competitive.

· · · · ·

> Jeremy has had some major, persistent problems with weakness and loss of coordination. When he was a year off therapy (9 years old), he still could not catch a ball. When he ran, he was like a robot, and the trunk of his body stayed straight. Some kids made fun of him, and he got very frustrated with himself. He had five years of physical therapy, and now, three years off chemo, his skills have improved, but he still has to work harder than the other kids. We put him into martial arts in hopes of further increasing his motor skills and his confidence.

# Bed wetting

Bed wetting, although infrequent, can be a very upsetting side effect of chemotherapy. Some drugs increase thirst and others disrupt normal sleep patterns, both of which can make bed wetting more likely. When bed wetting is caused by a specific drug or lots of IV fluids at night, time will cure the problem. Once the drug or fluids are no longer necessary, bed wetting will stop. Bed wetting may also be associated with tumor progression or post-operative problems with bladder tone and function.

There are also psychological reasons for bed wetting during chemotherapy. The trauma of the treatment for CNS tumors causes many children to regress to earlier behaviors, such as thumb sucking, baby talk, temper tantrums, and bed wetting. Punishment for this type of bed wetting only adds to the child's trauma and rarely solves the problem. The following are veteran parents' suggestions:

- Double-sheet the bed. Put down one plastic liner with fitted and flat sheets, then put on top another plastic liner with fitted and flat sheets. During the night, simply pull off the top sheets and plastic, and there are fresh sheets below.

- Keep a pile of extra-large or beach towels next to the bed. Cover the wet spot with towels, and save the bed change for the morning.

- Give the last drink two hours before bedtime, to allow your child's bladder to totally empty right before bed.

- Change sleeping arrangements.

    *Prednisone caused my daughter to have nightmares and frequent bed wetting. I felt if she could sleep through the night the bed wetting might stop. I told her she could sleep with me for the month that she was on prednisone, but that after that she would move back into her own bed. It calmed her to sleep with me. The nightmares and bed wetting decreased, and she moved back into her own bed without complaint when the time came.*

- Adopt an attitude that lets your child know that bed wetting is "no big deal." There should be no shaming or punishment.

- If your child or teen is extremely distressed by his bed wetting, ask him if he wants you to set the alarm for the middle of the night in order to help him get up to go the bathroom.

- Give extra love and reassurance.

*When my daughter started bed wetting, I didn't think it was the drugs. I thought long and hard about any additional worries that she might have, and I realized that because her dad had emotionally withdrawn from her during her illness, she might be worried that I would do the same. So I told her one night, "You know, I just realized that every day I tell you how much I love you. But I've never told you that no matter how hard life gets and no matter how mad we get at each other I will always love you. I love you now as a child, I will love you as a teenager, and I will love you when you are all grown up." She started to sob and hugged and hugged me. She has never wet the bed again.*

# Dental problems

Both radiation and chemotherapy can cause changes in the mouth and teeth. Awareness of the potential problems coupled with good preventive care can help your child be more comfortable during treatment.

Some chemotherapy drugs and radiation can cause changes in children's ability to salivate. Plaque may build up rapidly on your child's teeth, increasing the chance of both cavities and gum infections. Take your child for a cleaning and checkup every three to four months, as long as her counts are good (ANC above 1,000 and platelets above 100,000/mm$^3$). If your child has a central venous catheter (Hickman or port) or a shunt, she should be given antibiotics before and after each visit to the dentist. Ask your dentist to refer to the current issue of the *Pediatric Dentistry Reference Manual* to formulate a dental plan.

*When Kevin (diagnosed with posterior fossa ependymoma) turned 2, I asked our oncologists if they thought he should see a dentist, that I was worried about his teeth. They tried to take a peek at his teeth but Kevin was like Fort Knox. They both said that he shouldn't have any problems because of his illness and that we could bring him to our regular dentist when he turned 3. When Kevin was a little over 2½, I suspected that he had a few cavities. I brought him to a local pediatric dentist. After a horrible exam of three people holding him down, the dentist said he had four cavities. He wanted to fill them all without putting Kevin under anesthesia.*

*After talking to our pediatrician, she said, "Why don't you go to a Children's Hospital dentist?" So we did, and the exam was much better. Anyway, they thought he had more than four cavities and that two*

*of them would have to be removed. They wouldn't know for sure until*
*they did an x-ray during surgery. He was put under for his surgery*
*and they removed two teeth and filled five cavities. We were told that the*
*cavities were probably due to radiation. He also had a right paralyzed*
*vocal cord and right facial paralysis. He always chewed his food on the*
*left side of his mouth. But the cavities were on both sides. And he hated to*
*have his teeth brushed! After his cavities were filled, the Children's dentist*
*wanted to see him every three months for a cleaning and checkup.*

Get recommendations from your child's oncologist and dentist for advice on teeth care when counts are very low. Often parents are advised to use a sponge or damp gauze to gently wipe off their child's teeth after meals instead of brushing.

*My daughter had problems with thick yellow saliva during the entire*
*time she was treated. It coated her teeth and formed a lot of plaque. I*
*brought her to an excellent pediatric dentist every three months to have*
*the plaque removed. She took antibiotics half an hour before treatment*
*and then again six hours afterward. He also put sealants on all of her*
*molars and, even though there were many weeks when her teeth could*
*not be brushed, she never got a cavity.*

Some parents report delays in the arrival of their child's permanent teeth. Children who receive chemotherapy or cranial radiation therapy may have poorly developed or absent permanent teeth, as well as blunted tooth roots, increasing the possibility of premature tooth loss.

# Mouth and throat sores

The mouth, throat, and intestines are lined with cells that divide rapidly and can be severely damaged by chemotherapy drugs. This is more common for children on very intensive protocols and those having bone marrow transplants. The sores that develop (mucositis) are very painful and can prevent eating and drinking. Check your child's mouth periodically for sores, and if any are present, ask advice from the oncologist. Some parent suggestions are:

- To prevent infection, the mouth needs to be kept as clean and free of bacteria as possible. After eating, have your child gently brush teeth, gums, and tongue with a soft, clean toothbrush.

- Serve bland food, baby food, or meals put through the blender.

- Use a straw with drinks or blender-processed food.

- Keep an accurate record of your child's fluid intake. If oral intake is poor, pain may be the cause; your child may need prescription pain medication to allow him to swallow and take adequate fluids.

- If your child is old enough, the doctor may recommend a rinse to decrease the amount of bacteria in your child's mouth. This may help prevent mouth sores.

> When David was told to use Peridex, I asked the doctor if we could substitute 0.63% stannous fluoride rinse. He said yes. As a dentist I knew Peridex killed bacteria and lasts up to eight hours, but it tastes terrible and stains teeth. Patients did not like using it. The 0.63% stannous fluoride had the same bacterial killing properties and also lasts up to eight hours, but has a better taste and does not stain as badly. The fluoride also helps prevent cavities and makes the teeth less sensitive. It comes in a variety of flavors like mint, tropical, or cinnamon. It is a prescription drug that a lot of dentists dispense.
>
> One mixes 1/8 oz. of concentrate with warm water, making 1 oz. A measuring cup comes with the bottle. I have David swish with half the mixture for one minute (time it because it's longer than you think!). This can only be used by kids who are old enough to not accidentally swallow it. Six-year-old David has no problem taking this once a day before he goes to bed. If and when he starts developing mouth sores, he will take it A.M. and P.M. It's important not to eat or drink for 30 minutes after rinsing. That is why David rinses before bedtime, after he has taken his meds and brushed his teeth.

Glutamine, a nutritional supplement available at most drug and health food stores, may be helpful in preventing or minimizing mouth sores in some children. If your child is receiving chemotherapy with a high probability of causing mouth sores, you may want to try glutamine as a prophylactic measure. The powder can be mixed in juice and should be started one or two days before your child receives a cycle of chemotherapy. Be sure to get your oncologist's approval prior to starting this treatment.

> Roger just began his second round of chemo. He is on Lomustine, procarbazine, and some intravenous chemo. He seemed to be tolerating it fairly well until he started breaking out in terrible sores all through his mouth and under his tongue, very painful to him. He couldn't even eat. I decided to get him to gargle and swish 100% pure aloe vera juice all

*through his mouth. He held the aloe vera in his mouth for five minutes before swallowing it that night before he went to bed. Strangely enough, the sores were almost all gone by morning. Roger woke up the next morning and said, "Wow that stuff works fast!"*

# Changes in taste and smell

Chemotherapy can cause changes in the taste buds, altering the brain's perception of how food tastes. Meats often taste bitter, and sweets can taste unpleasant. Even foods that children crave taste badly. Coupled with altered taste, the sense of smell is also impacted by chemotherapy. The sense of smell can be heightened so that smells that other family members are unaware of can cause nausea in a child on chemotherapy.

A child's ability to smell and taste can take months to return to normal after chemotherapy ends.

> *Once Katy begged me to make her my special double chocolate sour cream cake. Surprisingly, it smelled really good to her as it baked. She took a big bite, spit it out all over the table, and ran back to her room sobbing. She cried for a long time. She told me later that it had tasted "bitter and horrible."*

# Skin and nail problems

Minor skin problems are frequent while on chemotherapy. The most common problems are rashes, redness, itching, peeling, dry skin, and acne. The following are suggestions for preventing and treating skin problems:

- Avoid hot showers or baths, because these can dry the skin.

- Use moisturizing soap such as Basic or Aveeno.

- Apply a water-based moisturizer after bathing.

- Avoid scratchy materials such as wool. Your child will feel more comfortable in loose cotton clothing.

- Have your child use sunscreen with a sun protection factor (SPF) of at least 30. This is especially important for areas that have been irradiated.

- If your child is bald, and especially if she has had cranial radiation, insist on head coverings or sunscreen every time she goes outdoors.

- Buy your child lip gloss with sunscreen.

  *Matthew's lips would get very dry and eventually start to peel. It irritated him and he developed a habit of biting on his lips. To minimize the problem I learned that wiping a cool, wet cloth over his mouth many times a day worked well. I would then apply a light coating of Vaseline to his lips to keep them moist.*

- Rub cornstarch on itchy skin. This is often soothing.

- Many chemotherapy drugs can cause dry, contact dermatitis, especially during the winter months. With your oncologist's permission, over-the-counter cortisone cream usually alleviates this problem.

If your child has chemotherapy drugs injected into the veins (rather than a central catheter), you may notice a darkening along the vein. This will fade after chemotherapy ends. However, skin and underlying tissues can be damaged or destroyed by drugs that leak out of a vein. If your child feels a stinging or burning sensation or if you notice swelling at the IV site, call a nurse immediately.

Call the doctor anytime your child gets a severe rash or is very itchy. Scratching rashes can cause infections, so you need to get medications to control the itching.

Chemotherapy affects the growing portion of nails located under the cuticle. After chemotherapy, you may notice a white band or ridge across the nail as it grows out. These brittle bands are sometimes elevated and feel bumpy. As the white ridge grows out toward the end of the finger, the nail may break. Keeping your child's fingernails trimmed can help prevent breakage.

# Eating problems

Most children have major nutritional problems while on chemotherapy. Chapter 17 is devoted to explaining eating problems, such as anorexia (lack of appetite), food aversions, overeating, and the myriad other problems induced by chemotherapy and radiation.

*Alan (age 8) is currently finished with chemo and radiation therapy for medulloblastoma, but needs to gain weight back. He has never been big on milkshakes since he started treatment. When he was in radiation his teeth were very sensitive to hot and cold. He does get Pedisure through a G-tube, but we found a juice called Nestle NuBasic which is a 5 oz. can of calories and nutrition. The small size is great because it isn't overwhelming for Al, and he has put on almost four pounds after two weeks. (He is drinking three cans a day in addition to the Pedisure at night, but not eating much "real" food yet.) Incidentally, my "healthy" 6-year-old loves Pedisure, and would drink it all the time.*

# Steroid problems

Many children with CNS tumors require therapy with steroid medications at intervals throughout treatment. Prednisone, dexamethasone, hydrocortisone, and others in this category can cause many unpleasant side effects, including fluid retention, high blood pressure, elevated blood sugar, sleep disturbances, muscle weakness, cataracts, and bone weakening. Many children experience profound mood swings and are very emotional. If you are having problems in this area, consult your oncologist to see if the dose of steroid medication can be adjusted or if a different type of steroid with fewer side effects is appropriate. For more information on steroids, see Chapter 12, *Chemotherapy.*

> *My 3-year-old niece was on Decadron during treatment for a brainstem anaplastic astrocytoma. She had localized radiation, then later whole brain and spinal radiation, plus various chemos, but nothing whacked her out like Decadron. She was on a high dose during radiation, and we were waiting to see her head turn all the way round or for her to start vomiting great gobs of green stuff. When the Decadron was reduced, sanity returned to the household.*

# Seizures

Seizures can be compared to an electrical storm in the brain. A seizure begins in a damaged or malfunctioning area of the brain, which is called a seizure focus. Anyone can have a seizure under certain conditions. Having a single seizure does not indicate that a person has a seizure disorder. Seizure disorders are defined as repeated episodes of seizure activity. A number of children with brain tumors experience seizure activity.

Around 40 different types of seizures or seizure disorders have been identified. The three main kinds are:

- **Absence seizure.** The child may blink and may not be aware that he has lost awareness for a few seconds.

- Partial seizure (also known as petit mal seizure). The child has longer periods of loss of awareness, but without loss of consciousness. She may have strange sensations and make involuntary grunts or noises.

- Tonic clonic (or grand mal). These seizures include loss of consciousness and visible arm/leg tremors or whole body convulsions.

Seizures can happen anytime, but most commonly occur during the year following surgery and during treatment. Seizure activity may happen just once, occasionally, or regularly, depending on the individual nature of your child's disease.

For more information on local and national support and on seizure management at school and home, contact the Epilepsy Foundation at (800) 332-1000 or see their web site at: *http://www.efa.org*.

*There were times during my son's protocol that I felt he suffered more from the side effects of treatment than from the disease. It was emotionally painful for me to watch him go through so much. I think one of the hardest moments for me was the day he lost all his hair. Up until that point I had been living in a semi-state of denial. His bald head was more proof of our reality—he really did have cancer.*

*I had to learn how to accept our situation, because I needed to be strong for my child. To get through, I reminded myself every day that the treatments were necessary and that without them he would die. It was a struggle, but the unpleasant side effects soon passed and he was able to resume some of his normal activities. I was constantly amazed at his resilience.*

# CHAPTER 14

# Bone Marrow and Stem Cell Transplantation

BONE MARROW TRANSPLANTATION (BMT) and peripheral blood stem cell transplantation (PBSCT) are complicated procedures used to treat some types of CNS tumors. These procedures are still in the experimental phase as treatment for CNS tumors.

During a bone marrow or stem cell transplant, the child receives high-dose chemotherapy to kill tumor cells. Normal bone marrow or peripheral blood stem cells (free of tumor cells) are then infused into the child's veins through a central venous catheter. The marrow or stem cells migrate to the cavities inside the bones, where new, healthy blood cells are produced.

Transplants, although possibly life-saving, are expensive, technically complex, and potentially life-threatening. Understanding the procedures and their ramifications at a time of crisis can be tremendously difficult. This chapter presents the basics of bone marrow and stem cell transplantation in simple terms and shares the experiences of several families.

## When are transplants necessary?

At present, some types of CNS tumors cannot be cured with conventional doses of chemotherapy, radiation, or surgery. Such tumors may be sensitive to extremely high doses of chemotherapy, but these doses permanently damage normal bone marrow. Transplants can replace damaged or destroyed marrow.

Many studies using high-dose chemotherapy, with or without radiation therapy, followed by rescue with bone marrow or peripheral blood stem cells from the child (autologous transplants), are ongoing. High-dose chemotherapy with autologous stem cell rescue is incorporated in some cooperative group and institutional studies for treating high-risk infant CNS tumors, glioblastoma multiforme, anaplastic astrocytoma, high-risk or recurrent medulloblastoma, primitive neuroectodermal tumor (PNET), high-risk embryonal CNS tumors, and anaplastic ependymoma. Tandem transplants (also called serial transplants, sequential transplants, and mini transplants), in which high-dose chemotherapy is repeatedly followed by stem cell rescue, are also being studied. Preliminary data from some of these studies is encouraging.

If a transplant has been recommended for your child or teenager, you may want to get a second opinion before proceeding. Chapter 22, *Relapse,* and Chapter 7, *Forming a Partnership with the Medical Team,* give several methods for obtaining an educated second opinion. In addition, to fully understand the issues, you may want to ask the oncologist some or all of the following questions:

• What are all the treatment options?

• For my child's type of tumor, history, and physical condition, what chance for survival does he have with a transplant? What are his chances with other treatment?

• What are the risks? Explain the statistical chance of each risk.

• What are the benefits of this type of transplant?

• What will be my child's short-term and long-term quality of life after the transplant?

• What is the institution's procedure for this type of transplant?

• What portion of the procedure will be outpatient versus inpatient?

• What is the average length of stay for children undergoing this procedure?

• What are the anticipated and rare complications of this type of transplant?

• Will she have to take medicines after the transplant? For how long?

• What are the side effects of these medicines?

• Is this transplant considered to be experimental, or is it accepted clinical practice?

# Types of transplants

It is important to understand the type of transplant being recommended to enable you to better evaluate what has been proposed for your child.

## Bone marrow transplant

During an autologous bone marrow transplant, the child's own marrow is withdrawn (harvested) from the large bones of the hips. While the child is under general anesthesia in the operating room, the doctor inserts a large needle into the bones and withdraws bone marrow. Marrow is withdrawn up to 50 times to obtain a total of one to two pints, depending on the child's weight. The entire process usually takes less than one hour.

Because the amount of marrow that is removed contains less than 5 percent of the child's developing blood cells, it takes only a few days for the body to replace the marrow. The child is usually sore for a day or two and may feel a bit tired for several days. Recovery time varies from child to child. A red blood cell transfusion may be necessary following the procedure.

> We had an autologous bone marrow transplant four months ago for high-risk PNET. Sean (age 3) went through the transplant fine. He had to be fed through an IV because he didn't eat much and he did get some bouts of diarrhea but he never got many of the problems that they say they will have like mouth sores. All our problems were from the central line, one infection after another with each one more serious than the last. His last infection we actually almost lost him. There was an infected clot in his line and when they accessed it the clot was pushed out into his bloodstream causing him to crash. His lungs filled with fluid and he had to be put on a ventilator and we spent a very difficult week in the PICU. I don't want to scare you but just be careful to not let anything go. If you think something isn't right make sure they listen to you. They are so open to infection with no immune system, so I say any temperature increase is something to check out.

After the marrow is harvested and treated, it is cryopreserved (a type of freezing). The child then undergoes high-dose chemotherapy to kill the remaining tumor cells. The frozen marrow is then thawed and reinfused into the child or teen intravenously.

> What helped me the most were the decorations and having a positive attitude. My mom decorated the area outside the transplant room with balloons, cards, and posters. It was hard to take the medicine, so my mom made a huge poster to mark off how well I did. Every time I took my medicine, I got a sticker. When I got one hundred stickers, I got some roller blades.

## Peripheral blood stem cell transplant (PBSCT)

When doctors aspirate liquid bone marrow from the cavities in bones, it is full of stem cells—cells from which all other blood cell types evolve (for example, white blood cells, red blood cells, and platelets). Stem cells are also found in the circulating (also called peripheral) blood, although in a much less concentrated form.

In a peripheral blood stem cell transplant (PBSCT), the child's own stem cells are harvested in a procedure called apheresis or leukapheresis. The child's bone marrow is "primed" using bone marrow growth factors, such as granulocyte colony stimulating factor (e.g., Neupogen), for several days prior to the procedure. Usually a moderate to high-dose of cyclophosphamide with or without other chemotherapy drugs is given in order to get the child's ANC to 0. This helps the child to generate adequate numbers of circulating stem cells.

> Six-year-old Ethan had a stem cell harvest after his recovery from the first cytoxan doses he got. He was on Neupogen (G-CSF), which is an injectable med that stimulates white cell release from the marrow. Neupogen has been a piece of cake for Ethan, doesn't hurt, partly because we have desensitized him to needles. Once he had enough of the stem cells in his bloodstream, he had a femoral PICC line placed because they needed a larger catheter to do this. The only down side was that he had to lay completely flat for about six hours, and collection took two days, so he had limited movement over night between collections. Plan a lot of quiet activities! Videos, books on tape, handheld games, cards. He hated the no bathroom privileges and refused to use a urinal at all. Ethan sailed through this, and we have no regrets having put those cells in the bank for him.

When the child's peripheral blood counts rise, blood is removed through a central venous catheter (specially equipped for pheresis) or a special temporary pheresis catheter placed in a vein. The blood circulates through a machine that extracts the stem cells and is then returned to the child. Each pheresis session lasts two to eight hours. Children with recent high-dose chemotherapy or radiation usually take longer for an adequate number of stem cells to be collected. In rare cases, it is impossible to get enough stem cells from children who have recently undergone extensive chemotherapy and/or radiation.

The number of sessions required is variable. Infants may need only one session, but children who have received extensive treatment may need six or eight.

Potential complications of peripheral blood stem cell apheresis include:

- **Hypocalcemia (low calcium in the blood).** Your child may experience muscle cramps, chills, tremors, tingling of the fingers and toes, dizziness, and occasionally chest pain. He will be closely monitored during the procedure, and IV or oral calcium supplements will be administered to prevent this problem.

- **Thrombocytopenia (low platelets).** This can occur if platelets stick to the inside of the apheresis machine. Your child's platelet count will be checked before and after the apheresis, and a platelet transfusion will be given if needed.

- **Hypovolemia (low blood volume).** This can occur at any time during the procedure and is more common in small children. Symptoms can include low blood pressure, rapid heart rate, lightheadedness, and sweating. To prevent this problem, the apheresis machine is generally "primed" with a unit of blood prior to the procedure.

- **Infection.** In many cases, a new and larger central venous catheter is placed prior to the apheresis procedure because infection is possible. If your child develops fever, chills, or low blood pressure, blood cultures will be obtained and IV antibiotics given.

Most apheresis procedures are safely performed on an outpatient or short-stay basis, so you and your child can go home each evening. Some institutions, however, do require hospitalization throughout the procedure.

There are two types of peripheral stem cell transplants used in children with CNS tumors:

- **Myeloablative chemotherapy.** This uses doses of medicine high enough so that marrow cells are totally destroyed and will not recover without infusion of new stem cells. This is the traditional BMT employed for leukemia or diseases that often harbor tumor cells within the marrow (i.e., neuroblastoma).

- **Myelosuppressive high-dose chemotherapy.** This uses doses of medicine high enough so that marrow cell production is severely suppressed, but would eventually return over a protracted period of time (6 to 12 weeks). PBSC is infused in this situation in order to shorten the recovery time to about 2 weeks (the time it normally takes with more conventional doses of chemotherapy). This treatment allows doctors to expose the tumor cells to higher doses of chemotherapy than could be achieved with conventional dosing (yet somewhat less than in BMT), while limiting the toxicity and potential high risk of death due to infection that would ordinarily be associated with simply allowing the child to recover on her own. This procedure is called serial transplant, sequential transplant, or mini-transplant.

Although myeloablative regimens are used in CNS tumors, the more common approach now is the use of the myelosuppressive regimens in sequence (2 or 3 cycles), each followed by PBSC infusion.

*Joshua was diagnosed in March of 1998 with a supratentorial*
*ependymoblastoma (aka anaplastic ependymoma grade IV). He had a 90%*
*resection and underwent five rounds of high-dose chemo and then an auto*
*stem cell transplant. It was our hope and the goal of the protocol to delay*
*radiation by a couple of years if possible, as he was only 27 months at*
*diagnosis and only turned 3 during his stem cell transplant. However, it*
*wasn't meant to be, as he had bulk tumor remaining at the start of*
*transplant and therefore needed radiation following the chemo to be sure*
*we did all we could do to stop the beast. He is now 3.5 years out from*
*diagnosis and 2.3 years out from end of treatment. We have been told*
*repeatedly that kids with this type of tumor will almost always recur within*
*the first 2 years, so we feel a slight bit of relief. But, which of us out there*
*will ever completely relax with this cloud hanging over our child's head.*
*Getting past the 2-year mark was a huge milestone, not only for my son,*
*but for me too. Now I let him do boy things. Climb the jungle gym, jump off*
*of rocks, and swing on things that shouldn't be swung on.*

## Other transplants

Allogeneic transplants use donor marrow from a family member or an unrelated person. Placental transplants use stem cells from the cord blood of a sibling or unrelated donor. Syngeneic bone marrow transplants are those in which the patient's donor is an identical twin. Because these types of transplants are rarely, if ever, used to treat children with CNS tumors, they are not covered here.

For more information on types of transplants, write or phone BMT Infonet, 2900 Skokie Valley Road, Suite B, Highland Park, IL 60035, (888) 597-7674. The *BMT Newsletter* is also electronically published on the Internet at *http://www.bmtinfonet.org*.

# Choosing a transplant center

Choosing a transplant center is a very important decision. Institutions may just be starting a marrow or stem cell program, or they may have vast experience. Some may be excellent for adults, but have limited pediatric experience. Some may allow you to room in with your child; others may isolate the patient for weeks. Protocols vary among institutions as well. The center closest to your home may not provide the best medical care available for your child or allow the necessary quality of life (rooming in, social workers, etc.) that you need. Additionally, your insurance plan may require you and your child to go to a transplant center with which they have an existing contract.

The Autologous Blood and Marrow Transplant Registry (ABMTR) collects patient data on autologous blood and marrow transplants performed in North and South America. More than 450 transplant centers from 48 countries are listed on their web site at *http://www.ibmtr.org* (click on transplant centers). You can contact them by phone at (414) 456-8325.

To help you learn about the policies of different transplant centers, here are some questions that you might ask:

* How many pediatric transplants did the institution do last year? How many of the type recommended for my child?

* How successful is your program? What are the one-, two-, and five-year survival rates? (Remember that some institutions accept very high-risk patients, and their statistics would not compare to a place that performs less risky transplants.)

* What is the nurse-to-patient ratio? Do all the staff members have pediatric training and experience?

* What support staff is available (educator, social worker, child life therapist, chaplain, etc.)?

* Will my child be on a pediatric or combined adult-pediatric unit?

* What are the institution's rules on parents staying in the child's hospital room?

* What on-site or close housing is available for families of children undergoing transplant? What are the costs for this housing?

* What are the institution's anti-infection requirements? Isolation? Gown and gloves? Washing hands?

* Describe the BMT procedure in detail, including anticipated complications.

* Explain the risks and benefits of this procedure.

* Assuming all goes well, how soon could my child leave the hospital? Leave the area to go home?

* What will his life be like, assuming all goes perfectly? If there are problems?

* What are the long-term side effects of this type of transplant?

* What long-term follow-up is available?

* Explain the waiting list requirements.

* How much will this procedure cost? How much will my insurance cover? (This is not applicable in Canada, where the cost of the procedure is covered by provincial health programs.)

Many transplant centers have videos and booklets for patients and their families that explain services and describe what to expect before, during, and after transplant. Call any transplant center that you are considering and ask them to send you all available materials.

To explore more fully what questions to ask various transplant centers, obtain the *Candlelighter's Guide to Bone Marrow Transplants in Children*. This excellent book has an entire chapter devoted to questions to ask to find the best transplant center for your child.

> *The head of oncology from a major center comes to our city every two months to follow up on the kids who have been treated there. It was a big draw to us to have post-transplant follow-up at home, rather than having to travel a great distance to get back to the center. The other thing was that children are not put in laminar air flow, and families weren't required to cap and gown, only scrub their hands. Since I'm allergic to those hospital gloves, this allowed me to stay with my daughter throughout. We did, however, call around to several centers to compare facilities, costs, and insurance coverage.*

Making an informed consent is a serious decision when considering a life-threatening procedure such as a bone marrow or stem cell transplant. It is very important to work closely with your oncologist and treatment team when making this decision. Do not hesitate to keep asking questions until you fully understand what is being proposed. Ask the doctor to use plain English if she has lapsed into medical jargon. Bring a tape recorder or friend to help remember the information. Many centers require the assent of children 7 to 18 years old in addition to the consent of the parent. Do not sign the consent form until you feel comfortable that you understand the procedure and have had every question answered.

# Paying for the transplant

Bone marrow and stem cell transplants are expensive. Some bone marrow transplants are considered standard of care, so insurers cover the procedure without problems. However, you will need to carefully research whether your insurance company considers the type of transplant proposed for your child to be experimental and therefore not covered. Most insurance plans have a lifetime cap, and many only pay 80 percent of the costs of the transplant up to the cap. Often, transplant centers will not perform the procedure without all of the money guaranteed. With time of the essence, this can cause great anguish for families who struggle to raise funds or mortgage all of their belongings to pay.

Most insurance companies will assign your child's care to a transplant coordinator or case manager, whose responsibility it is to make arrangements with the transplant center and handle financial issues. Getting to know your coordinator and letting him know your needs and concerns may provide an additional valuable resource for you during this stressful time.

If you are having difficulty getting your insurance company to pay for the transplant, contact the Childhood Cancer Ombudsman Program (contact information is in Appendix B, *Resources*) for help.

If you are not insured (or are underinsured) and must raise all or part of the necessary funds, you can contact the organizations that provide financial assistance listed in Appendix B. They may be able to offer financial help and can supply advice on how to quickly and effectively raise funds. Before working with any of these organizations, ask for all printed information available and ask questions about any fees or costs associated with their services. Make sure that, when the treatment is completed or the child dies, remaining funds are applied to outstanding medical debts.

In Canada, each province and territory has a provincial health plan that covers the medical costs of transplant. However, there are still expenses that will need to be covered by the family. Children will often have to travel long distances to facilities that are capable of performing a transplant. Travel, accommodations, and related costs have to be paid for by the parents. Bone marrow or peripheral blood stem cell transplants place financial burdens on Canadian families even though the country has a standardized healthcare system.

# The transplant

Prior to the actual transplant, the patient's bone marrow is suppressed using high-dose chemotherapy (radiation is generally not used for CNS tumors). This portion of treatment is called conditioning. The child in the following story had myeloablative chemotherapy including thiopeta. Children who receive thiopeta in a myelosuppressive serial transplant do not have such severe symptoms.

> *Our 2-year-old daughter had high-dose chemo and then a stem cell transplant to treat her medulloblastoma. The transplant was terribly hard. The thiotepa made her skin peel off, and she was wrapped in gauze like a*

*mummy. Her mucous membranes sloughed off in her mouth and down her
esophagus and she needed a morphine drip for pain. Her counts went to
zero and it was very scary. There was certainly a lot that could go wrong.
However, she recovered quickly and was back in preschool two months later.
She is 6 now, and has mostly happy memories of those days. Our family
sort of took over the room. We brought in a radio and we all danced. I'd
take her out of bed and put her on the floor on a blanket and we'd picnic.
We sang a lot. Now, she can't wait to go for her checkups.*

Conditioning regimens vary according to institution and protocol and also depend on
the medical condition and history of the child. For serial transplants, the chemotherapy is given for two to six days, and in many cases all or part of the therapy is given
in the outpatient setting. Your child may need IV fluids at night to provide proper
hydration. It is important to be sure you understand whom to call if problems occur
at night and what telephone number(s) to use in this event.

If your child receives conditioning chemotherapy as an outpatient, she will need to go
to the transplant unit no later than the evening before the procedure for hydration.
The transplant itself consists of simply infusing the marrow or stem cells through a
central venous catheter into the child, just like a blood transfusion. The marrow or
stem cells travel through the blood vessels, eventually settling in the long bones.

A transplant physician will monitor your child during the infusion. A variety of minor
to major complications may occur during the bone marrow or peripheral blood stem
cell transfusion. Possible complications are:

- Abdominal cramps
- Difficulty breathing
- Slow heartbeat
- Tightness in the chest
- Chills
- Cough
- Diarrhea
- Skin rash
- Fever
- Flushing
- Headache

- Changes in blood pressure
- Nausea and vomiting
- Unpleasant taste (usually relieved by sucking on hard candies or flavored liquids)

Now 13 years old, Andrew was diagnosed at age 11 with a pinealblastoma/germinoma. He had chemotherapy, cranial and spinal radiation, and a stem cell rescue. Andrew's mom, Melissa, and then Andrew, talk about the experience:

> Stem cell was a long haul. It was a time that we had absolutely no control over anything. You watch your child in the most horrible state. It was literally a time that we lived minute-by-minute and sometimes second by second. We're still dealing with the side effects. He doesn't have his energy or full strength. It's coming back, but it's a slow process. He missed about a year and a half of school.
>
> Stem cell was almost like a rebirthing for Andrew. He went from being so angry about his diagnosis to a much wiser, much more confident child. His insight is wise beyond his years. Andrew's involved in quite a bit of public speaking. He's gone before elementary, middle school, and high school groups and DARE groups, talking about how important life is, and why it's important to enjoy life, and how it feels to almost lose your life.

Andrew adds:

> Public speaking started with my teacher. He asked me if I'd do a high school class, and I said sure, if someone can learn from what I've been through, I'm all for it. I consider myself blessed with a tumor, not diagnosed with it. So many good things have come from it. Treatment feels like a never-ending battle, but it's not. You can't be afraid to die, thinking like that will bring you down as fast as anything. You need to have faith in something. I had faith in God, but you need to believe you're going to make it. Treatment is painful, but you have to think of the outcome and keep your eye on the goal. It's difficult, but not impossible.

# Emotional responses

The transplant experience can take a heavy emotional toll on the child, the siblings, and the parents. It can be a physically and mentally grueling procedure, with the possibility of months or years of aftereffects. Most transplant team members are extensively trained to meet the needs of the child and family during the transplant itself and the long convalescence that follows. The team usually includes physicians, nurses, social workers, educators, nutritionists, and physical, occupational, speech, and child-life therapists.

> *Levi's transplant experience was like watching someone wake up from a deep sleep. For the two weeks he was flat on his back, suffering greatly from mucositis and a tummy bug that caused diarrhea for days straight. It was a real horror. Then one evening he sat up and said, "What's all that stuff?" He was referring to all the gifts that had piled up in the corner of his room. He opened every toy, got down on the floor, and drew pictures of all the foods he was craving, and he never looked back. It was like an instant transformation. I think my own recovery was longer. I believe part of me froze in order to survive the transplant, and it took a long time to thaw.*

## Complications after transplant

Some children have a smooth journey through the transplant process, while others bounce from one life-threatening complication to another. Some children live, and some children die.

There is no way to predict which children will develop problems, nor is there any way to anticipate whether the new development will be a mere inconvenience or a catastrophe. This section presents some of the major complications that can develop post-transplant and the experiences of several families who faced these problems.

> *The transplant center was very clear about all of the potential problems. That was good, for it prepared me. My attitude is watch for them, hope they don't happen, if they do, then live with them. She had an easy time with the transplant, she's a happy third grader, she's alive, and we feel so, so very lucky.*

## Infections

Most infections following transplant come from organisms within the body (e.g., cytomegalovirus, mouth, and gut bacteria). Good hand washing can help prevent infections with bacteria and fungi.

The immune system of healthy children quickly destroys any foreign invaders; this is not so for children who have undergone a transplant. The immune systems of children undergoing bone marrow or peripheral blood stem cell transplantation have been temporarily impaired by chemotherapy. Until the new marrow or stem cells engraft and begin to produce large numbers of white cells (two to four weeks), post-transplant children are in danger of developing serious infections.

To prevent and combat bacterial infections, children receive large doses of several kinds of antibiotics if they develop a fever any time in the first weeks after transplant. Fungal infections can also occur. Fortunately, the use of bone marrow growth factors, such as Neupogen, that stimulate and accelerate white blood cell recovery has decreased the overall time to engraftment, thus decreasing the incidence of serious infections in many children. Your child will begin receiving this medication one to two days following the transplant procedure. Additionally, your child will be carefully evaluated each day for signs and symptoms of infection. Potential sites of problems include the skin, mouth, perirectal area, and central venous catheter exit site. Report any new symptoms, such as cough, shortness of breath, abdominal pain, diarrhea, pain on urination, vaginal discharge, or mental confusion to your nurses promptly.

In the first year post-transplant, children are also susceptible to serious viral infections, most commonly herpes simplex virus, cytomegalovirus, and varicella zoster virus. Viral infections are notoriously hard to treat, although a few are sensitive to the antiviral agents acyclovir and ganciclovir. Many centers use prophylactic acyclovir, ganciclovir, or immunoglobulin to prevent these infections.

CMV is usually preventable if your child is CMV negative and all transfused blood products are CMV negative or filtered to remove white blood cells.

> Our daughter (age 9) had a peripheral blood stem cell transplant. It's been several months and her white blood cell count is still low, but we have come to the conclusion that we can't make her live in a bubble anymore. We are careful to avoid potential risks, though, such as being around large crowds of people.

Preventing infections is the best policy for those children who have had a bone marrow or stem cell transplant. The following are suggestions to minimize exposure to bacteria, viruses, and fungi:

- Medical staff and all family members must wash their hands before touching the child.

- Keep your child away from crowds and people with infections.

- Do not let your child receive live virus inoculations until the immune system has fully recovered; your oncologist will determine the appropriate date for reinitiating immunizations.

- Keep your child away from anyone who has recently been inoculated with a live virus (chicken pox, polio).

- Keep your child away from barnyard animals and all animal feces.

- Avoid remodeling your home while your child is recovering.

- Have all carpets shampooed prior to child's return home from transplant.

- Family pets should be shampooed prior to your child's return home.

- Call the doctor at the first sign of a fever or infection.

> *After Hunter's double stem cell transplant, we had to follow many precautions. We had to be careful when we took him out, avoiding large crowds or public places (especially those indoors). He needed to wear a mask when we took him to his doctor's visits. We would take him to plenty of outdoor places for fun. I found the precautions easy to follow.*

## Venoocclusive disease

Venoocclusive disease (VOD) is a complication that can occur after bone marrow or stem cell transplantation in which the flow of blood through the liver becomes obstructed. Children who have had more than one transplant, previous liver problems, or past exposure to certain chemotherapy drugs (such as thioguanine) are more at risk to develop VOD. It can occur gradually or very quickly. Symptoms of VOD include jaundice (yellowing of the skin), an enlarged liver, pain in the upper right abdomen, fluid in the abdomen, unexplained weight gain, and poor response to platelet transfusions.

## Bleeding

Bleeding may occur throughout your child's post-transplant recovery phase until adequate bone marrow engraftment has occurred. Bruising, bleeding from the gums, urinary, or gastrointestinal tract, and nosebleeds are all common problems and are generally handled easily with platelet transfusions. Serious bleeding can occur in the lungs, gut, or brain. Your child is at increased risk for intracranial bleeding because he has a CNS tumor and especially if he has undergone recent surgery or radiation therapy. Most transplant centers strive to keep children's platelet counts at a safe level until bone marrow recovery has occurred. Generally speaking, platelets are the last type of blood cell to fully recover following bone marrow or peripheral blood stem cell transplant.

## Hemorrhagic cystitis

Hemorrhagic cystitis (bleeding from the bladder) may result from administration of certain chemotherapy drugs used in your child's conditioning regimen. Occasionally, it is caused by a bacterial or viral bladder infection. Symptoms of hemorrhagic cystitis include blood in the urine (which may be obvious to the eye or microscopic), blood clots in the urine, pain on urination, and bladder discomfort. If your child receives a chemotherapy drug that has the potential to cause this problem, she will probably also receive the drug Mesna to help coat the bladder lining. If your child develops hemorrhagic cystitis or a urinary tract infection, she will receive antibiotics, intravenous fluids, and pain medication as needed.

## Mucositis

Mucositis (inflammation of the mucous membranes lining the mouth and gastrointestinal tract) and stomatitis (mouth sores) are common complications following bone marrow or peripheral blood stem cell transplants. Symptoms include reddened, discolored, or ulcerated membranes of the mouth, pain, difficulty swallowing, taste alterations, and difficulty speaking. The majority of children undergoing transplant experience this problem.

Your child will require frequent mouth care, modifications in diet, and pain medications. It is very important to try and coordinate your child's required mouth care with the administration of appropriate pain medications. Likewise, making sure your child receives pain medication prior to eating often helps. When white blood cells return, your child's mouth will heal.

Andrew talks about having mucositis after his stem cell transplant:

> High-dose chemo kills your taste buds, and I wanted to only eat sweet or spicy food, anything else tasted like cardboard. I'd eat ribs with BBQ sauce. KFC mash potatoes and gravy was great. Drinking was hard. I used to suck on ice cubes. It's gross when the lining of your mouth comes out. It just pulls out, it's white, it doesn't hurt. It comes out during bowel movements, too, but you don't realize it. But, you can't swallow because of the sores, so you have to spit a lot.

## Eating difficulties

The vast majority of children undergoing bone marrow or peripheral blood stem cell transplants require intravenous nutrition during their convalescence. A variety of factors contribute to this problem, including preexisting nutritional problems, side effects of conditioning chemotherapy, nausea and vomiting, mouth sores, and infections of the gastrointestinal tract. Your child may experience a few, some, or all of these problems before engraftment occurs. Most transplant centers initiate intravenous nutrition promptly after transplant and continue until your child's appetite and ability to take in adequate calories by mouth have returned.

Your child may require prophylactic ulcer medications to coat the lining of the stomach or to decrease the amount of stomach acid produced. He may experience ongoing nausea, in spite of the fact that he is long past his conditioning chemotherapy. Ask to speak to the transplant unit dietician and keep accurate records of your child's eating. As with mucositis, your child's ability to eat and drink more normally is closely correlated with the recovery of blood counts.

## Pulmonary edema

Pulmonary edema (collection of fluid in lung tissue) is sometimes seen in children who undergo bone marrow or peripheral blood stem cell transplants. It may occur from injury to lung tissue caused by infections, chemotherapy, and, rarely, bone marrow growth factors, such as Neupogen. Symptoms include shortness of breath, productive cough, bloody sputum, fever, sweating, chest pain, and swelling of the hands and feet. Your child may require oxygen, diuretic medications, corticosteroids, and a temporary fluid restriction until the problem resolves. Rarely, mechanical ventilation is necessary to maintain adequate oxygenation.

## Neurological complications

Children with CNS tumors are at increased risk of developing neurological complications after transplant. Mental confusion, acute hearing loss, and expressive and receptive communication problems may occur. Fortunately, these are usually temporary. Your child may need assistance with communicating his needs and wants. In many cases, a communication board or other pictorial device is helpful until more normal function returns. Speech therapy helps, and you should request this service if your treatment team does not suggest it. Patience and a supportive attitude are very important and will reassure your child should this complication occur.

# Long-term side effects

Increasing numbers of children are being cured of their disease and surviving years after a bone marrow or peripheral blood stem cell transplant. The intensity of the treatment prior to, during, and after transplant can cause major effects not apparent for months or years. This section describes a few of the major long-term side effects that sometimes develop after a transplant.

## Recurrence

Despite the intensive chemotherapy given prior to the bone marrow or stem cell transplant, some children suffer a recurrence of the original disease. Recurrence is most likely to occur in the first two years after the transplant.

## Dental development

Certain chemotherapy drugs, administered in high doses prior to transplant, may result in improper tooth development and blunted or absent tooth roots in children less than 5 years of age. Your child will likely have a comprehensive dental examination prior to the transplant and should have dental follow-up after recovery has occurred.

## Thyroid function

Children who receive only chemotherapy do not develop thyroid deficiency as a result of treatment. If, however, your child receives radiation therapy to the brain and spinal cord, either before or following recovery from a transplant, she should be monitored for the development of thyroid deficiency. Tablets containing thyroid hormone are usually effective in treating the problem.

## Growth and development

Children who receive total body radiation or radiation to the brain may have altered growth and development. All children who have had a bone marrow or stem cell transplant should get periodic evaluations from a pediatric endocrinologist to monitor growth and development. Growth hormone is sometimes necessary for children who received radiation therapy.

## Puberty and sterility

Children who had only chemotherapy during the conditioning regimen usually have normal sexual development, though not always. If your child receives cranial radiation, either before or following recovery from a transplant, delays in puberty and sexual development may occur. Any child who had a transplant should be followed closely by a pediatric endocrinologist, who can prescribe hormones (testosterone for boys, estrogen and progesterone for girls) to assist in normal pubertal development. Girls are more likely to need hormonal replacement; boys usually produce testosterone but not sperm.

> *Our 4-year-old son had focal point and cranial/spinal radiation for medulloblastoma after high-dose cytoxan for his stem cell transplant. It took about a year for his counts to normalize and he was sick a lot during that time. He takes growth hormone and thyroid replacement. He has severe, high frequency hearing loss. But these are nothing compared to the learning difficulties.*

Your child's ability to have a normal sex life is not affected. Some children treated only with chemotherapy have remained fertile, and to date all offspring have been normal.

## Second cancers

Children who receive a BMT or stem cell transplant have a theoretical risk of developing a second malignancy (cancer). Because transplants are relatively new treatments for children and teens with CNS tumors, the overall impact and long-term effects are not yet clear. Your doctor can explain known risks given your child's disease and treatment.

> *My first piece of advice is to find a way to have a computer in the room. The care partners at our hospital actually provided one. It helped me maintain my sanity as I could post to listservs and have others help me through my bad days and laugh with me at the good. Hard to believe it's been over three years. The second thing: movies, books, games, puzzles. Anything to keep from staring at the walls, although it's sometimes nice to just "veg." My other advice is to try to keep things on a schedule. Get up every day at whatever hour strikes your fancy and take a shower, find some fresh clothes. And, as hard as it is, I recommend fresh air and sunshine for you as often as possible, at least once a day! That way you can share your experiences outside the room as a distraction for your child. Personally, I was so sick of the TV after we went into BMT that I wanted to rip it out of the wall.*

CHAPTER 15

# Feelings, Communication, and Behavior

UNDER THE BEST OF CIRCUMSTANCES, child rearing is a daunting task. When parenting is complicated by an overwhelming crisis such as cancer, communication within the family may suffer. Prior to the diagnosis, children know the family rules and understand the limits for their behavior. Afterward, normal family life is disrupted, and all sorts of confusing and distressing feelings appear. Parenting must change in response to the frequently shifting needs of the ill child and affected siblings.

This chapter begins with a discussion about talking over the illness and treatment with your child. It then reviews some feelings that many children have about their disease. Next, it examines some emotional and behavioral changes in both children and parents, and presents suggestions on how to maintain effective communication and appropriate behavior within the family.

## Telling your child

In the first harrowing days after a diagnosis of a CNS tumor, parents must decide when and what to tell their children about the illness. Because parents are coping with a bewildering array of emotions themselves, sharing information and providing reassurance and hope may be difficult. In the past, shielding children from the painful reality was the norm. Most experts now agree that children feel less anxiety and cope with treatments better if they have a clear understanding of the disease. It is important to provide age-appropriate information soon after diagnosis and to create a supportive climate so that children feel comfortable asking questions both of parents and the medical team.

> We felt we had to tell Jessica the truth from the very beginning. She
> needed to know that she could trust us. Talking about it helped her
> understand why the treatments were necessary. We told her that her hair
> would fall out, but that it didn't matter. She would still be beautiful to us,

301

*with or without hair. We told her when something would hurt and when it*
*wouldn't. We told her we were all in this together and that we would*
*discuss everything every step of the way.*

## When should you tell your child?

Tell your child as soon as possible. It is impossible to prevent a child from knowing that he is seriously ill. The child has been whisked to an unfamiliar hospital with frightened parents, endured painful tests, received drugs, and heard he needed surgery. Cards and presents begin to arrive, and friends and siblings are absent or behave in a strange manner.

> *Before Alissa's first surgery for spinal astrocytoma when she was 6*
> *years old, I took a little chalkboard, drew a stick figure with circles for*
> *vertebrae. I pointed to her back, and explained what the spinal cord does.*
> *I told her, "You have something growing in there that needs to be removed.*
> *The doctors need to cut your back and remove it." We didn't use any baby*
> *talk. We told her and her brother Nicholas exactly what was going on.*

Delay in providing age-appropriate information can escalate the child's fears. Well-meaning parents may cause great anguish by isolating their child in a conspiracy of silence. Parents may delude themselves into thinking that the diagnosis is a secret, but children are extraordinarily perceptive. They frequently keep their thoughts and feelings to themselves in order to protect their parents from more pain. In this case, not only must the child deal with having a CNS tumor, but must do it on her own with no one to console her. Lacking accurate information, children can imagine scenarios far more frightening than the reality.

> *We immediately told Ethan that he had a brain tumor. His father and*
> *I were crying and he knew something was wrong, so we felt this was the*
> *best approach. He was 6 years old at the time, and we told him he had*
> *something growing in his head that should not be there and he needed*
> *surgery to take it out. After the surgery, he was mute, so we had no idea*
> *what he wanted to know. We explained everything—that he was having*
> *radiation, that he would be asleep each time, that he would wake up and*
> *we would be there, that he had cancer and this was the treatment for it,*
> *and that we loved him very much. He knew about cancer before he had it,*
> *and he knew that it was a bad thing to have, but he has handled the*
> *knowledge that he had it very well.*

# Who should tell your child?

This is purely a personal decision, influenced by ease of communication within the family, age and temperament of the child, religious beliefs, and sometimes physician recommendations. Small children (ages 1 to 3) primarily fear separation from parents. The presence of strangers in an already unfamiliar situation may cause additional fear. Many parents tell their small children in private; others prefer to have family members, friends, a physician, nurse practitioner, clergyman, or social worker present.

> When we first found out that the MRI showed a moderately large
> tumor, we didn't tell Billy, who was 2 years old, until a few days later.
> I think we needed to be clear for ourselves what the plan was going to be.
> Over the next few days, we started to tell him that the MRI pictures
> showed that he had a boo-boo in his head, and soon we would take a trip
> to a hospital with Grammie where the boo-boo would be fixed. When the
> day came for surgery, Grammie was with us when we told him again
> about the boo-boo inside his head, that this was the day for it to be fixed,
> and that he would take a nap while the doctors fixed the boo-boo. He
> asked if we would be with him, and we each reassured him that we all
> would be there when he woke up. I had decided not to mention any pain
> or about bandages near his eyes, but I think now that we know a little
> better, we might have said something about that, too.

Older children (4 to 12) sometimes benefit from having the treatment team (physician, nurse practitioner, child life specialist, social worker, or psychologist) present. This can create a feeling that all present are working together to help him get well. Staff members can answer the child's questions and provide comfort for the entire family. Children in this age group frequently feel guilty and responsible for their illness. They may harbor fears that the cancer is punishment for something that they did wrong. Social workers and nurses can help explore unspoken questions, provide reassurance, and identify the needs of parents, the sick child, and siblings.

Adolescents' need for control and autonomy should be respected. Teenagers sometimes feel more comfortable discussing the diagnosis with the physician in private. At a time when teens' developmental tasks include becoming independent from their families, they are suddenly dependent on medical personnel to save their lives and parents to provide emotional support. In some families, a diagnosis of cancer produces an unwelcome dependence on parents and can add new stress to the already turbulent teen years. Other families report that the diagnosis creates closer bonds between teenagers and their parents.

*Just when I had expected her to become a rebellious teenager, Florence (15 years old) became even closer to me than before. She knew that I had believed her when she started having symptoms from the pituitary tumor and sometimes she said I'd saved her life.*

## What to tell your child

Children need to be told that they are seriously ill, that they will be spending time in the hospital, that the treatment will last for a long time and is sometimes painful, that treatments are usually successful, and that the doctors and nurses are experts and will provide the very best care available. Depending on the child's age, this could vary from saying, "You have a lump in your brain that is causing your headaches and we need to go to the hospital for an operation and medicine to make it better" to reading many books together and answering hundreds of questions.

Ill children need to be reassured that they did nothing to cause the disease. It is important that they understand the disease is not contagious and they cannot give it to their siblings or friends. They need to have procedures described realistically, so that they can trust their parents and the medical team.

*Our daughter was diagnosed as a preschooler. The older she gets, the more she asks: where's my tumor, why do I have it, what are all the medications for. She wants more of the details, and she needed to know the brain tumor wasn't her fault. We were talking about it recently, and she asked, "Why do I have it, mommy, was I bad?"*

Children should understand that it is expected they will have many questions throughout their treatment, and they should be assured they will be answered honestly. Parents need to let their children know that feeling frightened or upset is normal, indeed is felt by parents and children alike. Open and honest communication is essential for the child to feel loved, supported, and encouraged.

# Feelings

Chapter 1, *Diagnosis,* contains an extensive list of feelings that parents may experience after their child's cancer diagnosis. It is important to remember that children—both siblings and the ill child—are also overwhelmed by strong feelings, and they generally have fewer coping skills than do adults. At varying times and to varying degrees, children and teens may feel fearful, angry, resentful, powerless, violated, lonely, weird, inferior, incompetent, or betrayed.

Children have to learn strategies to deal with these strong feelings to prevent "acting out" behaviors (behavioral problems) or "acting in" behaviors (depression, withdrawal). For some children with cancer, the emotional impact of the disease is intensified by permanent changes to the body. This is especially true for children who have weakness in arms or legs, facial asymmetry, or communication problems.

> Eleven-year-old Zach has lower body weakness from his treatment for spinal spread. It was really hard for him to get used to a wheelchair. At first he liked using it to go bowling, but now he prefers his dad to help him stand and bowl without it. It's not something he talks about, but we know it makes him sad.

The emotional impact may be most pronounced during the teenage years. This is a time when appearance is particularly important. When adolescents look different from their peers, they may have feelings of sadness, anger, bewilderment, helplessness, and fear. Depression is common during and after treatment. Children and teens may go through a period of grieving. It is crucial that the teen receive support and counseling when needed.

> I had cancer when I was 15. I tried so hard as a freshman in college to put it all behind me and get on with my life. It just didn't work. Next to treatment, that was the worst year of my life. It showed me that if I didn't deal with it consciously, I was going to deal with it subconsciously. I had nightmares every night. I'd wake up feeling that I had needles in my arms. I decided to start taking better care of myself in a different kind of way. I do something fun every day. I try to see the positive side of situations. I read more and write a lot. I unplug from the cancer community whenever I feel overwhelmed. I try to explore my feelings rather than shove them in the back corner. Once I started dealing with these feelings, things really improved.

It's sometimes hard for children, and especially teens, to share the news about their cancer with friends. Each must work out a strategy that fits their circumstances.

> I'm going to talk about how you know who your real friends are. I was only 7 and in the first grade when I found out about my brain tumor. I don't remember how long I waited to tell my friends but I knew in my heart that it had to be soon. Well, first I told my closest friend at the time and she said, "No matter what you have we will always be BF4E!"(BF4E means Best Friends 4 Ever!). Then I told the rest of my friends. I was on the playground at school and I asked them would our friendship change if

*one of us were to get cancer? And they said "No." So I told them that I had
it and just like that I lost five to six good friends.*

*The next day at school no one would play let alone come near me (only
my best friend would play with me). I asked her why and she said, "The
kids you told yesterday went and told a lot of kids that if they played with
you (meaning me) that they would get cancer, too." So it took me a long
time to find a way to make them understand that you can't get it from
playing with someone who has it. So, I ran up to my best friend Loren,
and tapped her arm and jokingly told her, "Tag you have cancer now!!"
Loren and I and all of my friends sat down and I explained that you can
NOT get cancer from someone by playing with them!!! Then a few months
later my mom came to my class and explained to my class about what I
had. That day at lunch all my friends that would not play with me the
day before were playing with me.*

*Now I'm in high school and high schoolers can be more unaccepting
than grade school kids. So I think now before I tell about my cancer.*

Good communication is the first step toward helping your family identify how child
behavior and family functioning are being impacted. Talking things over helps family
members and professionals work together to restore order and a nurturing climate.

# Communication

Communicating with your child or teen is the foundation for trust. Children need to
know from the beginning that you will answer questions truthfully and take the time
to talk about feelings. Discussion of several aspects of good communication follows.

## Honesty

Above all else, children need to be able to trust their parents. They can face almost
anything, as long as they know that their parents will be at their side. Trust requires
honesty. For your ill child and her brothers and sisters to feel secure, they must always
know that they can depend on you to tell them the truth, be it good news or bad. This
reduces isolation and a sense of disconnection within the family.

*We were always very honest. We felt that she needed to know that she
could trust us to tell her the truth, however scary that would be. I saw a
few incidents in the clinic of people with totally different styles who didn't
tell their kids the truth. I have run into the bathroom at the clinic crying*

*after overhearing a mother who had deceived her child into coming to the clinic. Then he found out he needed a back poke and completely lost it. It makes me cringe. Children just have to be prepared. If they can't trust their parents, who can they trust?*

## Listening

Just trying to get through each day consumes most parents' time, attention, and energy. Consequently, one of the greatest gifts they can give their children is their time: a special time when they really focus on what their child is saying, when they listen to not only the words, but the feelings that generate them.

> *When my daughter was 7, three years after her treatment ended, I realized how important it was to keep listening. She was complaining about a hangnail and I told her that I would cut it for her. She started to yell that I would hurt her. I asked her, "When have I ever hurt you?" and she said, "In the hospital." I sat down with her in my arms, rocked her, and explained what had happened in the hospital during her treatment, why we had to bring her, and how we felt about it. I told her that I cried along with her when she was hurt by procedures. I asked her to tell me her feelings about being there. We cleared the air that day, and I expect we will need to talk about it many more times in the future. Then she held out her hand so that I could cut off her hangnail.*

It is also helpful for you to talk with your child, the school, and his healthcare providers about strategies for dealing with friendships.

## Talking

If you are not in the habit of talking to your children about how you are feeling, it is hard to start in a crisis. But now, more than ever, it's important to try. Parents can provide an opening for discussion by simply stating how much they miss their other children—for example, "I really miss you when I have to take your sister to the hospital. I'll call you every night just so I can hear your voice," or "Sometimes I really get mad at the cancer. I wish the family didn't have to be separated so much."

It is also helpful to tell your child with cancer how the illness is affecting her siblings—for example, "It is very hard for Jim to stay at home with a babysitter when I bring you to the hospital. Let's try to think of something nice to do for him." These statements not only reassure children of your continued love for them and distress about being separated from them, but creates an opportunity for them to share with you how they feel about what is happening to the family.

> *My daughter, diagnosed when 1 year old and now entering fifth grade, has three older siblings, so we have been through many developmental stages as far as communication goes. I try to answer their questions honestly, but only tell them what I think they can understand without overwhelming them with information. I remember one of my boys, soon after her diagnosis, asked me if she was going to die, and I said "no" emphatically. I regretted it immediately, and realized that I would have to deal with my fears about the possibility of her dying, then go back and tell him the truth. So, later, I told him that I hadn't given an accurate answer because I was scared; that we didn't know if she was going to die, we hoped not, but we would have to wait and see.*

> *I have found that as their understanding deepens, they come back with more questions, needing more detailed answers. So, my motto is, be honest but don't scare them. If you say everything is okay but you are crying, they know something is wrong, and they can't trust you for the truth.*

## Common behavioral changes of children

Discipline under the best of circumstances is difficult. But when one child has a tumor, parents are stressed, siblings are angry, and the situation may become unmanageable. First, you need to decide whether the ill child is going to be treated as if he only has a few months to live, or as if he will survive and needs to learn strategies for how to self-regulate difficult emotions. Then examine your own behavior to see if you are modeling the conduct that you expect from your children. Also, develop a consistent response to the angry or destructive child, which will then help the child develop social and emotional competence.

Barbara Sourkes, an experienced child psychologist, wrote the following in her book *Armfuls of Time: The Psychological Experience of the Child with a Life-Threatening Illness*:

> *While loss of control extends over emotional issues, and ultimately over life itself, its emergence is most vivid in the child's day-to-day experience of the illness, in the barrage of intrusive, uncomfortable or painful procedures that he or she must endure. The child strives desperately to regain a measure of control, often expressed through resistant,*

*noncompliant behavior or aggressive outbursts. Too often, the source of the anger—the loss of control—goes unrecognized by parents and caregivers. However, once its meaning is acknowledged, an explicit distinction may be drawn for the child between what he or she can or cannot dictate. In order to maximize the child's sense of control, the environment can be structured to allow for as much choice as is feasible. Even options that appear small or inconsequential serve as an antidote to loss, and their impact is often reflected in dramatic improvements in behavior.*

In the following sections, parents share how they handled various behaviors of their ill child.

## Anger

Parents respond to the diagnosis of cancer with anger, and so do children. Not only is the child angry at the disease, but also at the parents for bringing her in to be hurt, at having to take medicine that makes her feel terrible, at losing her hair, at losing her friends, and on and on. Children with cancer have good reasons to be angry.

> *We have a case of the halo or the horns. Our son is either very defiant or an absolute angel. He argues about every single thing. I really think that it is because he has had so little control in his life. I have very clear rules, am very firm, and put my foot down. But I also try to choose my battles wisely, so that we can have good times, too. My husband reminds me when I get aggravated, that if he wasn't this type of tough kid, he wouldn't have made it through so many setbacks. Then I am just glad to still have him with us.*

· · · · ·

> *If you talk to Ezra (age 13), he'd tell you he's angry that everything is so hard now. Because of the medulloblastoma and because of treatment, his life is hard every day. Even eating and drinking are work for him.*

## Tantrums

Healthy children have tantrums when they are overwhelmed by strong feelings, and so do children with cancer. In some cases, tantrums can be predicted by parents' paying close attention to what triggers the outburst. This knowledge helps parents prevent tantrums by avoiding situations that create overload for their child. In other cases, there is no warning of the impending tantrum.

*We never knew what would set off 3-year-old Rachel, and to tell the truth, she didn't know what the problem was herself. She was very verbal and aware in many ways, but she had no idea what was bothering her and causing the anger. I would just hold her with her blanket, hug her, and rock until she calmed down. Later she would say, "I was out of control," but she still didn't know why.*

Of course, if the child is destructive, he needs help learning other ways to vent his anger. For a child who is frequently destructive, professional counseling is necessary. *The Misunderstood Child* by Larry Silver has a chapter that explains in detail how parents can initiate a behavior modification program at home.

*My son had frequent, violent rages that sometimes caused damage (toys thrown at the walls, books ripped up). He was small, but strong. I talked to him when he was calm about how the tantrums would be handled. Tantrums with no damage would be ignored; afterwards we would cuddle and talk about what prompted the anger and other ways for him to handle the anger. If he began to break things or hurt people, I would wrap him in a blanket and rock him until he relaxed. I would tell him, "I need to hold you because you are out of control. Soon you will learn how to control yourself." All of the tantrums ended after he went off treatment, but, dealing with his destructive anger was one of the hardest things that I have ever experienced.*

· · · · ·

*My 5-year-old's behavior always intensified at clinic during treatment. He was hyperactive and defiant, to put it nicely. On his very last chemo day, he was hooked up to an infusion pump with a low battery, so his movement was limited to the bed. By the end of the session, he was so mad at being unable to move around, he was screaming at the top of his lungs, and throwing toys. First I tried to calm him, but then I got angry: I told him that he could just forget about the balloon we had in the car, it was gone. Of course, that just made it worse. We were both out of control, and they'll remember us there for quite some time, I'm sure.*

## Withdrawal

Some children deal with their feelings by withdrawing rather than blowing up in anger. Like denial, withdrawal can be temporarily helpful as a way to come to grips with strong feelings. However, too much withdrawal is not good for children. It can also be a sign of the kind of depression that some children suffer. Parents or counselors need to find ways to allow withdrawn children to gently express how they are feeling.

> *The day for our family band gig started out badly. Ez (age 13) was downhearted, green, looked very small, felt nauseated, and hadn't eaten much breakfast. He just sorta sat and stared for an hour as Hannah and I bustled around practicing, writing up the set list and deciding on introductions, and putting gear in the car. I kept asking him did he want to play trumpet a bit with us and he said no. We got to the site, it was a glorious day, the band before us was wonderful, everybody was smiling, but Ez sat hunched on a bench. I was in despair. I also was, practically, fearing he might throw up on stage. So we got up there and this is what happened: he played badly, but he was a good presence. He introduced some of the songs and was so funny the audience howled. He was relaxed and smiling even as at one point he dropped the bomb, saying through the microphone: "I just want you to know I used to play trumpet better than this before I had cancer." He rallied for the last couple songs, and nailed the ending of the last piece wonderfully. The most amazing thing, though, was that he was instantly in a wonderful smiley proud mood as we got off stage and had a huge appetite after.*

## Regression

Children with CNS tumors sometimes experience times of regression, which may appear during treatment or can be triggered by post-traumatic stress once treatment is over.

> *Jimmy used baby talk and reverted to infantile behavior for a while after surgery for debulking the brain tumor. He's almost 6, and he still sometimes asks to be wrapped like a baby and held as if taking a bottle. So we smile and laugh, and talk to him like a baby.*

## Comfort objects

Many parents worry when, after diagnosis, young children regress to using a special comfort object. Many young children ask to return to using a bottle or they cling to a favorite toy or blanket, and some children feel safer when they have a parent sleeping in the same room. It is reasonable to allow your child to use whatever he can to find comfort against the terrible realities of treatment. The behaviors usually stop either when the child starts feeling better or when treatment ends.

*Matthew had a special teddy bear that a friend had bought for him while visiting Germany. Mr. Bear, as he was called, went through everything Matthew went through. When he received cranial radiation, Mr. Bear had his skull irradiated, too. If Matthew needed oxygen, they both got a mask. That little teddy bear even had surgery a few times. Each time my son was admitted to the hospital, Mr. Bear went along and got his own hospital identification bracelet. They went through a lot together. It's amazing how much comfort he received from a stuffed toy.*

· · · · ·

*When Ayla (32 months) finally came home from the hospital after treatment for medulloblastoma, I decided to sleep with her. We were crammed into a small bed but I got to spend more time with her (you never know what the future may hold) and she knew that if she needed love all she had to do was open her eyes and see me there. Love has healing qualities. I think that the physical closeness somehow transfers the love. As we sleep and our body lets down its defenses, the love can flow back and forth much easier. So despite what our American culture believes, I think that if your child wants you to sleep right beside them, you should.*

## Talking about death

Part of effective parenting is allowing children to talk about topics that cause discomfort. In many cultures, the subject of death has become taboo. A diagnosis of a CNS tumor forces both parents and children to acknowledge that death is a very real possibility. Even children as young as 3 years old think about death and what it means.

*Eighteen months into treatment, 5-year-old Katy said, "Mommy, sometimes I think about my spirit leaving my body. I think my spirit is here (gesturing to the back of her head) and my body is here (pointing to her bellybutton). I just wanted you to know that I think about it sometimes."*

· · · · ·

*My son is a teenager and has to face some difficult issues with death. Just as my son finished treatment for medulloblastoma, another boy a year ahead of my son in our school was diagnosed with a glioblastoma multiforme brain tumor and died within nine months. It was very hard for my son and one of his teachers even said to him after the death, "I guess this puts things into perspective for you." Like he needed to be reminded. Also, three of his roommates from cancer camp have died in the past year and they were all brain tumor kids. It is like they are being put face-to-face with their own mortality. These kids are extremely intuitive, they know the score. All you can do is be there for them, to listen, to support them, to hold and love them.*

## Trusting your child

Sometimes, if parents listen to their children, they will say what they need to do to persevere. It may not be the way the parents cope; it may make them nervous. But, it is the child or teen's way to make peace with the day to day reality of diagnosis and treatment.

> *Early one summer morning, 12-year-old Preston and I left the hospital after a week-long stay. He had been heavily sedated, and was groggy and shaky on his feet. My husband and daughter were getting ready to go on a boat trip, and I felt Preston was too sick to go. We sadly saw them off, then returned to the car. Preston said, "Mom, I really need to go fishing. I know you don't understand, but I really need to do this."*
>
> *It made me very uncomfortable, but we went home to get his equipment. We then drove up to the mountains to a very deserted spot on the river, and Preston said that he needed to be out of my sight. So, I watched him put on his waders, walk into the swift river and disappear around a bend upstream. I went out into the river and sat on a rock. I waited for two hours before Preston came back. He said, "That's what I needed; I feel much better now."*

There is a fine line between providing adequate protection for our children or teens and becoming overly controlling because of worry about the disease. You might ask yourself, "If she didn't have cancer, would I let her do this?"

## Coping well

Many children develop emotional competence from facing and coping with the difficulties of cancer. Others, because of both temperament and the environments in which they have lived, are blessed with good coping abilities. They understand what is required, and they do it. A young adult survivor offers his thoughts:

> *I'll be finishing my last round of radiation today. I have an oligodendroglioma tumor on my right temporal lobe. I've been having some crazy feeling aura seizures. I do feel like I'm losing it at times.*

*I definitely feel it's okay to worry. Believe me, I have my times for sure! I like to get together with as many friends as I can and go to the beach and check out the waves and smell the air. Definitely have to be listening to music. Talk to as many people as I can surround myself with and of course be alone to hit up the computer and sleep. The telephone seems to be a good friend too. I feel that I have too many lives to touch before I'm all said and done.*

Many parents expressed great admiration for their child's strength and grace in the face of adversity.

*Stephan has not had any behavior problems while being treated for his initial diagnosis (age 5) or his relapse (age 7). He has never complained about going to the hospital and views the medical staff as his friends. He has never argued or fought about painful treatments. Unlike many of the parents in the support group, we've never had to deal with any emotional issues. We are fortunate that he has that confident personality. He just says, "We've got to do it, so let's just get it done."*

# Common behavioral changes of parents

It's impossible to talk about children's behavior without discussing parental behavior. Children's development does not occur in a vacuum, but rather in the context of their family. At different times during their child's treatment, parents may be under physical, emotional, financial, and existential stress. Their worries are endless. The crisis can cause them to behave in ways of which they are not always proud.

Some of the problem behaviors mentioned by veteran parents follow.

## Dishonesty

Children feel safe when their parents are honest with them. If the parents start to keep secrets from the child or "protect" him from bad news, the child feels isolated and fearful. He thinks, "If mom and dad won't tell me, it must be really bad," or "Mom won't talk about it. I guess there's nobody that I can tell about how scared I am."

Denial is a type of "unconscious" dishonesty. This occurs when parents say things to children such as, "Everything will be just fine" or "It won't hurt a bit." This type of pretending just increases the distance between child and parent, leaving children with no support. However horrible the truth, it seldom is as terrifying to a child as a half-truth upon which his imagination builds.

*I try so hard to be honest with my 5-year-old son, but blood draws, which he thinks of as "shots," are just so hard for him. Every doctor's visit, that's his first question, "I'm going to get a shot?" and you just want to say no. My husband's the one who started saying, "It'll be fine," but the anxiety that came up later at the appointment was so much worse, I put an end to that pretty quickly. Now I say, "Yes, but just once," because if I say, "I don't know," it just makes him worry.*

## Depression

Feelings of sadness or depression may occur in parents of children with brain or spinal cord tumors. If you are consistently experiencing any of the following symptoms, get professional help: changes in sleeping patterns (sleeping too much, waking up frequently during the night, awakening in the early morning), appetite disturbances (eating too little or too much), decreased sex drive, fatigue, panic attacks, inability to experience pleasure, feelings of sadness and despair, poor concentration, social withdrawal, feelings of worthlessness, suicidal thoughts, and drug or alcohol abuse. If a parent becomes depressed, children may be neglected. Depression is very common and very treatable and should be dealt with early.

*Find a counselor you "click with." Stick with that person until you truly feel some peace about your experiences and strength for dealing with the ongoing stress of treatment or whatever else might come up. I regret that I toughed it out and didn't recognize the depression I was experiencing for such a long time. I think finding sources of support in a variety of ways at the earliest moment possible can greatly mitigate long-term difficulties in coping, such as depression.*

• • • • •

*It was two years after my son finished treatment that my depression became severe enough that I recognized it. I actually had a lot of suicidal thoughts and my husband urged me to see a doctor. He started me on Zoloft and it has helped me tremendously.*

## Losing your temper excessively

All parents lose their temper sometimes. They lose their tempers with spouses, healthy children, pets, and even strangers. But it is especially painful when the target of the anger is a very sick child. Abuse of spouses and children increases at times when either or both spouses feel incompetent and powerless. If you find yourself unable to control your temper, seek professional counseling.

*I had my share of temper tantrums. The worst was when he was having his radiation. I tried to make him eat because it would be so many hours before he could have any more food. He always threw up all over himself and me, several times, every morning. It seemed like we changed clothing at least three times before we even got out of the house each day. I remember one day just screaming at him, "Can't you even learn how to throw up? Can't you just bend over to barf?" I really flunked mother of the year that day. I can't believe that I was screaming at this sick little kid, who I love so much.*

· · · · ·

*I had always taught my children that feeling anger was okay, but we had to make good choices about what to do with it. Hitting other people or breaking things was a bad choice; hitting pillows, running around outside, or listening to music were good choices. But, as with everything else, they learned the most from watching how I handled my anger, and during the hard months of treatment my temper was short. When I found myself thinking of hitting them, I'd say, in a very loud voice, "I'm afraid I'm going to hurt somebody so I'm going in my room for a time-out." If my husband was home, I'd take a warm shower to calm down; if he wasn't, I'd just sit on the bed and take as many deep breaths as it took to calm down.*

## Unequal application of household rules

You will guarantee family problems if the ill child enjoys favored status while the siblings must do extra chores. Granted, it is hard to know the right time to insist that your ill child must resume making his bed or setting the table, but it must be done. Siblings need to know from the very beginning that any child in the family, if sick, will be excused from chores, but will have do them again as soon as he is physically able.

*I spoiled my sick daughter and tried to enforce the rules for my son. That didn't work, so I gave up on him and spoiled them both. He was really acting out at school. What he needed was structure and more attention, but what he got was more and more things. They both ended up thinking the whole world revolved around them, and it was my fault.*

A child life specialist comments:

*It's hard for parents to learn that saying "No" is okay, especially when there is only one child. One mom told me the other day that it's easier for her because there are two kids, and if it was just the child undergoing treatment, he'd get away with a lot more, but the sister has to do 'X, Y, and Z' and so her brother does, too. But it's hard to learn to say, "No, you don't get everything you want when we go to the grocery store," or "No, you don't get a new toy every single time you leave clinic."*

## Overindulgence of the ill child

Overindulgence is a very common behavior of parents toward their child with a tumor.

*I bought my daughter everything that I saw that was pretty and lovely. I kept thinking that if she died she would die happy because she'd be surrounded by all these beautiful things. Even when I couldn't really afford it, I kept buying. I realize now that I was doing it to make me feel better, not her. She needed cuddling and loving, not clothes and dolls.*

• • • • •

*Someone asked me once if I didn't want to spoil him rotten or baby him because he might not survive. I said, "No, because what would I do if he does survive? I'd have a raging brat." So we just try to be normal and discipline like we would if he didn't have cancer. We don't let him get away with murder. We don't believe in hitting, but we do use time-outs, loss of privileges, and loss of opportunities to do things he enjoys.*

One aspect of overindulgence that is quite common is the parent's reluctance to teach the sick child life skills. After years of dealing with a physically weak and sometimes emotionally demanding child, parents may forget to expect age-appropriate skills.

*I realized that I had formed a habit of treating my child as if she was still young and sick. I was still treating her like a 3-year-old, and she was 7. One day, when I was pouring her juice, I thought, "Why am I doing this? She's 7. She needs to learn to make her own sandwiches and pour her own drinks. She needs to be encouraged to grow up." Boy, it has been hard. But I've stuck to my guns, and made other extended family members do it, too. I want her to grow up to be an independent adult, not a demanding, overgrown kid.*

## Overprotection of sick child

For a child to feel normal, he needs to be treated as if she is normal. Ask the doctor what changes in physical activity are necessary for safety, and do not impose any additional restrictions that go beyond this on your child. Let the child be involved in sports or neighborhood play, and even though it is hard, stop yourself from issuing constant reminders to "be careful."

*Life seemed to be finally returning to "normal." Surgery to remove tumor regrowth went great, all visible tumor removed, still low-grade. Only slight peripheral vision deficit, off all the meds, physically growing like crazy. Life was great!*

*Then, Michael (now 16) goes off snowboarding with some adult friends a couple of hours away from home. Sent that insurance card along, just in case. Hardly an hour or two goes by and the phone rings. Michael has "wiped out" and is on the way to the hospital in an ambulance! (My stomach does one of those nosedives again, the kind I thought we could leave behind, at least for a while). He doesn't remember why he wiped out and of course the first aid attendants flipped out when they removed his helmet and saw that nice big scar. After an hour ride to the hospital and several hours sitting in waiting rooms (hasn't this poor boy done his lifetime's worth of doctor visits yet?), a CAT scan reveals no problems— ruled out a concussion and sent back to the slopes—too late to do any more snowboarding. But I am devastated. Here come the sleepless nights again. I will start worrying why he wiped out—was it a focal seizure? It's almost PMS (pre-MRI syndrome) time anyways; scan to be done at the end of the month. Perhaps we ditched the Dilantin too soon. Michael hates to be on it, so he pushes the doctor to get him off as soon as possible.*

*Can't life ever be normal for this family again? And Michael! The one time he gets a chance to leave the doctors and the tests and the waiting rooms and the crazy, nervous mom behind and now his special day is ruined.*

· · · · ·

*My 6-year-old son finished his radiation and is still on chemo for his medulloblastoma. I feel like I have to lighten up in order for life to go on. So I just let the nanny take all four kids on a four-hour drive to spend eight hours at Six Flags. It just about drove us nuts with worry, but they all came home safe and sound. They felt like they had a normal sibling outing.*

· · · · ·

*Alissa (age 8) has metal rods to support her spine following multiple operations for spinal astrocytoma. She uses a wheelchair right now. We don't protect Alissa like she's going to break. On Fourth of July, she sat in the middle of the stands with all her friends for the fireworks, and then she cruised the field later like everybody else. The mayor of our city gave her*

*an award for being the first and only person in a wheelchair to perform the*
*pledge of allegiance at the city council meeting (she went with her Brownie*
*troop), and she will be participating in a fashion show with her Brownie*
*troop to raise funds for our neurological institute.*

## Not spending enough time with the sibling(s)

Although they acknowledge that there are only so many hours in a day, the parents interviewed for this book felt guilty about the effect of the cancer on the siblings. They wished that they had asked family and friends to stay with the sick child more often, allowing them to use more of their precious time with the siblings. Many expressed pain that they didn't know how severely affected the siblings had been.

> *I try to find some time in each holiday/weekend/whenever it is just for*
> *Christopher and me. No matter how ill Michael is, someone else can cope*
> *with it for an hour or two, and nothing is allowed to interfere with that.*
> *We still go out, even if it is only him and me in McDonald's.*
>
> *Bottom line is that all mothers have to accept that along with the baby*
> *is delivered a large package of guilt, and whatever we do for one we will*
> *wish we had done it for the other.*
>
> *But I don't think you can put one child on hold for the duration of the*
> *other's illness, because the year that Christopher has lost while Michael*
> *has been ill won't ever come again. He'll only be 11 once, just as surely as*
> *Michael will only be 14 once (or possibly forever) and we owe it to our*
> *healthy kids to allow them to be just that.*

## Using substance abuse to cope

Some parents find themselves turning to alcohol or drugs to help them cope. Not only illegal drugs are abused; overuse of over-the-counter sleeping pills or other medications also occurs. If you find yourself drinking so that your behavior is affected or using drugs to get through the day or night, seek professional help.

## Coping

Some parents have no major problems adjusting to the diagnosis and treatment of their child with a CNS tumor. They find unexpected reserves of strength and are able to ask for help from their friends and family when they need it. They realize that different needs arise when there is a great stress to the family, and they alter their expectations and parenting accordingly. These families usually had strong and effective communication prior to the illness, and they pull together as a unit to deal with it.

The majority of families, however, have periods of calmness and other times when nerves are frayed and tempers short. But families usually survive intact and are often strengthened by the years of dealing with cancer.

> *After twelve years living with Jen's glioma, I have made my own peace with the fact that I may not be able to prevent or choose what Jen has to deal with. I can, however, make a difference in how we go through it so she finds peace and comfort.*

> *We have been truly blessed by most of the care Jen has received. We have felt the compassion of those who have been willing to recognize the feelings of this process as a part of the medicine and were willing to communicate and acknowledge that to Jen and to us. For her that makes a tremendous difference in how she responds.*

# Improving communication and discipline

Parents suggest the following ways to keep the family on a more even keel:

- Make sure that the family rules are clearly understood by all of the children. Stressed children feel safe in homes that are very structured with regular, predictable routines.

- Have all caretakers consistently enforce the family rules.

> *We kept the same household rules. I was determined that we needed to start with the expectation that Rachel was going to survive. I never wanted her to be treated like a "poor little sick kid" because I was afraid she would become one. We had to be careful about babysitters because we didn't want anyone to feel sorry for her or treat her differently. I do feel that we avoided many long-term behavior problems by adopting this attitude early.*

- Give all the kids some power by offering choices and letting them completely control some aspects of their lives, as appropriate.

> *For a few months we ignored Shawn's two brothers as we struggled to get a handle on the situation. We just shuttled them around with no consideration for their feelings. When we realized how unfair we were being, we made a list of places to stay, and let them choose each time we*

*had to go off to the hospital. We worked it out together, and things went much smoother.*

- Take control of the incoming gifts. Too many gifts make the ill child worry excessively ("If I'm getting all of these great presents, things must be really bad") and makes the siblings jealous. Be specific if you want people not to bring gifts, or if you want gifts for each child, not just the sick one.

    *Paige has a sister, Chelsea, who was 5 at diagnosis, and a brother, Dan, who was 4 months old. Chelsea had a very difficult time. She didn't like it that Paige was getting so many presents and she often felt left out. When I would try to do something special for her, she would get mad—she just wanted normalcy.*

- Recognize that some problems are caused solely by the drugs. It helps to remember that these children are not naturally defiant or destructive. They are feeling sick, powerless, and altered by massive doses of toxic drugs, and they need both sympathy and clear limits. Remember, when they get off the drugs, their real personalities will return.

    *In the beginning, my 2-year-old daughter was incredibly angry. She would have massive temper tantrums, and I would just hold her and tell her that I wouldn't let her hurt anybody. I would continue to hold her until she changed from angry to sad. When she was on the dexamethasone, she would either be hugging me or pinching, biting, or sucking my neck. It drove me crazy. Now she's not having as many fits, but she still pushes her sisters off swings or the trampoline. She has a general lack of control. Sometimes, when I can't stand it anymore, I swat her on the bottom, and then I feel really bad.*

- If your child likes to draw, paint, knit, or do collages or other artwork, encourage it. Art is both soothing and therapeutic, and it allows the child a positive outlet for feelings and creativity. Making something beautiful really helps raise children's spirits. Recognize, however, that powerful emotions may surface for both child and parents through the child's writing or artwork.

- Allow your child to be totally in charge of his art. Do not make suggestions or criticize (e.g., "stay inside the lines" or "skies need to be blue not orange"). Rather, encourage them and praise their efforts. Display the artwork in your home. Listen carefully if your child offers an explanation of the art, but do not pry if it is private. Above all, do not interpret it yourself or disagree with your child on what the art represents. Being supportive will allow your child to explore ways to soothe himself and clarify strong feelings.

> *Jody was continually making "projects." We kept him supplied with a fishing box full of materials, and he glued and taped and constructed all sorts of sculptures. He did beautiful drawings full of color, and every person he drew always had hands shaped like hearts. If we asked him what he was making, he always answered, "I'll show you when I'm done."*

- Come up with acceptable ways for your child to physically release anger. Some options are: ride a bike, run around the house, swing, play basketball or soccer, pound nails into wood, mold clay, punch pillows, yell, take a shower or bath, or draw angry pictures. In addition, teach your child to use words to express her anger—for example, "It makes me furious when you do that," or "I am so mad I feel like hitting you." Releasing anger physically and expressing anger verbally are both valuable life skills to master.

> *Shawn was very, very angry many times. We had clear rules that it was okay to be angry, but he couldn't hit people. We bought a punching bag which he really pounded sometimes. Play-Doh helped, too. We had a machine to make Play-Doh shapes which took a lot of effort. He would hit it, pound it, push it, roll it. Then he would press it through the machine and keep turning that handle. It seemed to really help him with his aggression.*

> • • • • •

> *Our therapist recommended that we have our 5-year-old daughter make an "angry sheet." She should be encouraged to draw or write what she felt like doing when she was angry, and encouraged to get it all out. It was pretty scary, because she drew pictures of stamping people, gouging their eyes out, shooting them, etc. It was amazing how much better she felt afterwards. Then we went through the pictures together and discussed which ones she could really do, and which ones she could only think about doing because really doing it would hurt someone.*

- Treat the ill child as normally as possible.

> *When Justin was in the hospital, I could never stand to see him in those little hospital gowns. I asked if we could dress him in his own outfits, and they said yes. So even when he was in the ICU with all the tubes coming out of his body, we dressed him every day in something cute. It just felt better to see him in his clothes. Several months later my mother said that she had really admired us for doing that because we were sending the*

*message to Justin that everything was going to be okay. That even though he couldn't breathe on his own, he was still going to get up every day and get dressed. Now I think it probably did communicate to him that things were going to be normal again.*

- Get professional help whenever you are concerned or run out of ideas on how to handle emotional problems. Mental healthcare professionals (see Chapter 19, *Sources of Support*) have spent years learning how to help resolve these kinds of problems, so let them help you.

    *My daughter and I both went to a wonderful therapist throughout most of her treatment for cancer. My daughter was a very sensitive, easily overwhelmed child, who withdrew more and more into a world of fantasy as cancer treatment progressed. The therapist was skilled at drawing out her feelings through artwork and play. She also helped me with very specific suggestions on parenting.*

Most emotional problems that children develop as a result of treatment for cancer can be resolved by professional counseling. However, some children may also need medications to get them through particularly rough times.

    *My daughter was doing really well throughout treatment until a combination of events occurred that was more than she could handle. Her grandmother died from cancer during the summer, one of her friends with cancer died on December 27, then another friend with cancer relapsed for the second time. She was fine during the day, but at night she constantly woke up stressed and upset. She had dreams about trapdoors, witches brewing potions to give to little children, and saw people coming into her room to take her away. She would wake up smelling smoke. She was awake three or four hours in the middle of the night, every night. Her doctor put her on sleeping pills and anti-anxiety medications, and the social worker came out to the house twice a month.*

- Teach children relaxation or visualization skills to help them cope better with strong feelings.

- Have reasonable expectations. If you are expecting a sick 4-year-old to act like a healthy 6-year-old, or a teenager to act like an adult, you are setting your child up to fail.

- As often as possible, try to end the day on a positive note. If your child is being disruptive or if your feelings toward your child are very negative, here's an exercise that can end the day in a pleasant way. At bedtime, parent and child each tell one another something they did that day that made them proud of themselves, something they like about themselves, and something they are looking forward to the next day. Then a hug and a sincere "I love you" bring the day to a calm and loving close.

- Try to maintain a sense of humor. Laughing at the silly things that happen provides new energy for dealing with the serious stuff.

> *I attended a talk by a PhD counselor, on facing life changes and transitions. I had no clue who he was or what his presentation would be like. Turns out he's a very popular speaker on coping skills and a slick comedian to boot. He had us laughing the whole time. I must've needed it, because I was laughing and crying at the same time, which I guess was the point.*

# Checklist for parenting stressed children

A group of veteran parents compiled the following checklist to help you parent your stressed child:

- Model the type of behavior you desire. If you talk respectfully and take time-outs when angry, you are teaching your children to do so. If you scream and hit, that is how your children will handle their anger.
- Seek professional help for any behaviors that trouble you.
- Teach your children to talk about their feelings.
- Listen to your children with understanding and empathy.
- Be honest and admit your mistakes.
- Help your children to examine why they are behaving as they are.
- Distinguish between feelings (always okay) and acting on strong feelings in destructive or hurtful ways (not okay).
- Have clear rules and consequences for violations.
- Teach children to recognize when they are losing control.
- Discuss acceptable outlets for anger.
- Give frequent reassurances of your love.
- Provide plenty of hugs and physical affection.
- Notice and compliment your child for good behavior.

- Recognize that the disturbing behaviors result from stress, pain, and drugs.

- Remember that with lots of structure, love, humor, and time the problems will become more manageable.

Our children look to us to learn how to handle adversity. They learn how to cope from us. Although it is extremely difficult to live through your child's diagnosis and treatment for a CNS tumor, it must be done. So we each need to reach deep into our hearts and minds to help our children endure and grow.

*Children Learn What They Live*

*If a child lives with criticism, he learns to condemn.*

*If a child lives with hostility, he learns to fight.*

*If a child lives with ridicule, he learns to be shy.*

*If a child lives with shame, he learns to feel guilty.*

*If a child lives with tolerance, he learns to be patient.*

*If a child lives with encouragement, he learns confidence.*

*If a child lives with praise, he learns to appreciate.*

*If a child lives with fairness, he learns justice.*

*If a child lives with security, he learns to have faith.*

*If a child lives with approval, he learns to like himself.*

*If a child lives with acceptance and friendship,*

*He learns to find love in the world.*

—Dorothy Law Nolte

# CHAPTER 16

# Siblings

A CHRONIC ILLNESS SUCH AS A CNS TUMOR OR CHILDHOOD CANCER touches all members of the family, with especially long-lasting effects on siblings. The diagnosis creates an array of conflicting emotions in siblings. Not only are the siblings concerned about their ill brother or sister, but they usually resent the turmoil that the family has been thrown into. They often feel jealous of the gifts and attention showered on the sick child, yet feel guilty for having these emotions. The days, months, and years after diagnosis can be difficult for the sibling of a child with cancer.

This chapter starts with ways to explain the diagnosis of a CNS tumor to the well siblings. It also discusses common emotions and behaviors of the siblings. Parents and siblings then share their experiences and ways that they cope.

## Telling the sibling

The diagnosis of a CNS tumor is traumatic for siblings. Family life is disrupted, time with parents decreases, and a large amount of attention is paid to the ill child. Brothers and sisters need as much knowledge as their sick sibling. Information provided should be age appropriate, and all questions should be answered honestly. Healthcare providers (physicians, nurse practitioners, child life specialists, and social workers) can assist parents in educating the well siblings. Siblings can be extremely cooperative if they understand the changes that occur in the family and their role in helping the family cope. Maintaining open communication and respecting their feelings helps siblings feel loved and secure.

> Our situation is different in that Mary Margaret has been having health problems since early infancy. She was diagnosed with neurofibromatosis when she was 13 months old, and with an optic glioma when she was 4. With us, it's been a matter of Rhys, who is four years older than his sister, always knowing there have been problems with MM, rather than coming home from the hospital and gravely saying, "Son, your sister has a brain

*tumor." We did have to inform him when, after a period of tumor growth, we were advised to start chemo. Obviously, this had a major impact on him as well as the rest of us: on our family dynamic, on the time we spent together. My husband already worked long hours, and most of the childcare falls to me, so I knew "chemo duty" would fall to me as well. We do have a lot of extended family and lots of friends who were more than willing to help us out with the nuts and bolts, keeping Rhys while we were gone for treatment, getting him to ball games and practices and school.*

Even with optimum communication and support, however, parents may see behavior changes such as anger, guilt, jealousy, sadness, regression, school problems, and symptoms of illness to gain attention. These result from the stress of living with a brother or sister diagnosed with a CNS tumor.

# Emotional and behavioral responses of the siblings

Brothers and sisters are shaken to the very core by cancer in the family. Parents often have no time, and little energy, to focus on the siblings. During this major crisis for the siblings—this time when their beings are flooded with anger and concern, jealousy and love, when they are in conflict as never before—they often have no one to turn to for help. They may feel utterly alone in their pain. If you recognize these strong emotions of siblings as normal, not pathological, you will be better able to help your child talk about and cope with her overpowering feelings.

Although the time after diagnosis is emotionally potent, stress levels associated with life-threatening illnesses tend to decrease over time. Siblings also tend to have good psychological outcomes. In many cases, siblings report the experience as life changing in many positive ways.

## Concern for sick brother or sister

Children really worry about their sick brother or sister. It is hard for them to watch someone they love physically change, be hurt by needles, sickened by medicines, gain or lose weight, and be bald. It is hard to feel so healthy and full of energy when the brother or sister has to stay indoors because of weakness or low blood counts. The siblings may also be old enough to understand that death is a possibility. There are plenty of reasons for concern.

> *My 10-year-old son Travis has had two brain bleeds since treatment for his tumor. It's hard for Travis' little brother Gregory. Here he had a big brother who took care of him and nurtured him, and now his brother can't talk, can't walk, and is totally disabled. The other night, I found Gregory sitting on the stairs crying. I asked him what was wrong, and he said, "I want all of us to watch TV together. I miss my brother watching TV with me."*

## Fear

It is very common for young siblings of children with cancer to think that the disease is contagious, that they can "catch it." Many also worry that one or both parents may get cancer. The diagnosis of a CNS tumor changes children's views that the world is a safe place. They feel vulnerable, and they are afraid. Some siblings develop symptoms of illness in an attempt to regain attention from the parents.

Fears of things other than cancer may emerge: fear of being hit by a car, fear of dogs, and fear of strangers. Many fears can be quieted by accurate and age-appropriate explanations from the parents or medical staff.

> *It's almost midnight, which means that it will be exactly 36 hours before my sister Kylie goes for her first MRI after radiation. I don't know what to expect, but I would really love to hear some positive words coming from the oncologist's mouth when we meet up with him to receive the results. I can hardly sleep because, although I am always hoping for a miracle, I constantly worry, to the extent of having nightmares, about hearing something that I don't want to hear.*

## Jealousy

Despite feeling concern for the ill brother or sister, almost all siblings also feel jealous. Presents and cards flood in for the sick child, Mom and Dad stay at the hospital with the sick child, and most conversations revolve around the sick child. When the siblings go out to play, the neighbors ask about the sick child. At school, teachers are concerned about the sick child. Is it any wonder that they feel jealous?

The siblings' lives are in turmoil, and, being human, they feel a need to blame someone. It's natural for them to think that if their brother didn't get sick, life would be back to normal.

> *Our 9-year-old son seemed to be dealing with things so well until one evening as I was tucking him in he confided that he had tried to break his leg*

*at school by jumping out of the swing. He began to cry and told me he
doesn't want his brother to be sick anymore; that he needs some attention,
too. I was always so concerned with our sick child that I didn't realize how
much our healthy child was suffering.*

## Guilt

Young children are egocentric; they feel that the world revolves around them. It is
logical to them to feel that, because their sister has cancer, they caused it. They may
have said in anger, "I hope you get sick and die," and then their sister got sick.

This notion should be dispelled right after diagnosis. Children really need to be told,
many times, that cancer just happens, and no one in the family caused it. They need
to understand that just because you think something or say something, it doesn't
make it happen.

Beyond feeling guilt for causing the cancer, most siblings feel shame for their normal
emotional responses to cancer, like anger and jealousy. They think, "How can I feel
this way about my brother when he's so sick?" Assure them that the many conflicting
feelings they are experiencing are normal and expected. As a parent, share some of
your conflicting feelings (anger at the behavior of a child on prednisone, guilt about
being angry).

Some children even feel guilt for being healthy! They think, "Why should I feel great
when he's so frail and sick?"

## Abandonment

When parental attention revolves around the sick child, siblings may feel isolated
and resentful. Even when parents make a conscious effort not to be so preoccupied
with the ill child, siblings still perceive that they are not getting their fair share of
attention and may feel rejected.

*Jay had undergone many surgeries as a child, besides treatment for an
anaplastic ependymoma. On a well-child visit, the doctor said he was
concerned about his left eye turning in, and surgery for stabismus repair was
recommended. This noncancer-related surgery unearthed memories. Jealous
feelings from Jay's numerous surgeries, from the cancer days, resurfaced in
our 15-year-old daughter, Vanessa. "It's not fair, when Jay has surgery,
nobody does anything special for me." Her anger is wholly that of the 10-
year-old girl she was when her brother suddenly developed a brain tumor.*

## Sadness

Siblings have many very good reasons to feel sad. They miss their parents and the time they used to spend together. They miss the life they used to have, the one they were comfortable with. They worry that their brother or sister may die. Some children show their sadness by crying often; others withdraw and become depressed. Often children confide in relatives or friends that they think their parents don't love them anymore.

> When Jeremy was very sick and hospitalized, we sent his older brother Jason to his grandparents for long periods of time. We thought that he understood the reasons, but a year after Jeremy finished treatment, Jason (9 years old) said, "Of course, I know that you love Jeremy more than me anyway. You were always sending me away so that you could spend time with him." It just broke my heart that every time he made that long drive over the mountains with his grandparents, he was thinking that he was being sent away.

## Anger

A brother or sister's diagnosis of cancer disrupts children's lives, and it can make siblings very angry. Questions such as "Why did this happen to us?" or "Why can't things be the way they used to be?" are common. Children's anger may be directed at their sick brother parents, relatives, friends, or doctor. Children's anger may have a variety of causes—for instance, being left with babysitters so often, unequal application of family rules, or additional responsibilities at home. Because each member of the family may have frayed nerves, explosions of temper can occur.

## Regression

Siblings may react by regressive behavior. This includes bedwetting or toileting accidents in preschool children who are toilet trained. Temper tantrums, thumb sucking, clinging to parents, and generally acting younger than their age are quite normal.

## School Problems

Siblings may experience difficulty in school after the diagnosis of a CNS tumor in their brother or sister. This may manifest in behavioral or social problems or decline in academic performance.

# Worrying about what happens at the hospital

Children have vivid imaginations, and when they are fueled by disrupted households and whispered conversations between teary parents, children can imagine truly horrible things. Seeing how their ill sister looks upon returning from a hospital stay can reinforce their fears that awful things happen at the clinic or hospital. Or, the sibling may think they are missing some grand parties when they see their sister and parent come home from the hospital with presents and balloons.

Age-appropriate, verbal explanations can help children understand what happens at the hospital, but nothing is as powerful as a visit. Of course the effectiveness of a visit depends on your child's age and temperament, but many parents said bringing the siblings along helps everyone. The sibling gains an accurate understanding of hospital procedures, the sick child is comforted by the presence of the sibling, and the parent gets to spend time with both (or more) children.

> We made sure that Jasmine (age 1) was with us for everything. She gave me love at a difficult time and her being with us always made her know that she was still a part of our family despite being involved in a tragic thing and despite that her sister Aylu (32 months) got so much attention. Hospitals can be fun playgrounds for kids.

Another way to minimize worry is reading age-appropriate books together. Many children's hospitals have coloring books for preschoolers that explain hospital procedures with pictures and clear language. Adolescents might be helped by seeing videos on the subject or joining a sibling support group.

Veteran parents suggest that another way to reduce siblings' worries is to allow even the youngest children to help the family in some way. As long as children have clear explanations of the situation and concrete jobs to do that will benefit the family, they tend to rise to the occasion. Make them feel they are a necessary and integral part of the family's effort to face cancer together.

> My younger kids have never known 11-year-old Zach as "normal." He had his first surgery at 5 years old, when Emily was 3 and Sarah was barely 1. Emily helped Zach go through three months of inpatient rehabilitation, when he relearned how to walk, talk, chew, swallow, etc.! Zach having a brain tumor is all they know.
>
> All Zach's life, they treated him normally. No one ever let him win at games or anything (although I tried to make them). When we found out

*about the relapse, something got back to Emily in third grade. She got off the bus one day and asked if Zach was dying. I was shocked! I told her that his tumor was back but we were taking him to the best brain tumor doctor and we would do everything we could so he wouldn't die. That seemed to totally satisfy her.*

*There was only one time that I remember Emily's and Sarah's teachers both telling me at parent conferences that the girls had been chatting a lot and not listening much. At the time, we were going through more surgery with Zach, so I think that is why.*

*Lauren is 4. This past summer, Zach took horseback riding for physical therapy. It was great! The girls would take turns coming to watch. Well, one day, Lauren was watching and she picked out this beautiful horse and said, "When I have my brain tumor, I'm going to ride that horse." Oh my gosh! Can you imagine? It's just so normal to them.*

*As far as I can tell, none of them have issues with embarrassment over Zach or anything like that. Often they think he is lucky because he can ride in the wheelchair (and they have to walk) or he was lucky because he got to ride horses. They all have a deep faith and pray a lot for Zach and other kids with brain tumors.*

*They also seem to reach out more to others. The oldest two belong to Chemo Angels where they volunteer to send out small cards or packages twice a week to a child with cancer.*

You can find out more about Chemo Angels at: *http://www.chemoangels.com.*

*Alissa's older brother Nicholas is her best friend. We are at the hospital for appointments and therapy three nights a week, every week. Nicholas helps Alissa with "hospital homework" and he also helps with her therapy. Nicholas is doing great at school. We include him on everything.*

## Concern about parents

Exhausted parents often are not aware of the strong feelings of their healthy children. They sometimes assume that children understand that they are loved and would be getting the same attention if they were the ones who had cancer. But siblings frequently do not share their powerful feelings of anger, jealousy, or worry because they love their parents and do not want to place additional burdens on them. It is all too common to hear siblings say, "I have to be the strong one. I don't want to cause my parents any more pain." But burdens are lighter if shared, and parents need to try to encourage all of their children to talk about how they are feeling.

## Sibling experiences

Simply understanding the depth of the pain and fears of your "healthy" children eases their path. Even if parents do not have large amounts time to spend with them, siblings need to hear that what they feel matters. If parents understand that these overwhelming emotions are normal, expected, and healthy, they can provide solace.

Brothers and sisters of children with cancer shared the following stories to illuminate the difficulties they face.

Erin Hall (18 years old) considers his brother "a legend" for surviving childhood cancer:

> I'm really proud of my brother Judson for handling everything so well. During those years there were times when I was jealous of him, not only for the attention he received, but for his courage as well. This little boy was going through so much and I still cowered at getting my finger pricked. As I look back, I wonder if I would have been able to make it through, not only physically, but emotionally as well.
>
> According to some people a person needs to be dead in order to be a legend, or to have been famous, or well liked. A legend to me though, is someone who has accomplished something incredible, enduring many hardships and pains, and still comes out of it smiling.
>
> Judd is a legend to me because he didn't give up in a time that he might have. He is a legend because he survived an illness that many do not. Now I look at him after being in remission for almost five years, and I hope that someday if I am ever faced with a challenge like his, I will have the same strength and courage he had.

Eight-year-old Amanda Moodie explains the ups and downs of having a brother with cancer:

> Sometimes having a brother with cancer is fun, like when my family goes on the Fantasy Flight to the North Pole, and going to the special summer camp, and getting special privileges at Disney World.
>
> But other times, it can be really hard, especially when William gets put in the hospital. Right now, he can't leave his room in the hospital, and the

*doctors wear masks when they come in. I HATE seeing that. And he stays in for very long periods of time. The first time, he was there for almost three weeks! It comes so suddenly. He has stayed out for five months, then BAM! He's back in. And the worst of it is, people are always pitying us. "Poor little boy." "Poor William." I guess they like pitying us.*

*So, cancer has ups and downs like everything else, but to me it's mostly downs.*

Eleven-year-old Jeff Pasowicz explains what happened when "My Sister had Cancer." (Reprinted from CCCF Canada CONTACT newsletter, Vol. XVI, No.2, Spring 1994.)

*My sister Jamie got cancer when she was 23 months old. I was 8, and my two other sisters were 6 and 4.*

*My sisters and I were scared that my sister was going to die. We weren't able to go to public places and also weren't allowed to have friends in my house. We missed a lot of school when there was chicken pox in our school. I got teased in school sometimes because my sister had no hair. Once an older kid called my sister a freak. My mom was sad most of the time. It was very hard.*

*We are all pleased that Jamie is doing well, and our lives are getting back to normal. It was an experience I'll never forget, and I hope it has made me a stronger person.*

Fifteen-year-old Sara McDonnall won first prize in the 1995 Candlelighters Creative Arts Contest with her essay, "From a Sibling":

*Childhood cancer—a topic most teens don't think much about. I know I didn't until it invaded our home.*

*Childhood cancer totally disrupts lives, not only of the patient, but also of those closest to him/her, including the siblings. First, I was numbed with unbelieving shock. "This can't be happening to me and my family." Along with this came a whole dictionary full of incomprehensible words and a total restructuring of our (up to that time) fairly normal life-style.*

*One day in July 1988, I was waiting for my parents to pick me up from summer camp and anticipating the start of our family vacation to Canada. When they arrived, they informed me that my older brother Danny was very sick, and we wouldn't be taking that trip after all. The following day the call came that confirmed the diagnosis. Instead of packing for vacation, we packed our bags and headed for Children's Hospital in Denver, 200 miles away, where Danny was scheduled for surgery and chemotherapy.*

I developed my own disease (perhaps from fear I would "catch" what Danny had), with symptoms similar to my brother's:

- *Sympathy pains.* I asked, "Why him?" when he came home from the hospital, exhausted from throwing up a life-saving drug for three days.

- *Fear.* "How much sicker is Danny going to get before he gets well? He is going to get well, isn't he?"

- *Resentment.* My parents seemed so worried about him all the time. They didn't seem to have time for me anymore.

- *Confusion.* Why couldn't Danny and I wrestle around like we used to? Why couldn't I slug him when he made me mad?

- *Jealousy.* I felt insignificant when I was holding down the fort at home.

The parts I hated the most were: not understanding what was being done to him; answering endless worried phone calls; and hearing the answers to my own questions when my parents talked to other people.

I was helped to sort out these feelings and identify with other siblings when I attended a program held just for teens who had siblings with cancer. We got together, tried to learn how to cross-country ski, and talked about our siblings and ourselves.

Perhaps you remember this story: "U.S. [speed skating] star Dan Jansen, 22, carrying a winning time into the back straightaway of the 1000 meter race, inexplicably fell. Two days earlier, after receiving word that his older sister, Jane, had died of cancer, Dan crashed in the 500 meter" (Life Magazine). Having a sibling with cancer can immobilize even an Olympic athlete. Dan was expected to bring home two gold medals, but cancer in a sibling intervened. He became, instead, the most famous cancer sibling of all time. He shared his grief before a television audience of two billion people. Dan later went on to win the World Cup in Norway and Germany, and capture the gold at the Olympics. He is the first to tell you the real champions can be found in the oncology wards of children's hospitals across our nation, and the siblings who are fighting the battle right along beside them.

One adult sibling of a cancer survivor wrote:

Twelve young people aged 7 to 29 met at the 25th Anniversary Candlelighters Conference to talk about what it is like having a sibling with cancer in the family. We talked about our families, our anger, jealousy, worries, and fears, and thought about what we wanted to tell others about our experiences. In fact, we made lists of things we wanted other people to know: one for parents, one for other children or young adults in our position, and one for the child who has been diagnosed with cancer.

Some parts of these lists reflect anger and bitterness, but that was not the overriding feeling in the session. I hope it isn't the only message you take away. If nothing else, the issues raised here may provide you with a good starting point for discussions in your own family.

To Parents:

- We know you are burdened and trying to be fair. But try harder.
- Give us equal time.
- Be tough on disciplining the child with cancer. No free rides.
- Put yourself in our shoes once in a while.
- If you are away from home a lot, at least call and tell us, "I love you."
- Tell us what is going on. Don't just sit us in front of a video (about cancer); talk with us about it.
- Keep special time with us like lunch once a week or something. Time for just us. And if you can't be with us, find someone who can.
- When you talk to family members, say how everyone is doing—what we are doing is important, too.
- Ask how we are feeling. Don't assume you know.

To siblings of newly diagnosed kids:

- Keep a diary if you don't want to talk to your parents.
- Expect to not get as much attention.
- Expect that your parents are going to be extra cautious about what your brother/sister does, who he/she hangs out with, etc.
- Hang in there. You're all you've got for now.
- Don't feel like you have to think about the illness all the time.
- Be understanding of your parents and stay involved.
- Tell someone how you are feeling—don't bottle it up.
- Go to the hospital to visit when you can.
- Make as many friends as possible at school.

*To our siblings who struggled or are struggling with cancer:*

- *The world does not revolve around you.*

- *Stop feeling sorry for yourself.*

- *Not everything is related to cancer. Stop using that as an excuse for everything.*

- *I'm jealous of you sometimes, but I'm not mad. I know it sometimes seems like I'm mad, but I'm not.*

- *Don't take advantage of all the extra attention you get.*

- *Tell mom and dad to pay attention to me sometimes, too.*

- *Now that you are feeling better, where's the gratitude for all those chores that I did?*

- *I really admire your strength and courage. I wouldn't have gotten through your illness without you.*

# Helping siblings cope

Simply understanding the depth of the pain and fears of your "healthy" children eases their path. Being available to listen, to say, "I hear how painful this is for you," or "You sound scared. I am, too," makes siblings feel that they are still valued members of the family, that even though their brother or sister is absorbing the lion's share of parents' time and care, they are still cherished. The following are the experiences and advice from several families on ways to help the brothers and sisters cope.

- Make sure that you explain cancer and its treatment to the siblings in terms that they understand. Create a climate of openness, so that they can ask questions and know that they will get answers. If you don't know the answer to a question, write it on your list to ask the doctor at the next appointment or ask your child if he would like to go to the appointment with you and ask the question himself.

    *We always, always explained everything that was happening to Brent's older brother Zac (8 years old). He never asked questions, but always listened intently. He would say, "Okay, I understand. Everything's all right." We tried to get him to talk about it, but through all these years, he just never has. So we just kept explaining things at a level that he could understand, and he has done very well through the whole ordeal. The times that he seemed sad, we would take him out of school, and let him stay at the Ronald McDonald House with us for a few days, and that seemed to help him.*

- Make sure that all the children clearly understand that cancer is not contagious. They cannot catch it, nor can their ill sister give it to anyone else. Impress upon them that nothing the parents or brothers and sisters did caused the cancer.

- Bring home a picture of the brother or sister in the hospital, and carry a tape recorder back and forth to relay songs and messages.

- It is very hard for mothers and babies or toddlers to be separated. Some families leave out family photo albums for the caregiver to show the toddler whenever he gets sad.

    *My daughter was 18 months old when her 3-year-old sister was diagnosed. Each member of the family flew in to stay at the house for two-week shifts, so she had a lot of caregivers. A friend of mine gave her a big key chain which held eight pictures. We put a picture of each member of the family (including pets) on her key chain, and she carried it around whenever we were away. It seemed to comfort her.*

- Try to spend time alone with each sibling.

    *We began a tradition during chemotherapy that really helped each member of our family. Every Saturday each parent would take one child for a two-hour special time. We scheduled it ahead of time to allow excitement and anticipation to grow. Each child picked what to do on their special day—such as going to the park, eating lunch at a restaurant, riding bikes. We tried to put aside our worries, have fun, and really listen.*

- If people only comment on the sick child, try to bring the conversation back to include the sibling. For example, if someone exclaims, "Oh look how good Lisa looks," you could say, "Yes, and Martha has an attractive new haircut, too. Don't you like it?"

- Share your feelings about the illness and its impact on the family. Say, "I'm sad that I have to bring your sister to the hospital a lot. I miss you when I'm gone." This allows the sibling an opportunity to tell you how she is feeling. Try to make the illness a family project by expressing how the family will stick together to beat it.

    *I never kept my feelings secret from Shawn's two older brothers (5 and 7 years old). If I was scared, I talked about it. Once, my stomach was so knotted up I could barely walk. Kevin said, "Mom, I'm really worried about Shawn." I told him that I was, too, and then we both just hugged and cried together. They really opened up when we didn't hide our feelings.*

- Include all siblings in decision making on such matters as how chores will be done or devise a schedule for parent time with the healthy children.

> We always gave the boys choices about where they would stay when Shawn had to be in the hospital. I felt like it gave them a sense of control to choose babysitters. They usually stayed at a close neighbor's house where there were younger children. It allowed them to ride the same bus to school and play with their neighborhood friends. Their lives were not too disrupted. They also really pitched in and helped with the younger kids. I think it helped them to help others.

· · · · ·

> Sometimes I think that my mom does not treat us equally. For example, if I left my snack garbage on the floor I would not get a snack the next night but Zach would get a snack if he left his garbage on the floor. I know he cannot walk but he could ask someone to take it out for him or he could say, "I need to take my garbage out so can somebody help me walk out so I can throw my garbage away."

- Allow siblings to be involved in the medical aspects of their sister or brother's illness, if they wish it. Often the reality of clinic visits and overnight stays are easier than what siblings imagine. Many siblings are a true comfort when they hold their sister or brother's hand during blood tests or MRIs.

- Give lots of hugs and kisses.

> We assumed everything was fine with Erin because she had her grandma, who adored her, staying with her. We made a conscious decision to spend lots of time with her and include her in everything. But we realized later that she felt very left out. My advice is to give triple the affection that you think they need, including lots of physical affection such as hugs and kisses. For years, Erin felt jealous. She thought her brother got more of everything: material things, time with parents, opportunities to do things she was not allowed to do. She finally worked it out while she was in college.

- Be sure to alert teachers of siblings about the tremendous stress at home. Many children respond to the worries about cancer by developing behavior or academic problems at school. Teachers should be vigilant for the warning signals, and provide extra support or tutoring for the stressed child or teen. Continue to communicate frequently with the teachers of the siblings to make sure you are aware of any developing problems.

- Offer the siblings a chance to meet other sibs who are coping with a sick brother or sister. Many institutions have weekend programs and/or for camps for siblings.

- Expect your other children to have some behavior problems as part of living with cancer in the family. This is a normal, not pathological, response.

- The child with cancer receives many toys and gifts, resulting in hurt feelings or jealousy in the siblings. Provide gifts and tokens of appreciation to the siblings for helping out during hard times, and encourage your sick child to share.

> *Matthew received many new toys during the course of his disease. We finally told family members that we would prefer it if they could bring a toy for Matthew and his brother and sister, or to bring nothing at all. We told them that Matthew was happy to see them whether they came bearing gifts or not. His siblings couldn't understand why he was getting so many new things while they didn't get anything. Matthew always shared his presents, though. He would come home from the hospital and dump his suitcase onto the living room floor for David and Kristina to pick their new toy. Those were happy days for all three of them. Not only did they have new toys to play with, but they were all together in their own home.*

- Encourage a close relationship between an adult relative or neighbor and your other children. Having a "someone special" when the parents are frequently absent can help prevent problems and help your child to feel cared for and loved.

- Take advantage of any workshops, support groups, or camps for siblings. These can be of tremendous value for siblings, providing fun and friendships with others who truly understand their feelings.

## Positive outcomes for the siblings

After stating all of the above potential troubles that your children might experience, it is important to note that many siblings exhibit great warmth and active caretaking while their brother or sister is being treated for cancer. Their empathy and compassion seem to grow with the crisis.

> *It's been six months since Kylie was diagnosed with GBM. A lot has happened since last summer. I've matured overnight and I've learned how important it is to live each day at a time. I used to be an extremely impatient person but now I'm in no hurry.*

Some brothers and sisters of children with cancer feel that they have benefited from the stressful experience in many ways, such as increased knowledge about disease, increased empathy for the sick or disabled, increased sense of responsibility, enhanced self-esteem, greater maturity and coping ability, and increased family closeness.

> *Christopher was at home with us from boarding school when we finally found out that Michael's condition was terminal, and he has been an absolute star. He has looked after Michael, filled in the words he couldn't remember, helped him across the road—and bullied him, played physical games with him, helped him do packing for our upcoming house move— oh, everything.*

Many of these siblings mature into adults interested in the caring professions, such as medicine, social work, or teaching. Character can grow from confronting personal crisis, and many parents speak of the siblings with admiration and pride.

> *I don't think it matters how old the siblings are—it's a reality that the healthy ones will not get their fair share for a while. From what I've been able to observe in my own and other families, the siblings do eventually take it in stride and even seem to benefit from the opportunity to learn compassion, selflessness, and responsibility. As they get older, they even take comfort in the realization that, had they been the sick one, THEY would have received all the necessary attention and that their parent(s) can cope (somehow) with whatever comes around. Libby added to her observations that she noted carefully how I reacted to Casey's illness at first (fell apart!) but that the next day I could gather my strength and do what had to be done. She likes to think she would also react similarly should the occasion arise (although, at her age, every blip in her universe is a catastrophe).*

# CHAPTER 17

# Nutrition

THE EATING HABITS of children with CNS tumors go haywire. If they do want to eat, it is usually not a food that is in the nutritious category. Parents know that eating the right types of food will help their child heal faster, feel better, and continue to grow. Moreover, the treatment itself increases the need for balanced nutrition. The child's body works hard to repair the damage to healthy cells caused by chemotherapy and radiation therapy and to break down and excrete the tumor cells killed by treatment. Just metabolizing chemotherapy drugs stresses children's systems.

Despite knowing that children need to eat nutritious meals, the reality is that sick children often do not want to eat. This chapter discusses eating problems, explains good nutrition, suggests ways to pack extra calories into small servings, and offers tips on how to make food more appealing to children.

## Treatment side effects and eating

Eating is tremendously impacted by most types of chemotherapy and radiation therapy. Listed below are several common side effects of treatment that can prevent good eating. Other common side effects, including nausea, vomiting, diarrhea, constipation, and mouth and throat sores, are covered in detail in Chapter 13, *Common Side Effects of Chemotherapy*.

### Loss of appetite

Anorexia, or loss of appetite, is one of the most common problems associated with chemotherapy and radiation therapy. Children suffering from nausea and vomiting, diarrhea or constipation, altered sense of smell and taste, mouth sores, and other unpleasant side effects understandably do not feel hungry. Loss of appetite is most pronounced during the most intensive periods of treatment.

> *My son looked like a skeleton several months into his protocol. I used to dress him in camouflage clothes—several layers thick. This kept him warm and prevented stares.*

If your child loses more than 10 to 15 percent of his body weight, he may need to be fed intravenously or by nasogastric tube. Sometimes this can be avoided by parents' learning how to increase calories in small amounts of food.

In addition to simple loss of appetite, your child may experience a side effect of chemotherapy called satiety. This means that the child has a sense of being full after only a few bites of food. If the child is suffering from early satiety and eats only when hungry, she may begin losing weight and become malnourished. This chapter will provide dozens of creative ways to encourage your child to eat more.

## Increased appetite and weight gain

When children are given high doses of steroids, such as prednisone or dexamethasone, they develop voracious appetites. They are hungry all the time, develop food obsessions, and frequently wake parents up during the night begging for another meal. Almost all children with CNS tumors receive steroids at some point during their treatment.

> Jamie's treatment for low-grade astrocytoma called for weekly dexamethasone given intravenously to combat nausea, so we didn't have ravenous hunger like some kids have, but we did have nighttime munch sessions. We'd all get up and pull everything out: drinks, snacks, leftover pizza or pasta or chicken, grocery-cut fruit, precut carrots, almonds or peanuts, crackers and cheese, whatever was quick.

Most parents become very concerned when their child consumes huge quantities of food and gains weight. A moon face with chubby cheeks and a rotund belly are classic features of a child on high-dose steroids. Much of the extra weight is fluid that steroids cause the body to retain. Avoid foods with increased salt that can contribute to fluid retention and high blood pressure. There are two important points for parents to remember about treatment with steroids. First, when the steroids stop, the extra fluid is excreted and weight drops. Second, the child's appetite may go from voracious to poor after the steroids stop.

Do not put your child on a diet when he is taking steroids. Instead, try to make the most of this brief time of good appetite to encourage consumption of a variety of nutritious foods. A well-balanced diet now will help your child withstand the rigors of treatment ahead.

If you are concerned about the weight gain, consult your child's oncologist. If the fluid retention is extreme, the doctor may have you restrict your child's salt intake. In some cases children are given drugs called diuretics to rid the body of excess fluid.

# Lactose intolerance

Lactose intolerance occurs when the body can't absorb the sugar (lactose) contained in milk and other dairy products. Both antibiotics and chemotherapy can cause lactose intolerance in some individuals. The part of children's intestines that breaks down lactose stops functioning properly, resulting in gas, abdominal pain, bloating, cramping, and diarrhea. If your child develops this problem, it is important to talk to a nutritionist to learn about low-lactose diets and alternate sources of protein. The following are suggestions for parents of lactose-intolerant children:

- Add enzyme tablets or drops to dairy products to make them digestible. Some of these are over-the-counter additives, while others require a prescription. Discuss these additives with the oncologist prior to using them.

- Replace milk with cheese, nonfat yogurt, buttermilk, cream cheese, or sour cream.

- Replace milk with lactose-free sliced cheese and milk products, acidophilus milk, or soymilk. These are easier to digest and come in a variety of flavors.

- A new product called Vitamite 100 (800-443-3930), is lactose-free, but not soymilk. Your child may like the taste of this milk replacement.

- Remember that milk is a common ingredient in other foods, even bread. Read ingredient lists carefully.

- If no dairy products are tolerated, calcium can be supplied by serving canned salmon, sardines, or calcium-fortified fruit juices. Consult your child's oncologist, neurologist, and nutritionist about the interaction of calcium supplements with your child's other medications.

    *Calcium supplements interfered with my son's seizure medications, as do antacid supplements (which are usually made from calcium carbonate). We also recently found out Dilantin may be affected by some chemo drugs. We allow a window of about two hours between giving our son his seizure medications and any other meds, including calcium.*

- Always be sure that products are pasteurized, not raw.

*Diet and Nutrition* and *Eating Hints* are free booklets available from the National Cancer Institute, (800) 4-CANCER. They both contain recipes and suggestions for lactose-restricted diets.

In addition, some children with seizure disorders also have intolerances to milk protein and gluten, which is found in wheat.

## Altered taste and smell

One common reason why children do not eat is because food has no taste or tastes bad as a result of chemotherapy or radiation therapy. If the problem is food having no taste, try serving highly seasoned food (e.g., Italian, Mexican, or curried foods). If foods taste bitter or metallic, avoid using metal pots, pans, and utensils. Serve the child's food with plastic knives, forks, and spoons. Replace red meat with tofu, chicken or turkey, eggs, and dairy products.

Some children's taste returns to normal a few months into treatment, some after treatment ends, and for a few children, it takes years before some foods taste pleasant again.

# What is a balanced diet?

A good diet includes sufficient calories to ensure a normal rate of growth, fuel the body's efforts to repair and replace damaged normal cells, and provide the energy the body needs to break down the various chemotherapy drugs and excrete their by-products. Research has shown that a well-nourished body will:

- Tolerate more treatment
- Tend to have fewer side effects
- Maintain weight
- Recover faster from treatment

When the body becomes malnourished, body fat and muscle decrease. This leads to:

- Weakness, lack of energy, weight loss
- Decreased ability to digest food
- Limited ability to heal and fight infection
- Possible increase in the toxicities of treatment.

To keep your child's body well-nourished, foods from all of the five basic food groups are needed. The five groups are breads and cereals, fruits, vegetables, dairy products, and meats and meat substitutes.

Examples of foods contained in each group are listed next, with a small child's serving size in parentheses beside each food. Consult a nutritionist to determine the serving size appropriate for your child.

**Meat and Meat Substitutes (2 or 3 servings per day)**

| | |
|---|---|
| Meat (1 ounce) | Eggs (1) |
| Fish (1 ounce) | Peanut butter (2 Tbsp.) |
| Poultry (1 ounce) | Dried beans, cooked ($\frac{1}{2}$ cup) |
| Cheese (1 ounce) | Dried peas, cooked ($\frac{1}{2}$ cup) |

These foods provide protein, which helps build and maintain body tissues, supplies energy, and forms enzymes, hormones, and antibodies. Some typical one-ounce servings of meat and meat substitutes are: a meatball one inch in diameter, a one-inch cube of meat, one slice of bologna, a one-inch cube of cheese, or one slice of processed cheese. As you can see, two to three meatballs a day provide all the protein needed by a school-aged child.

**Dairy Products (2 or 3 servings per day)**

| | |
|---|---|
| Milk ($\frac{1}{2}$ cup) | Tofu ($\frac{1}{2}$ cup) |
| Cheese (1 ounce) | Custard ($\frac{1}{2}$ cup) |
| Ice cream ($\frac{1}{2}$ cup) | Yogurt ($\frac{1}{2}$ cup) |

These foods provide calcium, vitamin D, and protein.

**Breads and Cereals (6 to 11 servings per day)**

| | |
|---|---|
| Bread ($\frac{1}{2}$ slice) | Dry cereal ($\frac{1}{2}$ cup) |
| Oatmeal ($\frac{1}{2}$ cup) | Granola ($\frac{1}{2}$ cup) |
| Cream of Wheat ($\frac{1}{2}$ cup) | Cooked pasta ($\frac{1}{2}$ cup) |
| Graham crackers (1 square) | Saltines (3 squares) |
| Rice ($\frac{1}{2}$ cup) | Potatoes (1 baked) |

These foods supply vitamins, minerals, fiber, and carbohydrates. Try to use only products made with whole-wheat flour and limited sugar to get more nutrients per serving. One sandwich made with two slices of bread provides four servings of this food group.

**Fruits (2 to 4 servings per day)**

| | |
|---|---|
| Fresh fruit (1 medium piece) | Dried fruits ($\frac{1}{4}$ cup) |
| Canned fruit ($\frac{1}{4}$ cup) | Fruit juice ($\frac{1}{4}$ cup) |

Fruits provide vitamins, minerals, and fiber. Fruits can be camouflaged by pureeing them with ice cream in the blender to make a tasty milkshake or by adding them to cookie and muffin recipes.

**Vegetables (3 to 5 servings per day)**

| Raw vegetables (1/4 cup) | Cooked vegetables (1/4 cup) |
|---|---|

Vegetables, like fruit, are excellent sources of vitamins, minerals, and fiber. If your child does not want vegetables, they can be grated or pureed and added to soups or spaghetti sauce. If you own a juicer, add a vegetable to fruits being juiced.

**Fats (several servings a day)**

| Butter or margarine | Cheese |
|---|---|
| Mayonnaise | Whipped cream |
| Peanut butter (or nuts) | Avocado |
| Meat fat (in gravy) | Olives |
| Ice cream | Chocolate |

Although the food pyramid calls for fats to be used sparingly, higher consumption of fats is needed for children receiving chemotherapy or radiation therapy. Experiment to find the fats that your child enjoys eating and serve them frequently.

# Vitamin supplements

Vitamin supplements are often necessary. The nutritional needs of kids undergoing chemotherapy and radiation therapy are higher than other children's, yet kids on treatment often eat less food. Most children and teens undergoing treatment are unable or unwilling to eat the variety of foods necessary for good health. In addition, damage to children's digestive systems from chemotherapy or radiation to the spinal axis alters the body's ability to absorb the nutrients contained in the food they do manage to eat.

Vitamin supplementation should be done only after consultation with your child's oncologist. Over-supplementation of some vitamins, folic acid for example, can make your child's chemotherapy or radiation therapy less effective. But providing other vitamins can make the difference between a child with dull hair, no energy, and dry peeling skin and one with stronger hair, clear skin, and a better attitude. Vitamin supplements should be individually tailored for your child in consultation with the oncologist and nutritionist.

> We struggled with eating and weight loss throughout Emily's treatment. We absolutely drove ourselves crazy trying to get her to eat. I remember a few times when I simply sat down and cried after she vomited something up that

*I had gotten her to finally eat. We did give a multivitamin, with the blessing of the doctors. It got to the point that Emily had to have some specific vitamins because one of the chemo drugs made her body excrete them.*

# Making eating fun

In some homes, mealtimes turn into battlegrounds, with worried parents resorting to threats or bribery to get their child to eat. After such scenes, parents, the ill child, and siblings are exhausted, and nutritious food still has not been consumed. The next several sections are full of methods used successfully by many veteran parents to make mealtimes fun and nutritious.

## How to make food more appealing

Many children are finicky eaters at the best of times. Chemotherapy and radiation can make eating especially difficult. The following are general suggestions to make eating more enjoyable for your child:

- Give small portions throughout the day rather than three large meals. Feed your child whenever she is hungry.

- Remember that your child knows best which foods he can tolerate.

- Explain clearly to your child the importance of eating a balanced diet.

- Make mealtimes pleasant and leisurely.

- Rearrange eating schedules to serve the main meal at the time of day when your child feels best. If she wakes up feeling well most days, make a high-protein, high-calorie breakfast.

- Praise and encourage eating well.

- Don't punish the child for not eating.

- Set a good example by eating a large variety of nutritious foods yourself.

- Have nutritious snacks available at all times. Carry them in the car, to all appointments, and packed in knapsacks for school.

- Serve clear fluids between meals rather than with meals to keep your child from feeling full after only a few bites of food.

    *My son hates to drink water. Watered down juice, Popsicles, frozen juice, Italian ice, freeze pops, ice tea, lemonade, and my kid's favorite, Gatorade, are all great clear fluids.*

- Limit the amount of less desirable foods in the house. Potato chips, corn chips, soda pop, and sweets with large amounts of sugar will fill your child up with empty calories.

- If your child is interested, include him when making a grocery list, shopping for favorite foods, and preparing food.

## Make mealtime fun

The following are suggestions on how to make mealtime more fun:

- Try to take the emphasis off eating food because it's good for you and focus instead on setting a mood of enjoying each other's company while sharing a meal. Encourage good conversation, tell stories and jokes, perhaps light some candles.

- Make one night a week restaurant night. Use a nice tablecloth and candles, allow the children to order from a menu, and pretend the family is out for a night on the town.

- Because any change in setting can encourage eating, consider having a picnic on the floor occasionally. Order pizza or other takeout, spread a tablecloth on the floor, and have an in-home picnic. Some parents even send lunch out to the tree house for a lark.

  *My son enjoyed eating in different places around the house and seemed to eat more when he was having fun. I sometimes fed the kids on their own picnic table outdoors in good weather, and at the same picnic table in the garage during the winter. They were thrilled to wear their coats and hats to eat. Occasionally I would let them eat off TV trays while watching a favorite program or tape.*

- Some families have theme meals, such as Mexican, Hawaiian, or Chinese. They use decorations, wear costumes, and cook foods with exotic spices.

- Some children seem to eat better if food is attractively arranged on the plate or is decorated in humorous ways. Preschoolers enjoy putting a smiling face on a casserole using strips of cheese, nuts, or raisins. Sandwiches can be cut into funny shapes using knives or cookie cutters.

  *My daughter liked to have food decorated. For example, we would make pancakes look like a clown face by using blueberries for eyes, strawberry for a nose, orange slices for ears, etc. She also enjoyed eating brightly colored food, so we would add a drop of food coloring to applesauce, yogurt, or whatever appealed to her.*

## How to serve more protein

Because many children and teens cannot tolerate eating meat while on chemotherapy, the following are suggestions for increasing protein consumption:

- Add one cup of dried milk powder to a quart of whole milk, then blend and chill. Use this extra-strength milk for drinking and cooking.

- Use extra-strength milk (above), whole milk, evaporated milk, or cream instead of water to make hot cereal, cocoa, soup, gravy, custards, or puddings.

- Add powdered milk to casseroles, meat loaf, cream soups, custards, and puddings.

- Add chopped meat to scrambled eggs, soups, and vegetables.

- Add chopped hard-cooked eggs to soups, salads, sauces, and casseroles.

- Add grated cheese to pizza, vegetables, salads, sauces, omelets, mashed potatoes, meat loaf, and casseroles.

- Serve bagels, English muffins, hamburgers, or hot dogs with a slice of cheese melted on top.

- Spread peanut butter on toast, crackers, and sandwiches. Dip fruit or raw vegetables into peanut butter for a quick snack.

- Spread peanut butter or cream cheese onto celery sticks or carrots.

- Serve nuts for snacks and mix nuts into salads and soups.

- Serve yogurt and granola bars for extra protein. Top pie, Jell-O, pudding, and fruit with ice cream or whipped cream.

- Use dried beans and peas to make soups, dips, and casseroles.

- Use tofu (bean curd) in stir-fried vegetable dishes.

- Add wheat germ to hamburgers, meat loaf, breads, muffins, pancakes, waffles, and vegetables and use it as a topping for casseroles.

## Guidelines for boosting calories

Parents need to alter their perceptions of what constitutes healthy food when they are struggling to feed a child on chemotherapy. Many parents have ingrained habits of low-fat cooking and food preparation. That habit must be replaced by methods that add calories to their child's food:

- Add butter or margarine to hot cereal, eggs, pasta, rice, cooked vegetables, mashed potatoes, and soups.

- Use melted butter as a dip for raw vegetables and cooked seafood, such as shrimp, crab, and lobster.

- Use sour cream to top meats, baked potatoes, and soups.

- Use mayonnaise instead of salad dressing on salads, sandwiches, and hard-cooked eggs.

- Add mayonnaise or sour cream when making hamburgers or meat loaf.

- Use cream instead of milk over cereal, puddings, Jell-O, and fruit.

- Make milkshakes, puddings, and custards with cream instead of milk.

- Serve your child whole milk instead of 2 percent milk to drink.

- Saute vegetables in butter.

- Serve bread hot so it will absorb more butter.

- Spread bagels, muffins, or crackers with cream cheese and jelly or honey.

- Make hot chocolate with cream, and add marshmallows.

- Add granola to cookie, bread, and muffin batters. Sprinkle granola on ice cream, pudding, and yogurt.

- Serve meat and vegetables with sauces made with cream and pan drippings.

- Combine cooked vegetables with dried fruit.

- Add dried fruits to recipes for cookies, breads, and muffins.

## Nutritious snacks

Try to get into the habit of always bringing a bag of nutritious snacks whenever you leave home with your child. This allows you to feed her whenever she is hungry and avoids stopping for non-nutritious junk food. The following are some examples of healthful snacks:

- Apples or applesauce
- Baby foods
- Burritos made from beans or meat
- Buttered popcorn
- Celery sticks stuffed with cheese or peanut butter
- Cookies made with wheat germ, oat meal, granola, fruits, or nuts
- Cereal

- Cheese
- Cheesecake
- Chocolate milk
- Cottage cheese
- Crackers with cheese, peanut butter, tuna salad
- Custards made with extra eggs and cream
- Dips made with cheese, avocado, butter, beans, or sour cream
- Dried fruit such as apples, raisins, apricots, or prunes
- Fresh fruit
- Granola mixed with dried fruit and nuts
- Hard-cooked and deviled eggs
- Ice cream (made with real cream)
- Juice (made from 100 percent fruit)
- Milkshakes (made with whole milk or cream)
- Muffins
- Nuts
- Peanut butter on crackers or whole wheat bread
- Pizza
- Puddings
- Sandwiches (with real mayonnaise or butter)
- Vegetables like carrot sticks or broccoli florets
- Yogurt, regular or frozen

## Ask for help

It is very helpful to consult the hospital nutritionist to obtain more information and ideas on how to add more protein and calories to your child's diet.

> I had two quite different experiences with hospital nutritionists. At the children's hospital, I couldn't get the doctors concerned about my daughter's dramatic weight loss. She was so weak she couldn't stand, and her muscles seemed to be wasting away. I finally asked the receptionist to please send in a nutritionist. A very young woman came in and talked to

*me about the major food groups. I felt my cheeks begin to flush, and my eyes glistened as I said, "I know what she is SUPPOSED to eat, I need to know how I can make her want to eat." I must have sounded a bit crazy, because she just handed me a booklet and backed out the door.*

*The next week when my daughter began her radiation, the radiation nurse took one look at her and called the nutritionist right down. This nutritionist was very warm and caring. She helped me to understand that I needed to think fat, protein, and calories, and she gave me lots of practical suggestions on how to boost calories. I think that she probably saved my daughter from tube feedings.*

Another resource is the American Institute for Cancer Research Nutrition Hotline, (800) 843-8114, Monday through Friday, 9 A.M. to 5 P.M. EST. A registered nutritionist will answer your questions about your child's nutrition.

# What kids really eat

The previous part of the chapter listed ideas for increasing calories and making food more appealing. What follows are accounts of what several kids really ate while on chemotherapy and radiation. You'll notice how varied the list is, so experiment to see what your child finds palatable. Remember also that children's tastes and aversions change as time passes while on treatment.

*Judd craved chicken chow mein and fried rice take out from a Chinese restaurant. He also loved spaghettiOs and hot dogs.*

· · · · ·

*I let Preston eat whatever tasted good to him which was usually lots of potatoes and eggs. He liked spicy food (especially Mexican).*

· · · · ·

*Katy typically only ate one food for days or weeks at a stretch. One time, she ate pesto sauce (made from olive oil, garlic, Parmesan cheese, and basil leaves) on pasta every meal for weeks. She also went through a spicy barbecue sauce phase, in which she wouldn't eat any food unless it was completely immersed in sauce. She ate no fruits, vegetables (except potatoes), or meat for the entire period of treatment. She ate mostly cereal and beans when she was feeling well, and mostly pureed baby food when she was really sick.*

· · · · ·

In the beginning when Meagan lost so much weight, we snuck Polycose (a powdered nutritional supplement) into everything. She finally got stuck on cans of mixed nuts. They are high calorie, and were instrumental in putting back on the weight. She also craved capers, and would eat them by the tablespoonful.

• • • • •

All Brent asks for are "peanut butter and jelly sandwiches, cut in fours, no crusts, with Fritos." The only fruit he has eaten for three years is an occasional banana, and he eats no vegetables. He always ate everything before his diagnosis at age 6.

• • • • •

The doctor told me to keep Kim on a low-salt, low-folic-acid diet. She wouldn't eat anything, so he eventually said he didn't care what she ate, as long as she ate. She liked spaghettiOs, Chick-fil-A nuggets, Chick-fil-A soup, and McDonald's sausage and pancakes.

• • • • •

All that Carl ate was dry cereal, dry waffles, oatmeal, and bacon. He ate no other meat or vegetables throughout treatment, but did drink milk. I thought that he would never be healthy, but he's 15 now (diagnosed when 2), eats little junk food, never gets sick, and looks great.

• • • • •

John (14 months old) craved creamed corn and pork and beans. I would just sit him on a potty chair at the table and let him eat, and it would go in one end and out the other. When on prednisone, he would sit at the table almost all day. He also drank a gallon of apple juice a day. He rarely eats meat to this day (two years off treatment).

• • • • •

I guess Carrie Beth is the exception that proves the rule, because she has an excellent appetite. She eats fruits, vegetables, and lots of meat.

# Parent advice

Parents whose children have completed therapy offer the following suggestions on how to handle the many eating problems children have during treatment.

Doctors sometimes reassure parents by saying, "His appetite will return to normal." Don't be surprised if this does not happen until long after the most intensive parts of treatment are completed.

• • • • •

*Let the child control what type of food and how much he wants. In the beginning, any food is good food.*

• • • • •

*Buy a juicer, and use it every day. This was the only way we got any fruits or vegetables into our daughter. Make apple juice and sneak in a carrot. Sometimes we would make the juice, then blend it in the blender with ice cubes to make an iced drink, which we would serve with a straw.*

• • • • •

*I solved my daughter's salt cravings by buying sea salt and letting her dip french fries in it once a week. For some reason, that satisfied her and stopped her from begging for regular table salt at every meal.*

• • • • •

*One magic word: butter, butter, butter. We would make Maddie peanut butter and jelly sandwiches with a layer of butter on each side of the bread first. Milkshakes are great and Häagen Dazs ice cream has the highest fat content. We also went to an "eat when she's hungry" mode. It was definitely more relaxing.*

• • • • •

*Try not to worry about your child's future eating habits. During treatment, you just have to let go of normal requirements and feed him whatever he wants, whenever he is hungry.*

• • • • •

*If you only keep good food in the house, and don't buy junk food, your child will eat more nutritious food.*

• • • • •

*Take good care of yourself by eating well. We are all under tremendous stress and need good nutrition. I gave my daughter healthy foods and glasses of juiced fresh fruits and vegetables while I was living on lattés (a coffee drink). I now have breast cancer and wish that I had eaten well during my daughter's treatment.*

• • • • •

*There is reason for hope. My daughter ate almost nothing while on treatment. After treatment ended, she ate more food but still no variety. She didn't turn the corner until a year off treatment, but now she is gradually trying new foods, including fruits and vegetables again. I'm glad I never made an issue of it.*

# Commercial nutritional supplements

Many children cannot tolerate solid food or can eat only small amounts each day. Liquid supplements can help provide the necessary calories. The following is a sampling of the variety of supplements that can be purchased at pharmacies or grocery stores. If you are unable to locate a particular brand, your pharmacist may be able to order it for you:

- **Sustacal.** Lactose-free liquid. Flavors are chocolate, vanilla, eggnog, and strawberry. Also comes in a high-protein or extra-fiber formula. (Mead Johnson)

- **Sustacal Pudding.** Sustacal in pudding form. Flavors are chocolate, vanilla, and butterscotch. (Mead Johnson)

- **Sustacal HC.** Concentrated liquid. Flavors are vanilla, chocolate, strawberry, and eggnog. (Mead Johnson)

- **Ensure.** Lactose-free liquid. Flavors are chocolate, vanilla, black walnut, coffee, butter pecan, banana, and strawberry. Other formulas are high protein or extra fiber. (Ross Laboratories)

- **Ensure Plus.** Concentrated liquid. (Ross Laboratories)

- **Isocal.** Lactose-free liquid. Vanilla. (Mead Johnson)

- **Enrich.** Liquid with fiber. Lactose free. (Ross Laboratories)

- **Instant Breakfast.** Powder, which is added to milk. Variety of flavors. (Carnation Co.)

- **Citrotein.** Powder, which is added to water or juice. Orange flavor. (Doyle Pharmaceutical)

- **Polycose.** Liquid or powder. Powder is added to milk, juice, gravy, or soups. Adds carbohydrates for extra calories. One tablespoon adds 30 calories. (Ross Laboratories)

- **Myoplex Lite.** Nutrition shake, which is added to water plus a little ice and mixed in a blender. It comes in a variety of flavors, including orange, piña colada, and banana cream pie as well as chocolate, strawberry, and vanilla. (EAS, Inc)

> We tried all the high calorie drinks: Pediasure in three flavors, Boost, and Scandi-shake. The one that Emily would drink is called Nutrashake (tastes like melted ice cream, and can also be eaten frozen). Of course Pediasure and Boost are available over the counter. We had to get Scandi-shake at the hospital (this is a powder that you mix with milk). I had to do some research to obtain the Nutrashake. It comes frozen and Kroger grocery stores carry it.

*Since there were no Krogers near us, I finally found an outfit called
American Medical Supply that would ship it.*

•  •  •  •  •

*The home heath agency I worked for did a study on nutritional content of
Ensure, Sustacal, and Carnation Instant Breakfast. All were basically the
same with Carnation much more palatable. The other two have a bit of a
medicinal smell and taste to them. You can add calories by throwing it in
a blender with ice cream, bananas, strawberries. My other two non-brain
tumor kids loved this stuff. Mandy (diagnosed with medulloblastoma) would
"sip" a tiny bit but would rather eat the hot spicy food: bologne, polish
sausage, tomatoes drowning in Catalina dressing. Reeses peanut butter cups
were breakfast for a long time (7 grams of protein!).*

# Feeding by tube and IV

Tube feedings or intravenous nutrition may be a necessity for some children undergoing treatment for CNS tumors. Poor nutrition may occur as a consequence of chemotherapy and radiation or because your child is unable to chew or swallow properly
because of the tumor or as a result of surgery. These types of feedings do not represent
a failure on the part of parents or children to "eat properly." Although feeding by tube
and IV may require additional hospitalization, parents should understand the benefits clearly. If your child becomes malnourished, events are set in motion that can
have grim consequences. As appetite and weight decrease, your child's ability to repair
cellular damage caused by treatment is impaired. Your child may become progres-
sively weaker, and his resistance to infection decreases. Infections and weakness may
require interruptions in treatment. This scenario needs to be prevented. Most protocols suggest tube or IV feeding after 10 percent of body weight is lost. There are two
types of supplemental feeding: total parenteral and enteral nutrition.

## Total parenteral nutrition (TPN)

Total parenteral nutrition, also known as hyperalimentation, is a form of intravenous
feeding used to prevent or treat malnutrition in children who cannot eat enough to
meet basic nutritional needs. Some of the many reasons why your child may require
TPN are:

• Severe mouth and throat sores that prevent swallowing

• Severe nausea and vomiting

• Severe diarrhea

- Inability to chew or swallow normally
- Loss of more than 10 percent of body weight

TPN ensures that the child receives all of the protein, carbohydrates, fats, vitamins, and minerals she needs. The TPN is administered through the central venous catheter, but children receiving TPN can also eat solids and drink fluids.

> My daughter needed TPN for two weeks after her stem cell transplant. They told us ahead of time that it would be necessary, and they were right. She got terrible sores throughout her GI tract and couldn't drink or eat. They just hooked the bag up to her broviac. After a couple of weeks, she started gingerly sipping small amounts of water and apple juice. For some reason, I just didn't worry about her eating. I assumed when she could, she would. She was a robust eater before her illness, so I thought that would help. Before we left for home, she asked for a hospital pizza (yuck!) and ate a few bites. Her eating at home quickly went back to normal, although it took some time to regain the weight she lost.

In most cases, TPN will be started in the hospital. Each day the concentrations of glucose, protein, and fat will be increased in a step-wise fashion, and your child will be assessed for tolerance to the preparation. The time of the total infusion will be consolidated so that administration at home will be feasible. Generally, TPN is given 8 to 12 hours per day, depending on your child's unique situation. The infusion may be delivered over the hours that work best for your family. If your child attends school, overnight infusions will probably work best. If your child is at home during the day, infusions during these hours will give the entire family a better night's sleep. Be sure to request a small portable infusion pump and backpack from your home care company so that the day's activities will not be limited by this therapy. Your child's oncologist may need to write a letter to your insurance company to verify your child's malnutrition so that this therapy is covered.

## Enteral nutrition

If your child requires supplemental feeding and the bowel and intestines are still functioning well, enteral nutrition may be recommended. Enteral feedings are preferred over IV when possible. Enteral nutrition is feeding via a tube placed through the nose into the stomach or small intestine (NG tube) or via a tube surgically placed directly into the stomach through the abdominal wall (see Chapter 4, *Coping with Procedures*). Nutritionally complete liquid formulas are fed through the tube. The appropriate formula for your child will be determined by your oncologist and nutritionist.

Infrequent side effects of enteral nutrition are irritated throat, nausea, diarrhea, or constipation.

> *Rachel (age 14) was diagnosed with PNET in 1997. She used a backpack to carry a G-tube pump and her bag of Ensure with her when she went out. When chemo was over, she worked for about a month with a psychiatrist who used hypnotherapy to get her to start eating normally again. After about three months, she was eating everything she used to. The tube was removed and the hole closed on its own.*

Enteral feedings will also generally be initiated in the hospital. If your child's malnutrition is profound, she may initially require continuous feeding at a slow rate. These feedings will be increased as tolerated, with the eventual goal being 4 to 6 bolus feedings per day. Your child may also be a candidate for enteral nutrition even though she is still obese from steroid therapy. Blood tests can help your oncologist determine whether your child is malnourished in spite of the obvious weight gain that results from steroid therapy.

> *Alan (age 8) is currently finished with chemo and radiation therapy for medulloblastoma, but has weight issues. Alan has never been big on milkshakes since he started treatment. When he was in radiation his teeth were very sensitive to hot and cold. He does get Pediasure through a G-tube, but we found a juice called Nestle NuBasic which is a 5 oz. can of calories and nutrition. The small size is great because it isn't overwhelming for Al to drink, and he has put on almost four pounds after two weeks. (He is drinking three cans a day in addition to the Pediasure at night, but not eating much "real" food yet.)*

> *I feel good nutrition is very important to good health, but the reality of the situation with our child was that he hated anything nutritious when he was on chemotherapy. I could doctor it up, add the best toppings, make it look terrific, season it just right, and it would still be rejected. So I decided since my son wasn't allowed to make any decisions in regards to the pills, treatments, tests, or hospital stays, he wouldn't be forced to eat everything nutritious if he didn't want to. Whether this was a right or wrong decision, I don't know. I just know that I served him a lot of processed foods during those years and he's a healthy and happy teen ten years later. After he was finished with chemotherapy, however, we did require that he eat healthier foods.*

CHAPTER 18

# Record Keeping and Finances

KEEPING TRACK OF voluminous paper work—both medical and financial—is a trial for every parent of a child with a CNS tumor. It is a necessary evil, however, because accurate records help to prevent medical errors and reduce insurance over-billings. Checking each report allows parents to identify changes in lab reports that might otherwise go unnoticed and untreated. Easy access to medical reports and proper organization of bills can mean less time spent in conflicts with insurance companies and collection agencies.

This chapter suggests simple systems for keeping both medical and financial records. Financial record keeping is most important in countries such as the United States. In countries with standardized healthcare, such as Canada, parents never receive a bill for their child's cancer treatment.

## Keeping medical records

Think of yourself as someone with two sets of books: the hospital's and yours. If the hospital loses your child's chart or misplaces lab results, you have yours. If your child's chart becomes a foot thick, you will still have your simple system to make it easy to spot trends and retrieve dosage information.

Information that you should record follows:

- Dates and results of all lab work
- Dates of chemotherapy, drugs given, and dose
- Copies of all chemotherapy roadmaps and treatment schemas
- All changes in dosages of medicine
- Any side effects from drugs
- Any fevers and acute illnesses
- Dates of all scheduled and unscheduled hospitalizations

- Dates for all medical appointments and name of the doctor seen
- Dates for any procedures performed (both surgical and non-surgical)
- Dates of radiation therapy, including total dose delivered and areas treated
- Dates of diagnosis, completion of therapy, and recurrences, if any
- Copies of all reports (e.g., MRI, echocardiogram)
- Child's sleeping patterns, appetite, and emotions

Keeping daily records of your child's health for many months or years is hard work. But remember that your child will be seen by pediatricians, oncologists, neuro-surgeons, neurologists, residents, radiation therapists, lab technicians, nutritionists, psychologists, social workers, and physical, occupational, and speech therapists. Your records will keep things organized and help pull all the information together. They will help you remember questions to ask, prevent mistakes, and notice trends. They will help busy doctors remember what happened the last time your child was given a certain drug. Your records will help the entire team provide your child with the best possible care.

There are as many good ways to record the above information as there are parents. Some of the methods used by veteran parents follow.

## Journal

Keeping a notebook works extremely well for people who like to write. Parents make entries every day about all pertinent medical information and often include personal information, such as their own feelings or memorable things that their child has said. Journals are easy to carry back and forth to the clinic and can be written in while waiting for appointments. They have unlimited space. Unfortunately, however, they can be misplaced.

In *You Don't Have To Die: One Family's Guide to Surviving Childhood Cancer,* Geralyn Gaes writes of the value of keeping a journal:

> Some days my entries consisted of only a few words: "Good day. No problems." Other times I had so many notes and questions to jot down that my handwriting spilled over into the next day's space. I must confess that I probably went overboard, documenting every minute detail of Jason's life down to what he ate for each meal. If he gets over this disease, I thought, maybe this information will be useful for cancer research.

*I'm not so sure I was wrong. Jason went two years without a blood
transfusion, unusual for a child receiving such aggressive chemotherapy.
Studying my journal, one of his physicians remarked, "This kid eats more
oatmeal than anybody I've ever seen." Which was true. Jason wolfed it down
for breakfast, after school, and before bedtime. The doctor speculated,
"Maybe that's why Jason's blood is so rich in iron and builds back up so fast."*

Many institutions provide families with a notebook containing information specific to
the individual program. You should receive such a notebook from your treatment
center soon after diagnosis, if one is available. If your treatment center does not have
a parent handbook, suggest they develop one. Better yet, offer to help develop one
after life has settled down a little bit for you!

*Record keeping—very important! My father came to the hospital soon
after diagnosis and brought a three-ring binder and three-hole punch. I
would punch lab reports, protocols, consent forms, drug information sheets
etc. and keep them in my binder. A mother at the clinic showed me her
weekly calendar book, and I adopted her idea for recording blood counts
and medications. Sometimes the clinic's records disagreed with mine as to
meds and where we were on the protocol. I was very glad that I kept good
records.*

## Calendar

Many parents report great success with the calendar system. They buy a new calendar
each year and hang it in a convenient place, such as next to the telephone. Parents can
record counts on the calendar while talking to the nurse or lab technician on the
phone and take it with them to all appointments.

*Each year I purchase a new calendar with large spaces on it. I write all
lab results, any symptoms or side effects, colds, fevers, and anything else
that happens. I bring it with me to the clinic each visit, as it helps immensely
when trying to relate some events or watch trends. I also use it like a mini
journal, recording our activities and quotes from Meagan. Now that she's off
treatment, I'm superstitious enough to still bring it to our monthly checkups.*

• • • • •

*I wrote the counts on a calendar or on little pieces of paper that got lost.
But, to be honest, I didn't keep the medical records very well. After four
years, I've got boxes and bags, and piles on every bureau and countertop!*

• • • • •

*For a long time I was unorganized, which is very unlike the way I usually am. I found that my usual excellent memory just wasn't working well. It all seemed to run together, and I began to forget if I had given her all of her pills. Then I began using a calendar for both counts and medications. I wrote every med on the correct days, then checked them off as I gave them.*

## Blood count charts

Many hospitals supply folders containing photocopied sheets for record keeping.

*The folder used by the hospital that my daughter went to contained four sheets with thirty lines per page. Each line had a space for the date, WBCs, ANC, Hct (hematocrit), platelets, chemotherapy given, and side effects. By the end of treatment I had to xerox more pages.*

· · · · ·

*My record-keeping system was given to me by the hospital on the first day. We were given a notebook with information about the illness and treatment. Also included were charts that we could use to keep all the information about the child's blood work, progress, reactions to drugs, etc. While we were at the hospital we were able to get the information off one of the computers on our floor each afternoon. My notebook holds records and notes for three years. Perhaps I was being compulsive with my record keeping, but it made me feel that I was part of the team working on bringing my boy back to health.*

· · · · ·

*I have several binders that contain Matthew's medical records. One binder contains a copy of every blood test he's ever received, all organized by date and test. CBCs are in the front, chemistries are in the back.*

Appendix A, *Blood Counts and What They Mean*, contains examples of actual lab sheets and a record-keeping sheet that you can use to keep track of your child's blood counts.

## Tape recorder

For parents who keep track of more information than a calendar can hold and who find writing a journal too time consuming, using a tape recorder works well. Small machines are very inexpensive and can be carried in a pocket.

*I started keeping a journal in the hospital, but I was just too upset and exhausted to write in it faithfully. A good friend who was a writer by*

*profession told me to use a tape recorder. It was a great idea and saved*
*a lot of time. I could say everything that had happened in just a few*
*minutes every day. I kept a separate notebook just for blood counts so that*
*I could check them at a glance.*

## Computer

For the computer literate, keeping all medical records on the computer is a good option. Parents can print out bar graphs of the blood counts in relation to chemotherapy and quickly spot trends. You can also keep a running narrative of your thoughts, feelings, and concerns during your child's treatment. As with all other computer records, keep a backup copy on a separate disc.

# Keeping financial records

You will not need a calendar or journal for financial records, just a big, well-organized file cabinet. It is essential to keep track of bills and payments. Dealing with financial records is a major headache for many parents, but keeping good records can prevent financial catastrophe.

The following are ideas on how to organize financial records:

- Set up a file cabinet just for medical records.

- Have hanging files for hospital bills, doctor bills, all other medical bills, insurance explanations of benefits (EOB), prescription receipts, tax-deductible receipts (tolls, parking, motels, meals), and correspondence.

- Whenever you open an envelope, file the contents immediately. Don't lay it on the desk or throw it in a drawer.

- Keep a notebook with a running log of all tax-deductible medical expenses, including the service, charge, bill paid, date paid, and check number.

- Keep a record of all account numbers by institution and care provider.

- Don't pay a bill unless you have checked over each item listed to make sure that it is correct.

- Start new files every year.

> *I bought an accordion-style file folder each year to hold everything to*
> *do with Stephan. It had a slot each for hospital bill printouts, insurance*

*explanation of benefits, receipts for all prescriptions, all Candlelighters newsletters, pediatrician bills, laboratory bills, and other information.*

. . . . .

*To be honest, the paper trail really gets me down. I can only deal with the stacks every few months. I open things and make sure that the insurance company is doing their part, and then I try to sort through and pay our part.*

. . . . .

*I started out organized, and I'm glad I did because the hospital billing was confusing and full of errors. I cleared out a file cabinet and put in folders for each type of bill and insurance papers. I filed each bill chronologically so I could always find the one I needed. I made copies of all letters sent to the insurance company and hospital billing department. I wrote on the back of each EOB any phone calls that I had to make about that bill. I wrote down the date of the call, the person's name that I spoke to, and what she said. It saved me a lot of grief.*

## Deductible medical expenses

It is estimated that families of children undergoing treatment for a CNS tumor can spend 25 percent or more of their income on items not covered by insurance. Examples of these expenses are gas, car repairs, motels, food away from home, health insurance deductibles, prescriptions, and dental work. Many of these items can be deducted on federal income tax. Often parents are too fatigued to go through stacks of bills at the end of the year to calculate their deductions. If a monthly total is kept in a notebook, then all that needs to be done at tax time is to add up the monthly totals.

Medical expenses that could be deducted on US taxes for 2000 were: acupuncture, ambulance, artificial limb, artificial teeth, expenses to modify your home to provide medical care for your child, crutches, dental treatment, HMO fees, hearing aids, hospital services, insurance premiums, laboratory fees, special school or tutor for child with learning disabilities, lodging costs for family when child is hospitalized, meals at hospital, physician's services, medicines, nursing care, operations, osteopath, oxygen, psychiatric care, psychological care, physical, occupational, and speech therapy, special schools and education, transplants, transportation to obtain medical care, wheelchair, and x rays.

To find out what can be legally deducted for the years your child is undergoing treatment, get IRS publication 502. This booklet is available at libraries and IRS offices or by calling (800) TAX-FORM, (800) 829-3676 from 8 A.M. to 5 P.M. weekdays and

9 A.M. to 3 P.M. Saturdays. You can also download this publication from the Internal Revenue Service web site at *http://www.irs.gov.*

Canadian families are able to deduct many of the same medical expenses as those living within the US. To find out what can be legally deducted in Canada for the years your child is undergoing cancer treatment, contact Revenue Canada and ask for IT-519R2—Medical Expense and Disability Tax Credits. Call Revenue Canada at (800) 959-8281 between the hours of 8:15 A.M. and 5 P.M. weekdays.

If you keep a calendar, an easy way to keep track of tax-deductible items is to glue an envelope inside its cover. Whenever you incur a tax-deductible expense, put the receipt in the envelope, and then file it when you get home.

## Dealing with hospital billing

Unfortunately, problems with billing are the norm rather than the exception for parents of children with CNS tumors. Here are two typical experiences:

> *Insurance was an absolute nightmare. It almost gave me a nervous breakdown. After all we go through with our children to have to deal with the messed-up hospital billing was just too much—it was the worst part of the whole experience.*

> *We would stack the bills up and try to go through them every two or three months. Our insurance was supposed to pay 100 percent, but the billing was so confusing that they refused to cover some things because it wasn't clear what they were being billed for. The hospital frequently double billed, especially for prescriptions. We just stopped getting our prescriptions there.*

> *We would call them to try to get the mess straightened out, but the billing department was just as confused as we were. They kept sending our account to collections. We did everything in our power to get it straight, but we never did.*

· · · · ·

> *We had two distinctly different experiences at the two institutions that we dealt with. The university hospital where my daughter received her radiation gave me a folder the first day. It included, among other things, a sheet from a financial counselor giving all the information needed for preventing and solving billing problems. I never needed to call her because the hospital billing was clear, prompt, and organized.*

*The children's hospital where she was a frequent inpatient and clinic*
*patient was another story altogether. They billed from three different*
*departments, put charges from the same visit on different bills, frequently*
*over-billed, continuously made errors, and constantly threatened to send*
*the account to collections. I never spoke to the same billing clerk twice.*
*It was a never-ending grind and a constant frustration.*

It is impossible to prevent billing errors, but necessary to deal with them. The following are step-by-step suggestions for solving billing problems:

- Keep all records filed in an organized fashion.

- Check every bill from the hospital to make sure there are no charges for treatments not given or such errors as double billing.

- Check to see if the hospital has financial counselors. If so, make contact early in your child's hospitalization. Counselors provide services in many areas, including help with understanding the hospital's billing system, billing insurance carriers, understanding explanations of benefits, hospital/insurance correspondence, dealing with Medicaid, working out a payment plan, designing a ledger system for tracking insurance claims, and resolving disputes.

- Keep a record of all account numbers by institution and provider. Make sure payments are applied to the correct account.

- If you find a billing error, call the hospital immediately. Write down the date, the name of the person you talk to, and the plan of action.

> *I often couldn't even get through to the billing representative, I was just*
> *put on hold forever. Then I tried to discuss the problems with the director*
> *of billing, but she was never in. After about twenty phone calls, I finally*
> *said to her secretary, "You know, I have a desperately sick child here, and*
> *I have more important things to do than call your boss every day. I've*
> *been as patient and polite as I can. What else can I do?" She said,*
> *"Honey, get irate. It works every time." I told her to put me through to*
> *somebody, anybody, and I would. She connected me to the person who*
> *mediates disputes, I got irate, and we went through all the bills line*
> *by line.*

- If the error is not corrected on your next bill, call and talk to the billing supervisor. Explain politely the steps you have already taken and how you would like the problem fixed.

> *The hospital billing was so bad, and I had to call so often, that I developed a telephone relationship with the supervisor. I always tried to be upbeat, we laughed a lot, and it worked out. She stopped investigating every problem and would just delete the charge from the computer.*

• If the problem is still not corrected, write a brief letter to the billing supervisor explaining the steps you have taken and requesting immediate action. Send a copy of this letter to the Chief Financial Officer of the institution. Keep a copy of each letter that you write.

• Every time you receive an explanation of benefits (EOB) from your insurance company, compare it to the hospital bill. Track down any discrepancies.

• If you are inundated with a constant stream of bills and there are major discrepancies between the hospital charges and what is being paid for by your insurance, ask both the hospital billing department and your insurance company, in writing, to audit the account. Insist on a line-by-line explanation for each charge.

> *Within five months of my daughter's diagnosis, the billing was so messed up that I despaired of ever getting it straight. When the hospital threatened to send the account to a collection agency, I took action. I wrote letters to the hospital and the insurance company demanding an audit. When both audits arrived, they were $9,000 apart. I met with our insurance representative, and she called the hospital, and we had a three-way showdown. We straightened it out that time, but every bill that I received for the duration of treatment had one or more errors, always in the hospital's favor.*

• If you are too tired or overwhelmed to deal with the bills, ask a family member or friend to help. She could come every other week, open and file all bills and insurance papers, make phone calls, and write all necessary letters. Some friends might even enter all your records on a computer for storage.

• Don't let billing problems accumulate. Your account may end up at a collection agency, which can quickly become a nightmare.

> *Our insurance was constantly months behind in paying our bills to the hospital. The hospital sent our account to collections, despite my assurances that I was doing everything I could to get the insurance to pay. We were hounded on the phone constantly by the collection people, often until we were in tears. We finally just took out a second mortgage and paid off the hospital, but now I don't know if we will be reimbursed by insurance.*

Not all stories are so grim. People who are in a socialized healthcare system or on public assistance never even see bills. Many people with insurance encounter no problems throughout their child's treatment.

> Our insurance paid 80 percent of everything, no questions asked and always paid us within a month. People shouldn't have to worry about finances or their insurance program at a difficult time like this.

· · · · ·

> We have a low income, so we are on the state plan. They give us coupons for each child, and we just hand over a coupon at each visit. I have never seen a bill.

· · · · ·

> Although hospital billing was not ever perfect anywhere we went, we did have an absolutely great relationship with our regional HMO for four years. Whenever an out-of-area appointment was needed, I called the pediatrician to start their paperwork, then immediately let our insurance nurse coordinators know. We also kept in touch through phone calls and cards. Michael and Gail were interested in our son and his progress, and we will never forget their support.

## Coping with insurance

Finding one's way through the insurance maze can be a difficult task. Understanding the benefits and claims procedures can help parents get the bills paid without undue stress. The following sections outline steps that will help prevent problems with insurance.

> First thing I do when talking on the phone with the insurance people is ask for that person's complete name and title. That lets them know that they will be held accountable later on if I need to pursue something. Then, I ask for what I need. When someone says, "Not us, call them" or any variation on that, I then ask them to send that to me in writing. As soon as they are required to commit their comments to paper, they will think about whether they are correct or not. If I get two departments telling me to see the other one, I ask to go to the next level, and speak to their superior.

# Understand your policy

As soon as possible after diagnosis, read your entire insurance manual. Make a list of any questions you have on terms or benefits.

- Learn who the "participating providers" are under the plan, for, in today's managed healthcare climate, there may be a limited network of providers and hefty penalties or no benefits if the patient goes outside the network. This is particularly important for outpatient testing and radiographic tests and may require that you obtain these evaluations at a different venue than the institution where your child receives treatment.

- Review your plan carefully to make sure that it covers the services of a pediatric neurosurgeon. If no pediatric neurosurgeon is listed in your provider list, insist that your plan allow a consultation and second opinion at a minimum. Once you have obtained this consultation, you will be in a better position to partner with the pediatric neurosurgical team in insurance negotiations.

- Determine if your physician needs to document specific requirements in order to qualify for coverage for expensive or extended services.

   > With our insurance, neuropsychological tests, outpatient occupational therapy, speech therapy, and physical therapy are covered, but the phrasing must be that it is a "medical necessity" due to diagnosis and treatments.
   >
   > • • • • •
   >
   > As far as getting neuropsychological testing covered, it is listed in my child's protocol, and since our insurance had agreed to put her on this protocol when she was diagnosed, they have to continue to provide what it calls for, or risk being liable for damages if they don't. This is how we get neuropsychological testing every two years, MRIs regularly, endocrinology, and an evaluation from an ophthalmologist. We insist that they provide everything listed on the protocol. Also, some learning deficits are caused by the tumor itself, not just by the treatments. That would indeed make neuropsychological testing a medical issue.

- Find out what your insurance co-pays are for different levels of service (i.e., office visit, outpatient surgery, outpatient testing).

- Find out what your outpatient prescription drug benefits are for generic and non-generic drugs.

- Find out what your deductible is.

- Find out if there is a point where coverage increases to 100 percent.

- Determine if there is a lifetime limit on benefits.

- Find out when a second opinion is required.

- Learn when you have to notify the company about hospitalizations or out-of-area appointments—many firms require pre-notification except in the case of emergency.

> *I had called the insurance carrier to see if they could tell me if they'd sent a precertification for our out-of-town follow-up visits on Monday, but it was Friday afternoon, and they had closed early, so I left a voice message. About 5:30, I got a call from someone from the insurance company who'd said she was the person who reviewed precertifications, and that she thought she remembered doing one for my daughter, but she wasn't sure. She said that since I had obviously made an effort to get the certification, she would give me an authorization number when I called on Monday. Then she asked some very nice questions about Mary Margaret, expressed shock and sympathy, realized we would still be out of town for doctor visits on Monday, and told me not to worry about it, that I could call on Tuesday to get the number. Then she told me she's the CEO of the company and anything they could do to help, they'd be glad to! Completely shocking. Somebody from an insurance company who is helpful and pleasant!*

Get a copy of every form that you may need to submit—claim forms for inpatient care, outpatient care, or prescriptions. You can cut down on paperwork by filling in all the subscriber information on one of each type of form (except date and signature) and then making many copies. You will have a form ready to send in with each bill.

Determine whether your policy has benefits for counseling. If so, find out how many visits are covered and the level of training required (sometimes only counseling by persons with an MA or PhD degree is covered).

Find out the names of approved providers for home infusion supplies (IV medications, central venous catheter supplies, and home intravenous nutrition) and home nursing care. These are often separate companies. Determine policy coverage for these services.

> *We changed to a new pediatrician, and he asked me if I thought it would be easier on my son to have visiting nurses come to our home to do the chemotherapy injections and some blood work. Since he had very low counts, it made a lot of sense not to have to go out. It also lessened his*

*fears to be able to stay at home and have the same nurse come to do the procedures. It was a pleasant surprise to find these services covered by our insurance.*

## Find a contact person

As soon as possible after diagnosis, call your insurance company and ask who will be handling your claims. Explain that there will be years of bills with frequent hospitalizations, and it would be helpful to always deal with the same person. Insurers may be able to offer parents a contact person for claim review or special needs. Ask the contact person to answer any questions that you have on benefits. Try to develop a cooperative relationship with your contact person, because he can really make your life easier. Some insurance companies may assign your child's account to a case manager, who will review your child's plan of care in detail and make suggestions designed to make proper use of your policy benefits. Also, your employer may have a benefits person who can operate as a liaison with the insurer.

## Negotiate

Don't be afraid to negotiate with the insurance company over benefits. Often, your contact person may be able to redefine a service that your child needs to allow it to be covered.

> *I did have to fight to get my HMO to cover Michael at an out-of-plan pediatric brain tumor center for surgery. I wrote a long letter, sent lots and lots of backup documentation, got help and support from the Cancer Advocacy Group, and in the end, my local, fantastic hometown neurologist called the director of the HMO, pushed hard on them and helped me out. We got approval and Michael's medical costs were covered fully in plan for all services.*

## Challenging a claim

The key to obtaining the maximum benefit from your insurance policy is to keep accurate records and to challenge any denied claims. Some tips on good record keeping are:

- Make photocopies of everything you send to your insurance company, including claims, letters, and bills.

- Pay bills by check, and keep all of your canceled checks.

- Keep all correspondence from billing companies and insurance.

- Write down the date, name of person contacted, and conversation of all phone calls concerning insurance.

- Keep accurate records of all medical expenses and claims submitted.

Policyholders have the right to appeal a claim denial by their insurance company. The following are suggested steps to contest a claim:

- Keep original documents in your files and send photocopies to the insurance company with a letter outlining why the claim should be covered. Make sure to get the reply in writing.

> We were making inquiries into hospice care, feeling it was time to explore that option. I found out that the only pediatric hospice provider in the state of Georgia was not on the preferred provider list. They would pay for benefits, but at a reduced rate; not a good thing since the lifetime maximum for hospice care was $7,500. With these benefits, we would get 78 days of hospice care. I felt like my only options were reduced pediatric care or full benefits using adult services. I wrote a letter of appeal stating that medically and ethically, neither of these were good choices. Well, we got a better outcome than I asked for. Not only will they cover the pediatric provider, but they have waived the lifetime maximum!

- If the insurance company is refusing coverage because they claim the procedure is "investigational" or "experimental" and therefore not covered, contact the Childhood Cancer Ombudsman Program for assistance. This organization offers a free service to help families maximize benefits or resolve disputes. In most cases, a detailed letter from your treating oncologist may help to resolve these issues.

- Contact your elected representative to the US Congress. All Senators and members of the House of Representatives have staff who help constituents with problems. You may also contact your state insurance board with concerns and complaints.

> When I ran into insurance company problems, I wrote a letter to the insurance company detailing the facts, the decisions the insurance company made, and a logical explanation on why the procedure needed to happen. I also noted on the letter that a copy was going to our state insurance commissioner, and sent both letters by certified mail. Within two days, the insurance company all of a sudden decided to cover the procedure. I later found out that the insurance commissioner's office started an investigation against them. Letters help, especially when sent by certified mail.

- If all of the above steps do not resolve the dispute, take your claim to small claims court or hire an attorney skilled in insurance matters to sue the insurance company.

Above all, don't be afraid to ask questions, and be persistent!

# Sources of financial assistance

Sources of financial assistance vary from state to state and province to province. To begin to track down possible sources, ask the hospital social worker for assistance. In addition, some hospitals have community outreach nurses or case workers who may point out potential sources of assistance. Out-of-area treatment needn't be out of reach.

> *We flew to a pediatric neuro-oncology center this time around (it was Michael's second craniotomy) and they did the surgery and the resection went great. It wasn't as expensive an undertaking as you would think. We used the Corporate Angel Network to get plane tickets. No free flight they had would work for us, but we got the cheapest rate available. The hospital provided us with the flight company information and also a list of hotels in the area that provided rooms at a reduced medical rate. We stayed at a hotel for $69 a night (there were cheaper ones) and this place included free van service to take you to the clinics, the hospital, the local mall, and restaurants. While Michael was in the hospital, we ate in the cafeteria with our parent discount. All together, our costs were under $2000 (there were three of us and we stayed in the area seven days). Michael checked into the hospital the day before surgery to be started on steroids, had surgery first thing the next morning, left the hospital three days later, hung out at the hotel until our follow-up visit two days after that (at the follow-up, stitches were removed and we were cleared to head home). It was probably the best $2000 I will spend this year. We kicked tumor butt!*

## Hospital policy

If you find yourself unable to pay your hospital bills, don't sell your house or let your account go to collections. Ask the social worker to set up an appointment for you with the appropriate person to discuss the hospital policy on financial assistance. Many hospitals write off a percentage of the cost of care if the patient is uninsured or under-insured. Be proactive and talk to the hospital about setting up a monthly payment plan.

## SSI (Supplemental Security Income)

SSI is a federal (US) program administered by the Social Security Administration and is an entitlement based on family income. Recipients must be blind or disabled and have a low family income and few assets. Children with cancer qualify as disabled for this program, making some of them eligible for monthly aid if the family income and assets are low enough. To find out if your child qualifies, look in the phone book under "United States Government" for "Social Security Administration." Call the nearest field office to determine if your child is eligible for SSI.

Additionally, there is a professional organization of attorneys and paralegals called the National Organization for Social Security Claimants' Representatives (NOSSCR). NOSSCR can refer you to a member in your geographic location. The phone number for NOSSCR is (800) 431-2804. NOSSCR has a web page at: *http://www.NOSSCR.org*.

## Medicaid

Medicaid is administered by state governments in the US, with the federal government providing a portion of the entitlement. Rules on eligibility vary, but families with private insurance sometimes are eligible if huge hospital bills are only partially covered. Call your local or county social service department to obtain the number for the Medicaid office in your area. If they tell you that your child is ineligible, ask if the state has an "Aged, Blind, Disabled, Medically Needy" program.

In addition to helping pay some or all hospital bills, Medicaid sometimes also pays transportation and prescription costs. Some states cover children under the age of 21 if they are hospitalized for more than 30 days, regardless of parental income.

## Free medicine programs

Many drug companies have programs to provide free medicines (including chemotherapy) to needy patients. Eligibility requirements vary, but most are available to those not covered by private or public insurance programs. You can get a free copy of the Directory of Pharmaceutical Patient Assistance from the Pharmaceutical Manufacturers Association in Washington, DC (toll-free hot line for physicians: (800) PMA-INFO; online at *http://www.pharma.org/patients*).

Although the cost of in-hospital treatment in Canada is covered by provincial governments, families have to pay for other medications at their own expense. For those without private insurance, this usually creates an extreme financial hardship. In many instances, the Department of Social Services can help pay for medications. The qualifications vary in each province, and the decision is based on financial need. Canadian parents should contact their provincial Department of Social Services for further information.

## State-sponsored supplemental insurance

Most states have supplemental insurance programs for families with children who are living with chronic conditions. These programs often help cover services, prescriptions, and co-payments that your primary insurance will not. You can get more information on the specific programs in your state from your medical team or hospital social worker or by calling the state department that regulates insurance.

> *In Michigan, besides my husband's insurance, we also have what is called Children's Special Health Care Services (CSHCS). It is a secondary insurance that pays for what our primary insurance doesn't: Jake's copays and prescriptions, trips back and forth to the hospital, doctor appointment and prescription copays for my husband and I, our stay at the Ronald McDonald House. Any expenses related to treatment that our primary insurance won't cover, this will. The amount you pay for this coverage is based on family income. It has been a lifesaver for us.*

## Service organizations

There are numerous service organizations that can help families in need. They provide all kinds of aid: transportation, wigs, special wheelchairs, housing for out-of-town patients, and food. Often, all a family has to do is describe their plight, and Good Samaritans appear. Some organizations that may exist in your community are: American Legion; Elks Club; fraternal organizations, such as the Masons, Jaycees, Kiwanis Club, Knights of Columbus, Lions, and Rotary clubs; United Way; Veterans of Foreign Wars; and churches of all denominations. In addition, local philanthropic organizations exist in many communities. The American Cancer Society often provides hotel vouchers for out-of-town patients when they must travel to the treatment center. To locate service and philanthropic organizations, call your local Health Department, speak to the social worker, and ask for help or speak to your hospital social worker.

## Organized fund raising

Many communities rally around a child with cancer by organizing a fund. Help is given in various ways, ranging from mason jars in local stores to an organized drive using all of the local media. There are many pitfalls to avoid in fund raising, and great care must be exercised to protect the privacy of the sick child as much as possible. If your child is on or seeking Social Security or Medicaid eligibility, funds must be held in a special needs trust and paid directly to providers. If the family receives the money or the child's Social Security number is used to open the bank account, the child can lose both Social Security and Medicaid.

## Miscellaneous insurance issues

Loss of insurance coverage is every parent's worst nightmare. If you must change jobs or move while your child is on treatment, speak to your employer's benefit manager promptly. It is advisable to continue your insurance coverage with your previous employer through the COBRA plan until you are certain that your new insurance coverage is in effect. Although this may impose some financial strain on your family for several months, continuation of your child's coverage without interruption is well worth the strain. Such expenditures are tax deductible.

Speak to your employer about whether participation in a 125-Plan is an option at your place of employment. Such plans generally allow you to have your employer withhold pre-tax dollars from your pay for such things as child-care expenses and non-reimbursed medical expenses. The amount you are allowed to withhold is determined by the size of the employee pool covered.

> We had excellent insurance coverage, so we never experienced any major financial difficulties during my son's treatment. However, insurance company literature can be so complicated that I felt I almost needed an advanced degree in rocket science to decipher our coverage. Our hospital has a financial counselor available for families that need help. Given the enormous stress that parents are under, I think it's an invaluable service.

# CHAPTER 19

# Sources of Support

EVERY PARENT of a child with a CNS tumor has a story to tell of lost or strained friendships. As social creatures, we rely on a web of support from family, friends, neighbors, and church. We need the presence of people who not only care for us, but try hard to understand what we are feeling. Many parents experience deep loneliness after the first rush of visits, cards, and phone calls ends, when the rest of the world goes back to normal life.

Members of families of children with CNS tumors—parents, the child patient, and siblings—are turning increasingly to support groups and various other methods of psychological help. Families join support groups to dispel isolation, share suggestions for dealing with the illness and its side effects, and talk to others who are living through the same crisis. Individual and family counseling can help address shifting responsibilities within the family, explore methods to improve communication, and help find ways to channel strong feelings constructively.

The various methods of support described in this chapter can help return to families a sense of control over their lives as well as provide a setting for making wonderful new friends.

## Hospital social workers

Although the need for skilled pediatric social workers is widely recognized, shrinking hospital budgets often prevent adequate staffing. If you bring your child to a children's hospital that is well-staffed with social workers, child life specialists, and psychologists, consider yourself lucky. Sadly, millions of dollars are spent on technology, but programs that help people cope emotionally are often the first to be discarded. If your pediatric center offers no support, explore the other methods described later in the chapter to get help in dealing with the challenges of caring for a child with a CNS tumor.

Pediatric social workers usually have a master's degree in social work, with additional training in oncology and pediatrics. They serve as guides through unfamiliar territory by mediating between doctors and families, helping with emotional or financial problems, locating resources, and easing the young patient back into school. Many social workers form close, long-lasting bonds with families and continue to answer questions and provide support long after treatment ends.

> Over the course of my son's treatment, I became very close to the hospital's social worker. I came to see her as not only a person who was very good at her job and providing me with wonderful support, but also as a friend. She was very much in tune with my personality, and seemed to sense when I was having a rough day, even if I had been doing my best to hide it. So many times she would stop by my son's room and invite me to join her for coffee in the cafeteria, her treat. And we would sit and talk about anything and everything. She seemed to have a natural talent for making me laugh when I really needed to most. And she never expressed discomfort when I needed to cry or curse the unfairness of the situation we were in. She was a very good listener.

· · · · ·

> We went to a children's hospital that was renowned in the pediatric cancer field. The medical treatment was excellent, but psychosocial support was nonexistent. The day after diagnosis, we were interviewed for twenty minutes by a psychiatric resident, and that was it. I never met a social worker, and the physicians were so busy, they never asked anything other than medical questions. If I started crying, they usually left the room. I didn't know Candlelighters existed; I didn't know that there was a local support group; I didn't know that there was a summer camp for the kids. I felt totally isolated.

In addition to social workers, some hospitals have on-staff child life specialists, psychiatric nurses, psychiatrists, psychiatric residents, and psychologists who can help deal with problems while your child is an inpatient.

## Support groups for parents

Support groups offer a special perspective for all parents of children with CNS tumors, as well as filling the void left by the withdrawal or misunderstanding of family and friends. Parents in similar circumstances can share practical information learned through personal experience, provide emotional support, give hope for the future, and truly listen.

Coping with life-threatening illness requires unique perspective—the ability to accept the gravity of the situation while balancing other aspects of living. Many families find this frame of reference in support groups, where there are always those with more severe problems than theirs, as well as families whose children have completed treatment and are thriving. Just meeting people who have lived through the same situation is profoundly reassuring.

> The group was a real lifeline for us, especially when Justin was so sick. We looked forward to the meetings and were there for every one. It was a real escape; it was a place to go where people were rooting for us. People from the group would always swing by to see us whenever they were bringing their own kids in for treatment. They always stopped by to visit and chat. We amassed a tremendous library of children's books that the group members would drop off. The support was wonderful. But it came from the people more than it came from the group experience itself.

· · · · ·

> I felt like I was always putting up a front for my family and friends. I acted like I was strong and in control. This act was draining and counterproductive. With the other parents, though, I really felt free to laugh as well as cry. I felt like I could tell them how bad things were without causing them any pain. I just couldn't do that with my family. If I told them what was really going on, they just looked stricken, because they didn't know what to do. But the other parents did.

Many people find comfort in formal support groups, while others get support from informal meetings, such as those in Ronald McDonald Houses, or from other parents who are frequently in the hospital or clinic at the same time. The diagnosis of a CNS tumor can be a very isolating experience. The issues of all the other moms on the street are light-years away from the mother of a child with a CNS tumor. But the moms in the kitchen at Ronald McDonald can just look at a child on prednisone wolfing down a complete second dinner and tell the new mom how fast the appetite goes when the prednisone is tapered. They understand each other's feelings and emotions because they are sharing the same experience. The understanding of a mother or father of a child with a CNS tumor cuts across all social, economic, and racial barriers.

> My 2-year-old daughter was diagnosed one week after I gave birth to a new baby girl. I remember early in her treatment, I was sitting with Gina on my lap, and my husband sat next to me, holding the new baby. The doctor breezed in and said in a cheerful voice, "How are you feeling?" I burst into sobs and could not stop. He said just a minute and dashed out.

*A few minutes later a woman came in with her 8-year-old daughter who had finished treatment and looked great. She put her arms around me and talked to me. She told me that everyone feels horrible in the beginning, and it might be hard to believe, but treatment would soon become a way of life for us. She was a great comfort, and of course, she was right.*

• • • • •

*Families from all over the world stay at the Children's Inn during treatment or follow-up. The kitchen areas, the large open-air playroom, and the computer room are frequently places to meet parents or their kids and siblings, and the Inn's supporters are always hosting game nights or family-style dinners. Everyone at the Inn, the managers and volunteers, shuttle drivers and house staff, make a real effort. Our son feels completely at home staying there.*

Many wonderful national and regional organizations exist to help families of children with brain and spinal cord tumors. Several of them are listed in Appendix B, *Resources*. In addition to these organizations, there are dozens of different types of support groups, ranging from those with hundreds of members and formal bylaws to three moms who meet for coffee once a week. Some groups deal with only the emotional aspects of the disease while others may focus on education, advocacy, social opportunities, or crisis intervention. Some groups are facilitated by trained mental health practitioners, and others are self-help groups of parents only. And, naturally, as older members drop out and new families join, the needs and interests of the group may shift.

*Parents are horrified by acute postoperative recovery and afraid for their child's life; disoriented by the "foreign land" of the hospital: new language, seemingly arbitrary rules, strange sounds and smells, rotating teams of doctors and nurses; confused by medical and treatment decisions that need to be made quickly; disheartened by their feeling of incompetence; isolated and alone; angry at God, at themselves and even at the sick child, for which they immediately feel guilty. A family whose child is newly diagnosed with a brain tumor is hit with these emotions almost immediately. Most parents don't realize these reactions are normal, and their sense of desperation is enhanced by the conviction that they aren't "doing a good job handling things."*

*Meeting other families who are going through the same thing, or who have already been through it successfully, can greatly relieve the stress of a family new to the world of pediatric brain tumors. The emotional benefits are obvious, and much needed information can be shared. Families who*

*belong to a support group have the means to reorient themselves to the new*
*world they find themselves in. More experienced families can help them*
*learn the language, rules and customs, and offer an example of a*
*functioning family unit that has successfully navigated diagnosis and*
*recovery. Firsthand, from-the-trenches strategies for dealing with this*
*disease can be invaluable, and what a relief to know that you are not alone!*

## Online support

Parents may sometimes have a difficult time finding a support group in their area that fits their needs. Many families have found that emotional support is possible via their computer. Several online discussion groups exist for families dealing with childhood CNS tumors. These groups provide parents with the understanding that only another parent of a child with this diagnosis can give. Topics might include coping skills that have been effective for families or other helpful medical information that you can use in your fight against the tumor.

> *The support that I have gained through online discussion groups is*
> *priceless. I have received a great deal of comfort from my participation in*
> *these groups. They have enabled me to connect with families from all over*
> *the world, many of which are fighting the exact same disease. I have often*
> *come to my computer in the middle of the night, when everyone else in the*
> *house is asleep. I can express my fears at 3 A.M., and know that someone*
> *will always be there to hold my hand and reassure me with the knowledge*
> *that they have felt these things, too. That's one of the most beautiful things*
> *about these groups. Someone is always there, even in the middle of the night.*

> • • • • •

> *Going online enabled me to find answers to many questions. I spent*
> *countless hours searching out hopeful stories about other kids who had been*
> *through what Leeann was dealing with, and walked away with more*
> *optimism. It didn't take me long to realize that I had to be choosy about*
> *what information I took to heart and what I should disregard. I found*
> *another mother who had posted to one of the groups with a daughter in the*
> *same circumstances as Leeann, and we began to write each other about*
> *their treatments, day-to-day lives, etc. We became very good friends and*
> *still write on a daily basis four years later. She's always picked me up when*
> *I've gone into a panic and her sense of humor and experience grounds me.*
> *We've never met in person even though we only live two states apart, but*
> *getting input from her means the world to me.*

In person-to-person support groups or those online, you need to exercise caution. If the information given sounds different from what you have been told or if it is distressing to you, you should discuss these issues with your child's doctor, nurse practitioner, or social worker for clarification.

To find brain tumor discussion groups (or electronic mailing list services), you can start by consulting the following web sites: *http://www.acor.org, http://www.braintrust.org, http://www.virtualtrials.com,* and *http://www.yahoogroups.com*. Electronic chat rooms often are not monitored, but some lists are carefully monitored by moderators. One of the largest lists, composed of almost 1,000 members and dedicated to brain tumor caregivers, health specialists, and patients, is the Braintmr list, which is sponsored by T.H.E. Braintrust and listed at *http://www.braintrust.org* and *http://www.virtualtrials.com*.

# Support groups for children

Many hospitals have ongoing support groups for children undergoing chemotherapy or radiation therapy. Often these are run by experienced pediatric social workers, who know how to balance fun with sharing feelings. For many children, these groups are the only place where they feel completely accepted, where most of the other kids are bald and have to take lots of medicine. The group is a place where children or adolescents can say how they really feel, without worrying that they are causing their parents more pain. Many children form wonderful and lasting friendships in peer groups.

> *All four of my kids have been going to the support groups for over seven years now. We have one group for the kids on treatment which is run by a social worker. The sibs group is run by a woman who specializes in early childhood development. Both groups do a lot of art therapy, relaxation therapy, playing, and talking. They meet twice a month, and I will continue to take them until they ask to stop. I think it has really helped all of them. We also have two teen nights out a year. All of the teenagers get together for an activity such as watching a hockey game or basketball game, or going bowling, to the movies, or out for pizza. They also see each other at our local camp for children surviving cancer (Camp Watcha-Wanna-Do) each year.*

For children who are too ill or shy to join a group, there are alternatives. There are hundreds of kids who use computers to contact and chat with other kids in similar situations. For more information, see Appendix C, *Books and Online Sites*.

# Support groups for siblings

Many hospitals have responded to the growing awareness of siblings' natural concerns and worries by creating hospital visiting days for them. This not only allows one-on-one parent time for the siblings, but also gives them the opportunity to explore and become familiar with the hospital environment. Sibling days allow interaction with staff, a time to have questions answered and concerns addressed. Some hospital staffs have expanded these one-day programs into ongoing support groups aimed not just at siblings who are having problems, but also at improving communication, education, and support for all siblings.

> Annie went to Club Goodtimes long after her brother stopped going and attended camp as many years as they would allow. She intends to be on the staff at camp next summer.
>
> . . . . .
>
> Our local brain tumor support group has just started a monthly meeting for siblings. They have pizza, there's a counselor involved, and parents attend their own meeting in another room.

# Parent-to-parent programs

Some hospitals, in conjunction with parent support groups, have developed parent-to-parent visitation programs. The purpose of these visits is for veteran parents to provide one-on-one support for newly diagnosed families. The services provided by the veteran parent can be informational, emotional, or logistical. The visiting parent can also:

- Empathize with the newly diagnosed parents.
- Help notify family and friends.
- Help overcome loneliness.
- Ease feelings of isolation.
- Provide hospital tours.
- Write down parents' questions for the medical team.
- Advise on sources of financial aid.
- Explain unfamiliar medical terms.
- Be available by phone for any problems that arise.
- Supply lots of smiles and hugs, but most of all, hope.

Newly diagnosed families can ask if the hospital has a parent-to-parent program. If not, ask to speak to the parent leader of the local support group. Often, this person will ask a veteran parent to visit you at the hospital. Many, many veteran parents are more than willing to visit, as they know only too well what those first weeks in the hospital are like. They are often accompanied by their child who has completed therapy, rosy-cheeked and full of energy—a living beacon of hope.

> *I am the parent consultant for our region. Among the services I provide are: meet with all newly diagnosed families; give a packet of info to each child or teen patient; continue to visit the families whenever they return to the hospital; educate families about the various local resources; provide moral support; stay with children during painful procedures if the parents can't; organize and present all the school programs; liaise with schools for school re-entry; organize and send out monthly reminders for meetings; send out birthday cards to kids on treatment; serve as activities director at the summer camp; and generally try to help out each new family in any way possible.*

For step-by-step suggestions on how to organize, recruit volunteers, and work with the hospital to create a parent-to-parent visitation program, obtain the booklet *Making Contact* from Candlelighters.

# Hospital resource rooms

Check with your hospital's medical library. They often allow families to do research on-site. Hospital resource rooms are now becoming more widely available, and they operate specifically for patients and their families to help them find information on specific conditions. Make a point on your next doctor visit to ask if your facility has one.

> *I think I first learned from a medical librarian about* http://www.nih.gov *and Medline where you can find current research on chemotherapy and other treatment. If your local hospital is a teaching facility, they often have all the major medical journals, so we were able to get full text versions of papers that we needed. Until we had our own home access to the Internet, most of our researching was done through our local hospital's medical library.*
>
> • • • • •
>
> *Patient resource rooms are wonderful places. They usually have basic information on your child's illness, listings of agencies and brain tumor organizations, online access, and volunteer staff or a counselor available to*

*answer questions, and help get you started if you're unfamiliar with doing Internet searches. It should be one of the first places that families are directed to.*

# Brain tumor conferences

Most of the major brain tumor organizations offer annual or biannual multi-day conferences for patients and families, and it may be worthwhile to attend one. These conferences often bring to one location a number of experts in brain tumor research, neurosurgery, and neuro-oncology, as well as presenting panel discussions by specialists, caregivers, and long-term survivors. They offer an opportunity to gather information, network with other families, and find hope.

Many pediatric cancer facilities also sponsor day-long workshops centered on such topics as long-term effects of treatment, school issues, and updates on brain tumor treatments. Check with your affiliated centers for information.

> *I would like to share my thoughts on the very first brain tumor conference that my family attended. The connection began with the people: I reached to others for feedback, asked for information and embraced the intellect, experience, wisdom, and courage of friends. I left the conference knowing that it is okay to continue to dream, and although we showed our hurt, and cried, we learned we need to search, and try. We smiled too: for every tear, every pain and suffering, we united and became electrified.*

A number of organizations and major facilities sponsor teleconferences and web-based conferences. Cancer Care, Inc., is one such organization; information about its teleconferences can be found at: *http://www.cancercare.org.*

Additionally, a number of grass root groups have formed to promote brain tumor awareness. From the walks that take place in your hometown to the national events taking place during Brain Tumor Awareness Week in Washington, DC, individuals are becoming involved. Contact your favorite brain tumor organization to learn more, or check out the web site for the North American Brain Tumor Coalition, a sponsor of national awareness events, at *http://www.nabtc.org.*

# Clergy and religious community

Religion is a source of strength for many people. Many parents and children find that their faith is strengthened by the ordeal of undergoing treatment for a CNS tumor, while some begin to question their beliefs. Others, who have not relied on religion in the past, turn to it now.

Most hospitals have staff chaplains who are available for counseling, religious services, prayer, and other types of spiritual guidance. Often, the chaplain visits families soon after diagnosis and is available on an on-call basis. As with any mental health encounter, approaches that work well for one family may not be helpful to others.

> *When Shawn was first diagnosed, Father Ron came in, and we all just really bonded with him. Shawn was in the hospital most of the first year, so we had a chance to become very close. Often Shawn would ask for Father Ron before he had to have a painful procedure. Father Ron would talk to him, give him a little stuffed animal and a big hug, and then Shawn would feel fine.*
>
> *When Shawn was very ill, I began to worry about the fact that he had never been baptized, and I asked Father Ron to baptize him in the chapel. We ended up going to his own little church nearby, and we had a private service with just godparents and family because Shawn's counts were so low. It was a wonderful, special service; I'll never forget it.*

Parents who were members of a church, synagogue, or mosque prior to the diagnosis of their child's tumor often derive great comfort from the clergy and members of their home church. Members of the congregation may rally around the family, providing meals, babysitting, prayers, and financial support. Regular visits from the priest, minister, or rabbi provide spiritual sustenance throughout the initial crisis and subsequent months or years of treatment.

> *We belong to a Bible study group that has met weekly for eight years. In our group during that time there have been three tumor diagnoses and one of multiple sclerosis. We have all become an incredibly supportive family, and we share the burdens. I cannot begin to list the many wonderful things these people have done for us. They consistently put their lives on hold to help. They fill the freezer, clean the house, support us financially, parent our children. They do the laundry covered with vomit. They quietly appear, help, then disappear. I can call any one of them at 3 A.M. in the depths of despair and find comfort.*

# Individual and family counseling

The diagnosis of a CNS tumor is a crisis of major proportions for even the strongest of families. Parents do not need to face this crisis alone and unassisted. Many find it helpful to seek out sensitive, objective mental health professionals to explore the difficult feelings—fear, anger, depression, anxiety, resentment, and guilt—that such a diagnosis arouses. Family responsibilities and authority undergo profound changes when a child is diagnosed with a CNS tumor. Sometimes members of the family have difficulty adjusting to the changes. Although some families discuss the uncomfortable changes and feelings openly and agree on how to proceed, many need help.

Seeking professional counseling is a sign of strength, not failure. When a child has a CNS tumor, problems often become too complex for families to deal with on their own. Seeking advice sends children a message that the parents care about what is happening to them and want to face it together.

One of the first questions that arise is, "Whom should we talk to?" There are numerous resource people in the community who can make referrals and valuable recommendations, including:

- Pediatrician

- Oncologist

- Nurse practitioner

- Clinic social worker

- School psychologist or counselor

- Health department social worker

- Other parents who have sought counseling

Ask each of the above for a short list of highly regarded mental health professionals who have experience working with your issues (for example, traumatized children, marital problems, stress reduction, or family therapy). Generally, the names of the most well-respected clinicians in the community will appear on several of the lists.

> *The whole treatment experience put an enormous strain on our marriage. My wife has always been easy to excite, whereas I've always been very "laid back." There were moments when I was afraid that it would completely fall apart. Counseling really helped. We managed to survive, and I think in many ways, it has even brought us closer together.*

In making your decision, it helps to understand the different levels of training and education of the various types of mental health professionals. You will be able to choose from individuals trained in one of these fields:

- Psychology (EdD, MA, PhD, PsyD). Marriage and family psychotherapists have a master's degree, clinical and research psychologists have a doctorate (in some states, the use of the title "psychologist" may also be allowed for those with only a master's degree).

- Social work (MSW, DSW, PhD). Clinical social workers have either a master's degree or a doctorate in a clinically emphasized program.

- Pastoral Care (MA, MDiv, DMin, PhD, DDiv). Some laymen and members of the clergy have received specialized training in counseling.

- Medicine (MD, RN). Psychiatrists are medical doctors (and only they can prescribe medications). In addition, some nurses obtain post-graduate training in psychotherapy.

The designations LCSW (Licensed Clinical Social Worker), LSW (Licensed Social Worker), LMFCC (Licensed Marriage and Family Child Counselor), LPC (Licensed Professional Counselor), LMFT (Licensed Marriage and Family Therapist) refer to licensure by state professional boards, not academic degrees. These initials usually follow others that indicate an academic degree. If they don't, inquire about the therapist's academic training.

You may hear all of the above professionals referred to as counselors or therapists. Many jurisdictions require licensure or certification in order for professionals to practice independently; unlicensed professionals are allowed to practice only under the supervision of a licensed professional (typically as an intern or assistant in a clinic or in a licensed professional's private practice).

When seeking a good counselor, ask the professional how long he has been in practice. A licensed marriage and family therapist who has been seeing patients for ten years may be a much finer clinician for your needs than a licensed psychologist or psychiatrist in their first year of practice.

Another way to find a suitable counselor is to call The American Association for Marriage and Family Therapy, in Washington, DC, (202) 452-0109. This is a national professional organization of licensed/certified marriage and family therapists. It has more than 20,000 members in the US and Canada, and its membership also includes licensed clinical social workers, pastoral counselors (who are MFCC/LMFTs), psychologists, and psychiatrists.

To find a therapist, a good first step is to call two or three therapists who appear on several of your lists of recommendations. During your telephone interview, the following are some suggested questions to ask:

• Are you accepting new clients?

• Do you charge for an initial consultation?

• What training and experience do you have working with ill or traumatized children?

• How many years have you been working with families?

• What is your approach to resolving the problems children develop from trauma? Do you use a brief or long-term approach?

• What evaluation and assessment procedures will be used to define the problem?

• How and when will treatment goals be set?

• How will both parents be involved in treatment?

• What are your fees? Will the insurance company be billed directly?

The next step should be to make an appointment with one or two of the therapists who you think might be able to best address your needs. Be honest about the fact that you are interviewing several therapists prior to making a decision. The purpose of the introductory meeting is to see if you feel comfortable with the therapist. After all, credentials do not guarantee that a given therapist will work for you. Compatibility, trust, and a feeling of genuine caring are essential. It is worth the effort to continue your search until you find a good match.

> *I called several therapists out of desperation about my daughter's withdrawal and violent tantrums. I made appointments with two. The first I just didn't feel comfortable with at all, but the second felt like an old friend after one hour. I have been to see her dozens of times over the years, and she has always helped me. I wasn't interested in theory; I wanted practical suggestions of how to deal with the behavior problems. My daughter asked why I was going to see the therapist, and I said that Hilda was a doctor, but instead of taking care of my body, she helped care for my feelings. She asked to go to the "feelings" doctor, but was concerned about whether her conversations would be private. I asked the counselor to explain about the limits of confidentiality. So that began a very helpful course of therapy for my very traumatized daughter. To this day I don't know what was said, nor*

*would I ever ask my daughter or Hilda. I do know that they did a lot of art therapy, and I know that it helped immensely.*

· · · · ·

*We went into family therapy because every member of my family experienced misdirected anger. When they were angry they aimed it at me—the nice person who took care of them and loved them no matter what. But I was dissolving. I needed to learn to say "ouch," and they needed to learn other ways to handle their angry feelings.*

Children need to be prepared for psychological intervention as for any unknown procedure. The following are several parents' suggestions on how to prepare your child:

- Explain who the therapist is and what you hope to accomplish. For instance, you might be taking the whole family to improve communication or resolve conflicts. If you are bringing your child in for therapy, explain why you think talking to an objective person might benefit her.

- Older children should be involved in the process of choosing a counselor. Younger children's likes and dislikes should be respected. If your young child does not get along well with one counselor, change.

- Make the experience positive rather than threatening.

- Reassure young children that the visit is for talking, drawing, or playing games, not for anything that is physically painful.

- Ask the therapist to explain the rules of confidentiality to both you and your child. Do not quiz your child after a visit to the therapist.

    *David had a very difficult time dealing with his brother's cancer. Realizing that we were unable to provide him with the help that he needed, we sought professional help for him. I think the reason that he feels so comfortable with his therapist is that he is aware of the rules of confidentiality. After his sessions, I'll always ask him how it went. Sometimes he'll just grin and say that it was fine, and other times he might share a little of his conversation with me. I never push or question him about it. If it is something he needs to discuss, I wait until he decides to broach the subject.*

- Make sure that your child does not think that he is being punished; instead, assure his that therapists help both adults and children understand and deal with feelings.

- Go yourself for counseling or to support group meetings to model the fact that all ages and types of people need help from time to time.

> *In the beginning of treatment, my son had terrible problems with going to sleep and then having nightmares, primarily about snakes. We took him to a counselor, who worked with him for several weeks and completely resolved the problem. The counselor had him befriend the snake, talk to it, and explain that it was keeping him awake. He would tell the snake, "I want you to stop bothering me because I need to go to sleep." The snake never returned.*

In *Armfuls of Time*, Barbara Sourkes quotes Jonathan, a boy who underwent treatment, who told her, "Thank you for giving me aliveness." She discusses the importance of psychotherapy for the child with a life-threatening illness:

> *Even when life itself cannot be guaranteed, psychotherapy can at least "give aliveness" to the child for however long that life may last. Through the extraordinary challenges posed by life-threatening illness, a precocious inner wisdom of life and its fragility emerges. Yet even in the struggle for survival, the spirit of childhood shines through.*

# Camps

Summer camps for children undergoing treatment for CNS tumors, and often their siblings as well, are becoming increasingly popular. These camps provide an opportunity for such children and their siblings to have fun, meet friends, and talk with others in the same situation. Counselors are typically volunteers, many of whom are survivors or their siblings. Sometimes oncology nurses, residents, social workers, and child life specialists are camp counselors. Supervised by experts, children can have their concerns addressed without involving their parents. These camps provide a carefree time away from the sadness of the family or the all too frequent hospital visits.

> *Of all the ways to get support, I think the camp really helps the most. You are all there together for enough time to break down the barriers. Although camp does not focus on "illness", many times we really got down to talking about how we really felt. I have been a counselor at the camp for eight summers now. Most of the campers know that I relapsed three times and I'm doing great many years later. They see the many other long-term survivors who are counselors, and it gives them what they need*

*the most—hope. The best support is meeting survivors, because nobody*
*else truly understands.*

Some camps are set up to accommodate not only the child who has undergone treatment, but their siblings and parents as well. Many camps offer separate weeklong camping experiences just for siblings.

> *There was not a chance my husband would have gone last summer, and*
> *all my exhortations about how much fun he could have with our children*
> *were in vain. He can't stand the thought of going to a place for fun where*
> *"cancer" is the binding element, so I went alone last year and had the best*
> *six days since diagnosis! In fact, it was the only time I was really happy*
> *since Danny's brain and spinal tumors were discovered in April. The staff*
> *went out of their way to ensure that parents had as much fun as kids,*
> *there was constant companionship for the kids, even at meals, and they*
> *created such a warm environment for everyone. It is a truly wonderful*
> *experience, and it was so hard to leave and come back to normal life and*
> *clinics, chemo, decisions. I have been looking forward to this coming*
> *summer since I left camp in August.*

Although the diagnosis of a CNS tumor can be an overwhelming experience for both children and their families, many useful and helpful support sources are available. Current technology allows you and your child to receive help in your hometown, at your treatment center, and online through the Internet. Each family's needs are unique, and you may need to browse around to find the types of support that works best for your family.

> *How ironic that we subscribed to this list in a moment of panic, with a*
> *black cloud lined with despair lingering above. But now we can say we*
> *have lassoed cyberspace, and here, among new friends, we have found*
> *and we have shared love, hope, support, disparity, informative*
> *information, mutual stories, mutual questions, thoughtful and sincere*
> *answers, honesty, disagreement, pain, inspiration, fundraising, friendship,*
> *humor, enjoyment, as well as understanding. This list reflects the roller*
> *coaster of life. Activity on this list enables an individual to place that*
> *initial black cloud in their back pocket, hold sunshine in their hand, and*
> *watch hope dance above.*

# CHAPTER 20

# School

CHILDREN WITH CNS TUMORS often experience disruptions in their education due to repeated hospitalizations, cycles of treatment and therapy, physical weakness and fatigue, and the cumulative effects of medications, surgery, chemotherapy, and radiation. In addition, many children also have neurological changes including seizures, behavior disorders, mood swings, short-term memory problems, and visual processing deficits. A child may want to go to school, but may not feel well enough to fully participate in daily school life. As their health improves and treatment allows, children with brain and spinal cord tumors may find both relief and challenges in school.

For many children, school is a refuge from the world of hospitals and procedures—a place for fun, friendship, and learning. Because school is the defining structure of every child's daily life, returning to school signals normalcy; indeed, expectations of school attendance impart a clear and reassuring message that there is a future. Other children, especially teens, may dread returning to school because of temporary or permanent changes to their appearance (from steroid medications such as Decadron) or concerns that prolonged absences may have changed their social standing with their friends.

Children with CNS tumors often have physical disabilities that prevent participation in games or other classroom activities. These physical impairments also require time out from the regular classroom work for physical, occupational, and speech therapies. Additionally, school can become a major source of frustration for children who learn differently as a result of the tumor and/or treatment. These learning differences, if handled in an insensitive or uninformed manner, can affect a child's confidence and self-esteem. Many children who survive CNS tumors require specialized education/ remediation as a result of deficits that develop, but not all children do.

The issues of educating children with a CNS tumor are complex, but most can be successfully managed through planning and good communication. In this chapter, parents and educational specialists share advice and experiences to help you meet the educational and rehabilitative needs of your child.

# Keeping the school informed

Communicating with the school often does not enter a parent's mind during the nightmarish days after diagnosis. Keeping the school informed, however, lays the foundation for the months or years of collaboration as the child goes through the rigors of treatment. Parents need to forge a strong alliance with school professionals to ensure that their child, who may be emotionally and/or physically fragile, continues to be welcomed and nurtured at school. Unlike other cancers, a CNS tumor often results in decline in the child's academic performance. For this reason, the school may already be aware of the tumor if the school problems led to the diagnosis.

As soon as your child is diagnosed, notify the principal in writing of the child's diagnosis and hospitalization. The next step in ensuring a good relationship is choosing a designated person or advocate to be the liaison among hospital, family, and school. This may be someone within the school, such as the child's teacher, guidance counselor, or special education staff. Often the advocate is the hospital social worker, but it may also be a hospital or school nurse, psychologist, principal, or other motivated individual. The advocate will work to keep information flowing between the hospital and school and will help pave the way for a successful school reentry for the sick child. The most important qualifications for this role are good communication skills, knowledge of educational programs and procedures, comfort in dealing with school issues, and organizational skills. It must be someone you trust to act fairly on your child's behalf.

You will need to sign a release form authorizing the school and hospital to exchange information. Schools have these forms. The school and hospital/medical personnel may not exchange any information about your child until they have received these signed documents. It is especially important for the school nurse to have copies of relevant medical information regarding the child's situation, as well as for the school psychologist and school counselor to have copies of any assessments completed by hospital psychologists or therapists.

The advocate should locate a contact person at the school (or hospital) and should provide frequent updates about the child's medical condition, treatment, emotional state, and tentative reentry date. The advocate should encourage questions and should address staff concerns about having a seriously ill child in school.

> Zach has a brain injury because of his treatment. While he is not
> impulsive, he is not his "age," either. But we expect that he should still be able
> to do his own best. We had an advocate who knew where the best place for
> school for him would be. She helps all brain-injured kids (not only ones with

*tumors). We also had a neuropsychological evaluation done on Zach and it was very, very detailed. It told his strengths, weaknesses, and the best ways for him to learn.*

## Keeping teacher and classmates involved

While your child is hospitalized, it is vital to her well-being to stay connected with her teacher and classmates. Children attend school not only for instruction, but also to develop communication and social skills.

It is important that both you and the school realize that many CNS tumors (especially those involving the cerebral hemispheres) significantly interfere with the child's cognitive functioning. For this reason, it is not realistic to expect that the child can keep up with the schoolwork. It is important, however, to maintain communication and participation in the social activities of the school as much as possible.

The teacher should be getting updates through the advocate and the parents periodically, by telephone or notes sent to the classroom. The following are suggestions for keeping the teacher and classmates involved:

* Give the teacher helpful written material. Visit *http://www.lapublishing.com* for a comprehensive list of appropriate, teacher-friendly information.

* Have the pediatric oncology nurse or social worker come to class to give a presentation about what is happening to their classmate and how he will look and feel when he returns. This should include a question and answer session to clear up misconceptions and allay fears. Teenagers should be involved in deciding what information should be given to classmates.

* Send pictures of your child on treatment to the school. Some families fill photo albums with pictures that are shared with the classmates.

* Encourage classmates to keep in touch by sending notes, calling on the phone, sending class pictures, or making a banner.

## Keeping involved with school work

A child who is out of school longer than two weeks for any medical reason is entitled by law to home or hospital instruction. As soon as your child is hospitalized is the ideal time to request this service. A letter is required from the physician stating the reason and expected length of time for this service.

If the child is in the hospital, the school district that the hospital is located in is responsible to provide the teacher. If the child is at home, the home school district must provide the teacher, and then that teacher is responsible for gathering materials from the school and judging how much the child is capable of handling. Children or teens with CNS tumors experience nausea, headaches, vision/hearing problems, and extreme fatigue, so the work must be adjusted accordingly. Ability to do schoolwork may improve and diminish before, during, and after treatments as well, so ability levels will not be consistent. Trying to keep up in school can cause a great deal of stress for children and that can interefere significantly with the recovery process.

# Siblings need help, too

The diagnosis of cancer catastrophically affects all members of the family. Siblings can be overlooked in the early months when the parents are spending most of their time caring for the ill child at the hospital or clinic or in the home. Many siblings keep their feelings bottled up inside to prevent placing additional burdens on their distraught parents. Often, the place where siblings act out the most is at school. It is very common for siblings to withdraw or become disruptive in the classroom, cry easily, become frustrated, fall behind in class work, bring home failing grades, cut classes, become rebellious toward authority, or have fistfights with classmates. Siblings, like parents, are overwhelmed by feelings, and they generally have fewer coping skills.

You should send a letter to the school principal of each sibling, asking the principal to alert teachers, counselors, and nurses about the tumor diagnosis in the family and ask for their help and support for the siblings.

> Lindsey was in kindergarten when Jesse was first diagnosed. Because we heard nothing from the kindergarten teacher, we assumed that things were going well. At the end of the year, the teacher told us that Lindsey frequently spent part of each day hiding under her desk. When I asked why we had never been told, the teacher said she thought that we already had enough to worry about dealing with Jesse's illness and treatment. She was wrong to make decisions for us, but I wish we had been more attentive. Lindsey needed help.

Remember to include the siblings' teachers in all conferences at school. If the siblings' teachers are in different schools or if the siblings have several teachers (e.g., in middle school and high school), ask the principal to send a school representative. They need to be aware of the stresses facing the family and to understand that feelings may bubble to the surface in their classroom. It is essential that parents advocate for the healthy child's emotional and educational needs as well as those of their sick child. Chapter 16, *Siblings,* deals exclusively with problems, feelings, and burdens and contains suggestions for coping.

# Returning to school

It is normal for parents not to even think about school during the early efforts to save their child's life, but a quick return to school is often strongly advised. Going to school helps children regain a sense of normalcy and provides a lifeline of hope for the future.

> *Kids are fantastic with Alissa (age 8) who has had multiple surgeries for spinal astrocytoma. They can also be brutally honest. The best therapy for Alissa is being around her friends. She just took her school's standardized test, and we think she's right with the top 25% of her class. School offered us home teaching when Alissa was diagnosed, but we said no. Alissa looks forward to school, it helps her. The people and the teachers rally around her. Alissa would be able to have a major back operation on a Friday, and she would be back to school by Tuesday. Going to school got her off pain medications and other medications much sooner. The most important thing is to get them back into real life as soon as possible.*

Preparation is the key to a successful reentry to school. Parents may want to prepare a written statement that covers the following concerns:

- A physician's statement regarding the student's health status and ability to return to school safely.

- Whether she will attend full or half days.

- Whether he can attend unrestricted general physical education classes or general physical education with restrictions (e.g., no running) or will require adaptive physical education.

- How much recess is allowed, if any.

- If a seizure may occur, what it may look like and what the treatment is. Parents should meet with the school nurse and the teacher to develop a seizure treatment plan for the child.

- A description of any changes in her physical appearance (e.g., weakness in face, arms, or legs, hair shaved or lost from treatment).

- His feelings about returning to school.

- Any anticipated behavioral changes resulting from medication or treatment (especially weight gain or mood swings from steroid or other medication).

- The possible effect of medications on her academic performance.

- When any medications or other health services need to be given at school.

- A reminder to never give any medication, especially aspirin, which can cause uncontrollable bleeding, without parental permission.

- Dietary restrictions (especially modifications for those with difficulty swallowing or on tube feedings).

- Any special considerations, such as extra snacks, rest periods, extra time to get from class to class, use of the nearest restroom (even if it's the teacher's), and the need to leave for the restroom without permission.

> There was a beanbag chair in the back of Brent's class, and he just
> curled up in it and went to sleep when he needed to.

- Concerns about exposure to communicable disease.

- A list of signs and symptoms requiring parent notification (e.g., fever, nausea, vomiting, pain, swelling, bruising, or nosebleeds). If parents are divorced, which parent to notify or which to notify first.

- A reminder that the teacher's job is to teach, and the parent and nurse will take care of all medical issues.

Request in writing a meeting that includes parents, your educational advocate, teachers, administrators, school nurse, school counselor and psychologist, and special education service providers. At this meeting, answer any questions about the information contained in your statement, pass out booklets regarding the return of children with CNS tumors to the classroom, formulate a communicable disease notification strategy (if necessary), discuss the ongoing need for appropriate discipline, and do your best to establish a rapport with the entire staff. Take this opportunity to express appreciation for the school's help and your hopes for close collaboration in the future to create a supportive climate for your child.

The following are additional parent suggestions on how to prevent problems through preparation and communication:

- Keep the school informed and involved from the beginning. This fosters a feeling that "we're all in this together."

- Reassure the staff that even if the child looks frail, he really needs to be in school.

- Reassure other children that your child poses no health threat to anyone. Tumors aren't contagious.

- Bring the pediatric oncology nurse/practitioner back into the class to talk about CNS tumors and answer questions whenever necessary. This should also be done at the beginning of each new year to prepare the new classmates.

- Develop a 504 plan (see section "Your legal rights" later in this chapter) to get exemptions to rules and policies if you think it will help your youngster. For example, wearing a hat can sometimes eliminate teasing, and leaving textbooks in the classroom can prevent the need to carry a heavy backpack.

    *My 16-year-old son was allowed to leave each textbook in his various classrooms. This prevented him from having to carry a heavy backpack all day. They also let him out of class a few minutes early because he was slower moving from room to room.*

- For elementary school children, enlist the aid of the hospital advocate or school counselor to help select the teacher for the upcoming year. Although this violates the policy at some schools, it can go a long way toward preventing problems. Although you have no legal right to this, you can ask nicely to have the policy modified for your child.

    *Because my son has had such a hard third-grade year, I have really researched the fourth-grade teachers. I sat in and observed three teachers. I sent a letter to the principal, outlining the issues, and requested a specific teacher. The principal called me and was very upset. He said, "You can't just request who you want. What would happen if all the parents did that? You'll have to give me three choices just like everybody else." I said, "My son has had three years of chemotherapy, has a seizure disorder, behavior problems, and learning disabilities. Can you think of a child who has greater need for special consideration?" My husband and I then requested a meeting with him, and at the meeting he finally agreed to honor our teacher request.*

- Prepare both teacher(s) and student for the upcoming year.

*I asked for a spring conference with the teacher selected for the next fall and explained what my child was going through, what his learning style was, and what type of classroom situation seemed to work best. Then I brought my son in to meet the teacher several times, and let him explore the classroom where he would be the next year. This helped my son and the future teacher adjust to one another.*

- Get professional help. The school counselor can talk with your child about problems with grades or classes. A mental health professional can help your child express emotions about what is happening in school and other areas in your child's life.

  *My daughter went to a psychotherapist for the years of treatment. It provided a safe haven for frank discussions of what was happening, and also provided a place to practice social skills, which was a big problem for her at school.*

- Realize that teachers and other school staff can be frightened, biased, overwhelmed, and discouraged by a child with a life-threatening illness in their classroom. Accurate information and words of appreciation can provide much-needed support.

# Avoiding communicable diseases

The dangers of communicable diseases to immunosuppressed children were discussed in Chapter 13, *Common Side Effects of Chemotherapy*. To prevent exposure, parents need to work closely with the school to develop a chicken pox, shingles, and measles outbreak plan. Check to see if your child's school already has an organized disease notification plan. Parents need to be notified immediately if their child has been exposed to chicken pox so that the child can receive the Varicella Zoster Immune Globulin (VZIG) injection within 72 hours of exposure.

There are several methods used to ensure prompt reporting of outbreaks. Some parents notify all the classmates' parents by letter to ask for help. If the parent has a good rapport with the teacher, she can have the teacher report any cases.

*My daughter's preschool was very concerned and organized about the chicken pox reporting. They noted on each child's folder whether he or she had already contracted chicken pox. They told each parent individually about the dangers to Katy, and then frequently reminded everyone in the monthly newsletters. The parents were absolutely great, and we always*

*had time to keep her out of school until there were no new cases. With the*
*help of these parents, teachers, our neighbors, and friends, Katy dodged*
*exposure for almost three years. She caught chicken pox seven months*
*after treatment ended and had a perfectly normal case.*

Other parents enlist the help of the office workers who answer the phone calls from parents of absent children.

*We asked the two ladies in the office to write down the illness of any*
*child in Mrs. Williams' class. That way the teacher could check daily and*
*call me if any of the kids in her class came down with chicken pox.*

## What about preschoolers?

A large proportion of children diagnosed with CNS tumors are preschoolers. Parents face the dilemma of continuing preschool through treatment, risking exposure to all the usual childhood viruses and diseases, or holding their child out, which denies them the opportunity for social growth and development. The decision is a purely personal one made after considering the following issues:

• Has the child already had chicken pox or received the chicken pox vaccine?

• Is the child already enrolled and comfortable in a preschool program?

• Are social needs being met by siblings and/or neighbors?

• Is preschool an option, given medical considerations?

*Elizabeth was in preschool at the time of her diagnosis. The manager*
*did a wonderful job of integrating her back into the fold. All of the other*
*children at the school were taught what was happening to Elizabeth and*
*what would be happening (such as hair loss). They learned that they had*
*to be gentle with her when playing. The manager was a former home*
*health nurse, so I was very confident that she would be able to take care*
*of my daughter in the event of an emergency. She was already familiar*
*with central lines and side effects from chemotherapy. She was a gem!*

• Does the child need special services, such as early childhood intervention, including physical, occupational, and speech therapy, that are available through the school system?

US federal law mandates early intervention services for disabled infants and toddlers and, in some cases, children at risk of having developmental delays. Infants, toddlers, or preschoolers with CNS tumors may be eligible for these services in order to avoid developmental delays caused by the tumor or treatments. These services are administered either by the school system or the state health department. You can find out which agency to contact by asking the hospital social worker or by calling the special education director for your school district.

The law requires services not only for the infant or preschooler, but for the family as well. Therefore, an Individualized Family Service Plan (IFSP) is developed. This plan includes:

- A description of the child's physical, cognitive, language, speech, psychosocial, and other developmental levels

- Goals and objectives for family and child

- The description, frequency, and delivery of services needed, such as:

    – Speech, vision, occupational, and physical therapy

    – Health and medical services

    – Family training and counseling

- A caseworker who locates and coordinates all necessary services

- Steps to support transition to other programs and services

> We have had an excellent experience with the school district throughout preschool and now in kindergarten. We went to them with the first neuropsychological results, which were dismal. They retested him, and suggested a special developmental preschool and occupational therapy. Both helped him enormously. He had an evaluation for special education services done, and now has a full-time aide in kindergarten. He is getting the help he needs.

# Rehabilitation

Rehabilitation services are necessary for the majority of children with CNS tumors. The tumor itself or the effects of treatments may impair use of or coordination in the arms or legs. Speech, language, and problems with understanding may also occur. Problems with swallowing and breathing difficulties sometimes happen. Your child should see a pediatric physiatrist—an MD who evaluates children's physical function and then writes the orders for physical, occupational, and/or speech therapy.

The initial evaluation occurs soon after surgery, and periodic re-evaluations focus on revising the long and short-term goals of therapy. Most children can receive rehabilitation on an outpatient basis. Occasionally an intensive inpatient rehabilitation program is needed for children with many deficits. Physical, occupational, and speech therapy are all components of rehabilitation.

> *I have made it quite clear what I think is best for my daughter. My approach is that I am the CEO of the company "My Tori has a Brain Tumor, Inc." and that essentially everyone else is consultant and that I do have options. I definitely don't know everything, but no one else knows my daughter, my family, or our ethos better than me, and that has to count for a lot. You may be bothersome, but guess what, it is your child, and you have that right.*

> *When my Tori came out of surgery for a multicentimeter, standard risk medulloblastoma, she was blind, mute, her right eye turned all the way in, had right facial droop, was unable to swallow, she was paralyzed in the right leg and both arms, incontinent, irritable and very hypotonic (floppy): essentially the severe end of cerebellar mutism with several regular neuro complications thrown in. They initially did not want to send her to a rehab facility and I got the feeling that they did not think that she was a promising rehab candidate.*

> *The rehab doc and our neuro-oncologist (independently) told us it would be about three years until she could walk again, and the rehab doc added that that might even be a little optimistic. Well, essentially we did a lot of stuff ourselves using the therapist as guides. We got tapes to play for her so she could listen to music and stories. We read books. We described everything going on in the halls. I brought in a little shopping cart from a local store (one of the heavy metal ones) that she could use as a walker when her left arm came back (she couldn't use a walker because her right side was too weak and she wouldn't tolerate the arm being strapped in). She was able to guide the shopping cart by putting her left arm in the middle of the bar and pushing.*

> *I actually had a box of sand in the room for her to dig through and find treasures (one with about 25 pounds of sand). Also had shaving cream to play with and we had syringe battles (like squirt guns). I got bath sponges and we made a shield from cardboard (that I velcroed on her arm). We had battles throwing the bath sponges. It is not quite 18 months later, and she has regained her sight and speech (albeit a little nasal and often slow). She is able to walk on just about any surface, play on a playground independently, swings, slides, and climbs ladders, she goes on the trapeze bar and she can do chin-ups and flip over. She finally*

*is not tube fed and she can write. Hospital staff need to believe that these kids can come back and go on to do normal kid things.*

## Physical therapy

Physical therapy involves using exercise and motion to improve the strength and movement in the arms or legs. In the arm or leg that is not moving at all, physical therapy provides range of motion to prevent the muscles from tightening during recovery. When the arm or leg begins to recover, the physical therapist devises strengthening exercises for the affected limb. Physical therapy uses equipment such as tilt tables, stationary bicycles, and treadmills. Pool therapy (also called aquatic therapy) is another form of physical therapy used to strengthen affected limbs.

> *Our son was diagnosed with medulloblastoma when he was two years old. He was inpatient for most of the first six months, then on outpatient chemo for 18 months. He had intensive rehab while in the hospital. When we were at home, I accessed the city early intervention program. He had physical therapy, occupational therapy, speech therapy, and an itinerant teacher each twice a week until he was five years old when he became ineligible. Now we get the services he needs through the school system.*

## Occupational therapy

Occupational therapy focuses on specific weaknesses and how they interfere with the activities of daily living. Occupational therapists work on the fine motor skills involved in such things as tying shoes, holding a pencil, eating, and dressing. They try to improve function of the limbs. They also evaluate the child's need for any special equipment to maximize independence in activities of daily living. For example, the occupational therapist may provide an adaptive holder to help the child write with a pencil or may recommend the use of a computer if handwriting is not a realistic goal.

One type of occupational therapy is sensory integration. It is based on teaching children and adults how to better integrate input from the senses. Each sense works with the others to form a composite picture of where we are and what is going on around us. Sensory integration is the brain interpreting and organizing all sensory input—touch, movement, awareness of the body in space, sight, and sound—for use in daily life. For more information on sensory integration, see organizations listed in Appendix B, *Resources*.

Ideas for helping create a sensory playground in your home are:

- Build a crash pad. Get foam remnants from an upholstery shop and make it yourself out of large sheets sewn together and then stuffed very full of the foam. Hold it against the wall and let your child run and crash onto it or lay it on the floor to roll on.

- Play in water (either the sink or tub) with different sized bottles/cups/measuring implements.

- Fill a huge bowl ¼ full with beans or rice. Give your child small toys to bury and then find.

- Push back the furniture and dance.

- Sculpt with clay or Play-Doh.

- Jump on the sofa with the cushions off.

- Teach the long jump. Have your child run and jump over a towel folded up. Slowly increase the length so that he is jumping farther.

- Roll on a therapy ball (available from occupational or physical therapy catalogs or stores).

- Build a tent out of blankets.

- Play dress up.

- Color, cut, glue, or make paper mache items.

> Alissa's had multiple operations for astrocytoma. One of her best friends at the hospital is Julie, a recreation therapist. One time, Julie came in with some paints. She just started painting, quietly, and then Alissa started painting. They've bonded and Julie always comes by now to work with Alissa. All the recreation therapists come to see Alissa when she's in for an operation. They come see her right before surgery and stay with her until she goes in. Alissa's taking oil painting, taught by adults, once a week. She is using her hands, using the parts of her body that work, and she is doing very well.

## Speech therapy

Speech therapy improves children's speech and language skills. Young children may need therapy because of delay in speech development. Older children require this therapy if the tumor or its treatment affects the speech and language center. Some survivors of CNS tumors have trouble interpreting speech or difficulty actually getting the words to come out. Children with slurred, halted (referred to as ataxic) speech benefit greatly from speech therapy. Speech therapists also work with children who have difficulties with swallowing.

## Accessing therapies in school

Once a child re-enters the school environment, it is best to negotiate the administration of rehabilitative services within the school. However, schools only provide educationally relevant therapies (i.e., speech therapy and occupational therapy) and not rehabilitation therapies. There are agencies in most states (in California it is California Children's Services) that provide the medically relevant therapies. These rehabilitation services are mentioned in the individual education plan (IEP) but are not provided by the school district. Your legal rights and the development of IEPs are discussed in detail later in the chapter.

> My son had problems as soon as he entered kindergarten while on treatment. He couldn't hold a pencil, and he developed difficulties with math and reading. By second grade, I was asking the school for extra help, and they tested him. They did an IEP, and gave him special attention in small remedial groups. The school system also provided weekly physical and occupational therapy, which really helped him.

In a time of insurance reductions (where a limited amount of funds is allocated from insurance companies for rehabilitation) it is extremely important to access this system to provide the best therapies for your child. For more information on insurance companies, see Chapter 18, *Record Keeping and Finances*.

Rehabilitation helps many children make a full or near full recovery. These children will have the rehab slowly phased out. Other children, however, have disabilities that require long-term rehab to maximize and maintain function. This may become an issue during the annual evaluation process in the school system. Parents and the child's educational advocate must lobby for the continuation of such services. This involves obtaining letters of medical necessity from individual therapists, the physiatrist, teachers, and the primary treating physician and presenting them as supporting documentation during the IEP meeting.

Formal rehabilitation in the outpatient or school setting is frequently enhanced by recreational activities. Community and school athletic teams are excellent therapy for those who can participate in them. Additionally, the arts, such as music, art, drama, and dance, are excellent therapy alternatives.

*Last Friday, Tori had her dance recital (tap and ballet). For me it was a completely overwhelming experience. In the fall, I looked around for a place that was willing to take her since she was fairly disabled from her treatment for medulloblastoma. Finally, I found that the YMCA would enroll her in their Saturday morning program. Although she was 6, I put her with the 4- and 5-year-olds. She is tiny and no one really knew the difference.*

*When we started she did most everything from a chair and often would just sit and watch. Later, I would kneel behind her and hold her waist as she tried to do the front and back points. Over winter, I had to decide whether she would be in the spring recital. It was hard: getting up to get there by 9 A.M. every Saturday, watching how hard it was for her, hoping that she would be able to go on stage and not be frustrated or embarrassed. During dress rehearsal the doubts multiplied. Would she be too cold in the skimpy outfit (beautiful but sleeveless and very, very short)? Would she slip and fall as she only wore the tap shoes once before? Would she go on in front of 200 people or so? Would the sound system bother her? Would the bright lights make her shield her eyes? When the curtain opened, there she was standing so poised and absolutely stunning. She did the entire routine. She didn't look different than any of the other kids. Most people in the audience had no idea how incredibly fantastic it was, how she could weight shift, point her toes, jump, move side to side and all in tap shoes! It was truly a moving moment.*

· · · · ·

*Our 6-year-old son has slower speed than his peers. He also has a visual field cut and partial seizures. Our local Jewish Community center has an excellent swimming and camp program. Our son was assigned an experienced counselor for a swimming buddy at camp. They also provided lessons in soccer, archery, and tennis. Our son sat out any activities when he was too tired. There was no pressure, and it was very supportive. The nurse handled the few partial seizures quite well.*

Many communities have formal or informal therapeutic activities. Some have sports teams for disabled youngsters. Other children participate in Special Olympics and Easter Seals programs. Many locales have therapeutic riding programs for children with medical challenges.

*A new girl approaches. The same lilting gait as my daughter who had a brain tumor removed three years ago. The new girl lifts her face to the horse. She turns her head to see him better. The child steps forward and wraps her arms around the middle of the horse, not the head of the horse.*

*She buries her face there and lingers. As a part of WE CAN, a parent support group for families of pediatric brain tumors, we invite other survivors to meet our horse and learn to ride.*

*"You brush the way the hair grows," my daughter says, showing her how to move her hand. "Before you can ride, you have to pick the horse's feet." She leaned over beginning below the knee, squeezing her fingers down the length of the horse's hock until he lifted his foot. The other child stood by the leg trying to mimic the movement. The leg wouldn't budge. This is common. A horse requires a certain feel, a confidence. Together they run their hands down the length of the horse's leg, which yields easily this time.*

*"I can't talk to her anymore you know, there's just so much stress. With all of the tests we've been through, and the surgeries. Sometimes it's difficult to be normal. Being here in the dirt, having something to talk about, feels like we are mending something between us."*

*I knew what her mother meant. I had also found that my daughter's riding, her self-induced therapy so to speak, gave her something that made her feel good about herself. In a way I felt the riding was re-circuiting her brain's functions, repairing the damage to the left side of her body, damage from the encroaching tumor and surgery. For her it was simply the smell of horse, the feel of it, the fact that he would be there to listen if she needed him.*

• • • • •

*My Anjuli, who had a diffuse brainstem glioma, had aquatherapy and it benefited her greatly. Not only did the water calm and soothe her, but it provided her with much needed freedom to move. The water pressure also helped her digestive system and lungs, too. Anjuli loved swimming and she worked hard at all of her games while in the pool.*

# Identifying cognitive problems

State-of-the-art treatment for childhood tumors has increasingly resulted in greater numbers of long-term survivors, but not without cost. This is especially true for children with CNS tumors. Survivors of CNS tumors sometimes suffer neurological late effects, which cause changes in their learning style as well as social behavior. Others are more fortunate.

*My daughter was treated for a cerebellar astrocytoma. She was recently accepted into the GATE (Gifted and Talented Education)*

*program at her school. She placed second in her district in the math*
*contest. At this time there does not appear to be any regrowth of her*
*tumor. Forty years ago this child who whispers her secrets to a horse*
*would not have lived. Ten years from now there may be a cure.*

Although many children with CNS tumors experience neurological changes early on because of the tumor itself or the initial surgical treatment, others develop these problems later, after radiation and/or chemotherapy.

*Matthew (now age 7, diagnosed in 1996 and in rehab after surgery for*
*medulloblastoma) begins to read! As he was once again going through the*
*program from Toy Story on Ice, he said to me, "Mom, does Woody start*
*with 'W'?" I said, "YES! YES! YES! Woody starts with W!" Oh, man, it felt*
*like those first steps he took a year ago, such a big deal! It was truly a*
*beautiful thing. He has spent hours and hours playing with Disney stuff*
*and "reading it" and watching it. Amen to Disney. Sometimes I feel like*
*Matt is like Helen Keller: it just takes the right time and right experiences*
*to start to learn. Once this starts, we are on our way.*

It is important that parents and educators remain vigilant for potential learning problems to allow for quick intervention. The signs of possible learning disabilities are problems with:

- Handwriting.
- Spelling.
- Reading or reading comprehension.
- Understanding math concepts, remembering math facts, comprehending math symbols, sequencing, working with columns and graphs, and difficulty using calculators or computers.
- Auditory or visual language processing, which cause trouble with vocabulary, blending sounds, and syntax.
- Attention deficits. Some children become either inattentive or hyperactive or both. These behaviors are indicative of neurologically based deficits in attention, which can cause children to be more impulsive and distractible than their peers.
- Short-term memory and information retrieval.
- Planning and organizational skills.
- Social maturity and social skills.

You should also suspect learning difficulties if:

- Your child was an A student prior to diagnosis, and she is working just as hard and getting Cs.

- Your child takes three hours to do homework that used to take one hour.

- Your child reads a story and then has trouble explaining the plot.

- Your child frequently comes home frustrated from school, saying he just doesn't understand things as well as the other kids.

- Your child's teacher complains that she "just doesn't pay attention" or "just needs to work harder."

- Your child complains that he can't hear the teacher.

All children with CNS tumors should be evaluated for the presence of these learning problems. That evaluation is incorporated into most treatment protocols beginning at diagnosis or shortly after surgical intervention. It is often hard to take this first step, because some children appear to reason well and think clearly and may be above average academically in several areas. As the time from surgery and other treatments passes, however, signs of late effects may appear. Children may fall behind their classmates on tasks that require fast processing skills, short-term memory, sequential operations, and organizational ability, especially visual. Once identified, these differences can be addressed by such strategies as utilizing resource services in memory enhancement, eliminating timed tests, improving organizational skills, and acquiring extra help in mathematics, spelling, reading, and speech.

Other children may exhibit weaknesses and learning problems prior to the actual diagnosis, and these symptoms only worsen with further treatment. Early evaluation and intervention, however, maximize the potential for learning for these children as well.

> When she entered adolescence, my daughter became very angry about her learning disabilities. She used to be gifted, and now does very well, but it is a struggle for her. We honestly explained that the choices were life with the possibility of some academic problems versus death, and we chose life.

Numerous online sources provide reliable information on learning styles and parents' rights under special education law, but one that many parents find especially useful is at *http://www.wrightslaw.com*.

# Your legal rights (United States)

The cornerstone of all federal special education legislation in the United States is Public Law 94-142, The Education for all Handicapped Children Act. It was amended in 1990 to PL 101-476 and called IDEA—The Individuals with Disabilities Education Act, and then re-authorized in 1997. The major provisions of this legislation are the following:

- All children, regardless of disability, are entitled to a free and appropriate public education (FAPE) and necessary related services.

- Children will receive fair testing to determine if they need special education services.

- Schools are required to provide a free and appropriate public education through an individually designed instructional program for every eligible child. An amendment to 94-142, called Public Law 99-457, requires early intervention programs for infants and toddlers at risk.

- Children with disabilities will be educated in the least restrictive environment (LRE), usually with children who are not disabled.

- The decisions of the school system can be challenged by parents, with disputes being resolved by an impartial third party.

- Parents of children with disabilities participate in the planning and decision-making for their child's special education.

Of course, each school district has different interpretations of the requirements of the law, and implementation varies, so you should contact the school superintendent, director of special education, or special education advisory committee to obtain a copy of the school system's procedures for special education ("Notice of Parents' Rights"). Depending on the district, this document may range from two to several hundred pages. Also write to your state Superintendent of Public Instruction to obtain a copy of the state rules governing special education. To get the address, ask the school principal or a reference librarian.

There is a time line for the referral process, although it varies in different states. Some school districts take advantage of parents who do not know the state regulations and they drag out the process. The "Notice of Parent's Rights" explains the time requirements for the referral process.

> *Our son has multiple late effects from his chemotherapy, radiation, and stem cell rescue. He has an FM unit to help him hear his teacher.*

*The school system was great about providing physical therapy, OT, and speech therapy. They wanted to put him in a special needs school, but I wanted him to have support in the classroom. They said they had no staff, so I put an ad in the newspaper at a university graduate school near his school. We found a 2nd year grad student in special ed to help him in the classroom. The school district refused to hire her, so we appealed and had a hearing. We won. The aide is wonderful and helps Michael stay on task, understand instructions, and keep organized. I'm an effective, but exhausted, advocate.*

Children on or off treatment may also be eligible for services and accommodations under the federal Rehabilitation Act, "Section 504." Section 504 applies when the child does not meet the eligibility requirements for specially designed instruction, but still needs accommodations to perform successfully in school. For example, a child who has difficulty walking and climbing stairs may need additional time to switch between classes. A child undergoing chemotherapy or radiation might need some special accommodations to address health needs (e.g., use of separate bathroom for neutropenic children, water bottle on desk, different medication administration policies, time for rest if fatigued, reduced homework during periods of frequent illness, and waiving regular attendance, tardy policies, and procedures). A child off therapy with cognitive impairments that do not meet the IDEA requirements might need to have accommodations that eliminate timed tests or provide more time to finish written assignments.

## Your legal rights (Canada)

The Canadian special education process is very similar to that used in the US. Provincial guidelines are set down by the national Ministry of Education and governed by the Education Act, but most decisions are made at the regional, district, or school level. Evaluations are done by a team that may include a school district psychologist, a behavioral specialist, a special education teacher, other school or district personnel, and in some cases a parent, although the latter is not required by law as it is in the US.

Children between the ages of 6 and 22 may qualify for special education assistance under the Designated Disabled Program (DDP), the Special Needs Program (SNP), or the Targeted Behavior Program (TBP), depending on the evaluation.

A full range of placement options is available for Canadian students, from home-based instruction to full inclusion. Students from rural or poorly served areas may receive funding to attend a day program outside of their home area.

# Referral for services

You will need to become an advocate for your child as she goes through the several steps necessary to determine what placement, modifications, and services will provide a free and appropriate public education. The steps in an IEP process are referral, evaluation, eligibility, developing an individual education plan (IEP), annual review, and 3-year assessment.

> My daughter was diagnosed with medulloblastoma, has had surgery, major rehabilitative intervention, chemotherapy, and radiation. It's been a fight to get the services she needs from the school district. You cannot assume the teachers are doing the best they can, and that the kids in the class will be good. It's not an easy thing.

Parents or teachers can make a referral by writing the school principal and requesting special education testing. Some school districts will automatically set up an IEP for any child who has had cranial radiation as part of his therapy; other school districts are extremely reluctant to even evaluate struggling children for possible learning disabilities. Therefore, it is best for the parent or physician to send a written request to the principal stating that the child is "health impaired" because of treatment for cancer, listing her problems, and requesting assessments and an IEP meeting.

Once the referral is made, an evaluation is necessary to find out if the school district agrees that the child needs additional help and, if so, what types of help would be most beneficial. Usually, a multidisciplinary team—consisting of at least the teacher, school nurse, district psychologist, speech and language therapist, resource specialist, medical advocate (whoever is serving as the hospital liaison with the school), and social worker—meets to administer and evaluate the testing. Areas usually included in the evaluation process are educational, medical, social, psychological, and others.

Sometimes if a child was assessed by hospital therapists or psychologists (or while in rehab), the district will accept those reports and just supplement their assessment with what was not done. In fact, it is important to watch for duplication of testing between the school and medical/rehab professionals.

Children with a history of chemotherapy and/or radiation to the brain require thorough neuropsychological testing, which is best administered by psychologists experienced in testing children with CNS tumors Most large children's hospitals have such personnel, but it sometimes takes very assertive parents to get the school system to use these experts. Your written consent is required prior to your child's evaluation, and you have the right to obtain an independent evaluation if you believe that the school's evaluation is biased or flawed in any way. However, you are responsible for this cost unless the district agrees or you follow the notice procedures.

> This past week we found out our daughter's test results from kindergarten. Although she missed more than $1/3$ of the time she is ready for first grade; except for math she was above the 50th percentile for all the other testing. She was in the 95th percentile for visual (identifying patterns). For math she was in the 5th percentile. We had really been working on visual stuff, obviously it paid off. I am not going to worry much about math yet as we just didn't work on things beside counting. My mom (a recently retired first grade teacher) was thrilled with the results, which were much better than expected. She was able to do practically all the beginning and ending sounds (identification) and got all the blends! Not bad considering we were also working on things like re-potty training, walking, and relearning how to eat when she started school in the fall.

After the evaluation, a conference is held to discuss the results and reach conclusions about what actions will be necessary in the future. Make sure that in all written correspondence with the school, you clearly express a wish to be present at all meetings and discussions concerning your child's special education needs. You know him best, and you and your spouse have the right to be there.

> Initially, the school was reluctant to test Gina because they thought she was too young (6 years old). But she had been getting occupational therapy at the hospital for two years, and I wanted the school to take over. I brought in articles from Candlelighters Childhood Cancer Foundation, and spoke to the teacher, principal, nurse, and counselor. She had a dynamite teacher who really listened, and she helped get permission to have Gina tested. Her tests showed her to be very strong in some areas, and very weak in others. Together, we put together an IEP that we have updated every spring. Originally, she received weekly occupational therapy and daily help from the special ed teacher. She's now in fourth grade and is doing so well that she no longer needs occupational therapy, and she only gets extra help during study hall. They even recommended her for the student council, which has been a tremendous boost for her self-confidence.

# Eligibility for special education

There are thirteen eligibility categories for special education under the federal law.

- Autism

- Deaf/blindness

- Deafness

- Emotional disturbance

- Hearing impairment

- Mental retardation

- Multiple disabilities

- Orthopedic impairment

- Other health impairment (OHI)

- Specific learning disability

- Speech or language impairment

- Traumatic brain injury (TBI)

- Visual impairment

Most children with brain tumors tend to fall under the category of OHI. The federal definition of OHI is:

Having limited strength, vitality, or alertness, including a heightened alertness to environmental stimuli, that results in limited alertness with respect to the educational environment, that is due to:

- Chronic or acute health problems such as asthma, attention deficit disorder or attention hyperactivity disorder, diabetes, epilepsy, a heart condition, hemophilia, lead poisoning, leukemia, nephritis, rheumatic fever and sickle cell anemia and

- Adversely affects a child's educational performance

Some school districts use traumatic brain injury (TBI) as an eligibility category for these children. The federal definition for TBI is:

Traumatic brain injury means an acquired injury to the brain caused by an external physical force, resulting in total or partial functional disability or psychosocial impairment, or both, that adversely affects a child's educational performance. The term applies to open or closed head injuries resulting in impairments in one or more areas such as cognition; language; memory; attention; reasoning; abstract thinking; judgment; problem-solving; sensory, perceptual , and motor abilities; psychosocial behavior; physical functions; information processing; and speech. The term does not apply to brain injuries that are congenital or degenerative, or to brain injuries induced by birth trauma.

Either of these categories leads to eligibility for the same services. Some children who have or had a brain or spinal cord tumor may end up with a specific disability (e.g. visual impairment) and they may fall under a category other than OHI or TBI. Some children with many disabilities as a result of the brain tumor, surgery, and radiation, may end up in the category of multiple disabilities. Do not allow your child to be placed in the mental retardation category. It's important that everyone involved realizes that it is an acquired brain injury.

## Special education in private schools

Children in private or religious schools have to be assessed by the home school district for consideration for special education services. If special ed services are deemed necessary, the child needs to enroll in her local public school. If the parents do not want to move the child from the private school, they attend a meeting to discuss a private school service plan (PSSP). This allows for the child to stay in his private school and receive one service equal to about $500.00 per school year. Examples of these services are speech therapy, occupational therapy, physical therapy, or special education teacher consultation. Also, private schools can but are not required to implement accommodations or a 504 plan.

## Individual Education Plan (IEP)

The Individual Education Plan describes the special education program and any other related services specifically designed to meet the individual needs of your child with learning differences. It is developed as a collaboration between parents and professional educators to determine what the student will be taught and how and when the school will teach it. Students with disabilities need to learn the same things as other students: reading, writing, mathematics, history, and other subjects in preparation for college or vocational training. The difference is that, with an IEP in place, many specialized services, such as small classes, home schooling (usually five hours per week), speech therapy, physical therapy, counseling, and instruction by special education teachers, are used.

The IEP has five parts:

1. **A description of the child.** Includes present levels of performance (PLOPs) regarding social, behavioral, and physical functioning, academic performance, and learning style, as well as the child's medical history.

2. **Goals, objectives, and benchmarks.** Lists skills and behaviors that your child can be expected to master in a specific period of time. These should not be vague like "John will learn to cooperate," but rather, "John will prepare and present an oral book report with two general education students by May 1." Each goal should answer the following questions: Who? What? How? Where? When? How often? When will the service start and end?

3. **Related services.** There are many specialized services that might be mandated by the IEP that will be provided at no cost to the family. These can include:

   - hearing assessment
   - speech therapy
   - social skills training
   - seizure log
   - mental health services
   - occupational therapy
   - vision/orientation and mobility services
   - assistive technology assessment
   - psychological and neuropsychological testing
   - behavioral plans and functional behavior assessment
   - recreational services
   - physical therapy and adaptive physical education
   - parent counseling and training
   - transportation to and from school and therapy sessions

   Attendance of in-services by all members of your child's team regarding your child's particular disability (childhood cancer workshops, seizure disorders, vision impairment) should be requested in your child's IEP and must be complied with under IDEA. For each of these services, the IEP should list the frequency, duration, start date, end date, for e.g., "Jane will receive physical therapy twice a week, for 60 minutes each, from September until December, when her needs will be reevaluated."

4. **Placement.** Describes the least restrictive setting in which the above goals and objectives can be met. For example, one student would be in the regular classroom all day with an aide present, and another might leave the classroom for part of each day to receive specialized instruction in the resource room or physical therapy. The IEP should state the percent of time the child will be in the regular education program and the frequency and duration of any related services.

5. **Evaluating the IEP.** A meeting of all the members of your child's team is held to review your child's progress toward attaining the short- and long-term goals and objectives of the IEP. In order to ensure that the IEP is working for your child, parents should make sure their child's IEP is reviewed at least once a year, and more frequently if needed to address parent or teacher concerns. Some states have limits on the number of IEP meetings per year.

Parents should come prepared to IEP meetings. Bring copies of all current testing and recommendations by specialists (or send ahead of time if possible), which will help support your requests for services. It is best to create a positive relationship with the school so that you are able to work together to promote your child's well-being. If, for whatever reason, communication deteriorates and you feel that your child's IEP is inadequate or not being followed, there are several facts you need to know:

- Changes to the IEP cannot be made without parental consent.

- If parents disagree about the content of the IEP, they can withdraw consent and request (in writing) a meeting to draft a new IEP, or they can consent only to the portions of the IEP with which they agree.

- Parents can request to have the disagreement settled by an independent mediator and hearing officer.

IEPs in Canada are almost identical to those used in the US. In Canada, the IEP is updated yearly or more frequently if needed. A formal review is required every three years. In Canada, if disputes arise between the school or the district and the parents, there is a School Division Decision Review process available to resolve them. The concept known as due process in the US is usually referred to as fundamental justice in Canada.

> We've set up goals and objectives in Victoria's IEP so that she succeeds at her level. She is graded against these requirements. We have two or three meetings each year to determine the appropriate level of her capabilities. We've negotiated for all her classwork to be done during school hours with one-to-one help in the resource room. Victoria, who has seizures and

*cognitive issues due to a hypothalamic hamartoma, is on her school's Honor Roll for grades! Her name was published in our town newspaper along with others who excelled and she received a nice certificate. This is how an IEP is supposed to work, grades being determined upon achievable goals outlined in an IEP, and hard work. She knows of course that grading for her is different than for other kids, and attempted to downplay her accomplishment, but secretly I think that she was quite proud and it has motivated her to work even harder.*

Having an IEP in place, however, does not guarantee the perfect education. It is also not a replacement for parental/teacher communication. Like children who are not ill, those with CNS tumors will have better academic years than others for various reasons. It may be related to a specific teacher, family stress, a move from inactive to active treatment, or for reasons no one can identify.

*This year (third grade) has been a nightmare. My son has an IEP that focuses on problems with short-term memory, concentration, writing, and reading comprehension. The teacher, even though she is special ed qualified, has been rigid and used lots of timed tests. She told me in one conference that she thought my son's behavior problems were because he was "spoiled." We asked her at the beginning of the year to please send a note home with my son if he has a seizure, and she has never done it. She even questions him when he tells her that he had a seizure at recess. I began communicating directly with the principal, and I finally received a written notice that he had a seizure. I learned that the IEP is only as valuable as the teacher who is applying it.*

## More on placement and modifications

IDEA intentionally falls short on detailing specific types of educational placement, modifications, and related services. Because options are open, your child's IEP should reflect those programs and services uniquely appropriate for his needs. Advocates, disability organizations, and your child's medical team, teachers, and therapists can assist you in determining which options best suit your child, although ultimately you know your child best. The following are placement options listed from the least restrictive to the most restrictive.

- Regular education and accommodations
- Regular education and support services and accommodations

- Reduced day regular education and accommodations
- Regular education in team-taught classes (special education monitoring)
- Regular education and resource room for weak areas
- Special education placement and mainstream elective
- Special education self-contained placement
- Homebound instruction and support services
- Residential placement

Possible accommodations available through a 504 plan or IEP include:

- Reduced day
- Personalized course selection
- Preferential seating
- Instruction of student in preferred learning mode
- Study groups with discussion for learning/memory
- Taping of classes for reinforcement
- Reduction in reading load
- Books on tape
- Technology supported reading
- Enlargement of print size
- Slant board for visual issues
- Visual tracking systems for dealing with print
- Copy of peer notes to increase listening in class and reduce writing
- Copy of teacher's planning notes prior to instruction
- Reduction in writing load
- Computer for written assignments
- Keyboard training (kindergartners are not too young to learn)
- Software for written language
- Use of preplanning organizers for written language
- Calculator use permitted after mastery demonstrated
- Extended time for tests

- Test questions written for recognition to facilitate retrieval
- Travel between classes with adult/responsible peer
- Elevator/wheelchair access
- Locker placement consideration
- Organizational notebook for tracking assignments
- Assignment check-off system
- Breakdown of large assignments into steps
- Daily one-to-one tutoring with a certified special education specialist

## Home schooling

Some parents prefer to home school their children. If you are thinking of doing this, check with your school district to find out their policies. This is especially important if your child requires special education services.

> Home schooling is not for everyone but it has worked for us. Home schooling is a life style that you grow accustomed to. You are not boxed in as to how you teach or when you teach. I am thankful that we home school because of what Jessica is going through right now. She has at least two or three doctor appointments a week on the average. So we can work school in before we go to the doctor appointments or after the appointments depending on when we have to be there. Most of the schoolwork she does is on the computer or she does orally with me.

> Jessica has had a major set back academically after being diagnosed with a brain tumor. She was on a second grade level last year and was almost to the third grade level where she was supposed to be, when she was diagnosed. Since that time, she is now on a first to second grade level and has to relearn a lot of very basic academics. She had to have radiation during the summer and I think this also affected her concentration and her overall functioning in an academic setting. I am able to get curriculum and testing materials from the varying resources that are on the Internet such as: Timberdoodle, Abeka, and Sonlight to name a few.

• • • • •

> We will be partially homeschooling our daughter next year while her dad takes a research position in another state. We've worked out a plan that keeps her in contact with her school. Her grandparents, who have educational backgrounds, will take on a large part of her homeschooling

*and we'll be incorporating trips to historical sites in Massachusetts, Washington, DC, and Virginia too.*

## Transition services

Transition planning should begin in the early years of middle school, when the student's peers are beginning to gain work skills and preparing for high school graduation. The law states that transition services should begin no later than age 14. Special education students have a right to be prepared for graduation, higher education, and employment in ways that fit their needs. For some survivors, extra support is needed to make the transition from high school to adulthood go smoothly.

# The terminally ill child and school

In the sad event that the child's health continues to deteriorate and all possible treatments have been exhausted, it is time for the students and staff to discuss ways to be supportive during her final days. Classmates need timely information about their ill classmate, so that they can deal with her declining health and prepare for her death. The possibility of death from cancer should have been sensitively raised in the initial class presentation prior to the student's return to school, but additional information is needed if the student's health declines. The following are suggestions on how to prepare for the death of a classmate:

- The entire school staff needs to be in continuous communication with parents and hospital. They need to be reassured that most likely the child will either die at home or in the hospital, not at school.

- Staff needs to be aware that participation at school is vital to a sick child's well-being. They should welcome and support the child's need to attend school as long as possible.

- Staff can design flexible programs for the ill student—for example, part-time school attendance and/or part-time home tutoring (if appropriate) for a child too weak to attend school all day.

- Staff can designate a "safe person" and "safe haven" in the school building so that the student can retreat if physically or emotionally overwhelmed.

- The hospital advocate should meet with school personnel and the student's class to answer questions about the student's health status and to address fears and misconceptions about death.

- It is helpful to provide reading materials on death and dying for the ill child's classmates, siblings' classmates, teachers, and staff.

- Extraordinary efforts should be made to keep in touch once the child can no longer attend school. Cards, banners, tapes, telephone calls, or conference calls (on the principal's speaker phone) from the entire class are good ways to share thoughts and best wishes.

- Visits to the hospital or child's home should be made, if appropriate. If the child is too sick to entertain visitors, the class could come wave at the front window and drop off cards or gifts.

- The class can send a book of jokes, a Walkman and tapes, or a basket of small gifts to the hospital.

- The class can decorate the family's front door, mailbox, and yard when the child is returning home from the hospital.

All of the above activities encourage empathy and concern in classmates, as well as helping them adjust to the decline and imminent death of their friend.

> *Jody was lucky because he went to a private school, and there were only sixteen children in his class. Whenever he could come to school, they made him welcome. Because children worked at their own pace, he never had the feeling that he was getting behind in his classwork. He really felt like he belonged there. Sometimes he could only manage to stay an hour, but he loved to go. Toward the end when he was in a wheelchair, the kids would fight over whose turn it was to push him. The teacher was wonderful, and the kids really helped him and supported him until the end.*

When the child dies, a memorial service at school gives students a chance to grieve. School counselors or psychologists should talk to the classmates to allow them to express their feelings.

Parents appreciate receiving stories or poems about their departed child from classmates, and having classmates attend the funeral also supports the grieving family.

# Record keeping

Other than medical record keeping, no records are more important to keep than those concerning your child's special education. Many parents recommend that you keep a yearly file that includes the name of the teacher, principal, and district psychologist, a copy of the IEP and all test results, all correspondence, a current copy of the local and state regulations, and all of your child's report cards. You should also include in the file a list of the medications taken by your child during the year. The thought of this may seem overwhelming, but try to think of it this way: appropriate schooling is what will enable your child to overcome the cancer experience and become a productive adult. Your child needs your help to secure that future.

Do not throw these records out—give them to your child when she reaches eighteen. These records can be crucial for college testing and college accommodations.

# On accepting disabilities

Children with CNS tumors often have visible physical disabilities and many invisible disabilities. To help children and teens reach their true potential, changes in intellectual functioning and social skills must be diagnosed early and addressed. Students whose style of learning has changed as a result of the tumor and/or treatment need their parents and teachers to explore the many excellent methods to enhance their ability to learn.

> *Josh's sister Nettie recently was tested for auditory processing disorder. She did very well with the testing, but the ability to score it only goes down to seven years and developmentally she is lower than that in some areas. Therefore, certain aspects of the test were unable to be administered. However, based upon what testing was done, Nettie does demonstrate a great deal of difficulty processing things presented auditorily. It was suggested that we try using a device called an "Easy Listener." She would wear a little box like a walkman with headphones. The teacher would wear a microphone which links right to the box Nettie is wearing. That would mean that no matter what the noise level in the room, or where the teacher is, the teacher's voice will always sound only six inches away from Nettie's ears. We are also going to try using a computer program called Earobics to try and retrain parts of her brain to "listen" better. Auditory processing disorder is sort of like having dyslexia of the ears. The ears hear fine, but the brain doesn't receive the message properly. So we'll see if any of these things help her.*

Location of the tumor plays an important role in what types of disabilities may occur. Unlike with other childhood cancers, issues related to school occur in the majority of children who have CNS tumors. Many parents of CNS survivors have learned to look beyond the disabilities and to focus on advocating for an appropriate educational support system for their child, with the hope that he not only achieves his full learning potential, but develops a strong and positive sense of self.

*Mary Margaret (age 10) was diagnosed at 4 years of age with neurofibromatosis, and later on with a related optic glioma. She has skin tumors and a skull-based tumor because of NF. Mary Margaret has won the citizenship award at school every year, including kindergarten. I've been especially impressed with her this year. There's a boy in her class who is being mainstreamed after being in an alternative class for several years. He was a challenge for the teachers and for the other students, because of his temper, outbursts, and repetitive behavior. None of the kids were friends with him and would tease him terribly; they'd throw sand on him on the playground, stuff like that. Mary Margaret would make them stop, saying "Stop picking on him. How would you feel if you were him and people were doing this to you?" She told me once that this boy was sitting by himself at lunch, because no one would sit with him, and she went and sat with him, even though her girlfriends were saving her a seat. She could miss 100 math awards and I'd be more proud to hear stories like that and see her get recognized for THAT kind of behavior. Being nice is way more important than being good at math, that's our family motto.*

# CHAPTER 21

# End of Treatment

THE LAST DAY OF TREATMENT is a time of both celebration and fear. Some children and teens quickly return to excellent physical and mental health; others have lingering or permanent effects from the tumor and/or treatment.

End of treatment for children with CNS tumors is best defined as completing a specific treatment protocol and moving to a period of observation. Sometimes no more treatment is needed, but, for many, another phase will become necessary. Despite the possibility of regrowth, most families are thrilled that the days of hospital stays and procedures have ended. However, many fear a future without surgery, radiation, or drugs to keep the tumor from returning.

When treatment ends, concerns about recurrence or growth are an almost universal parental worry, and for a significant number of families, periodic scans and assessments are a constant reminder of the diagnosis. Those children who have no evidence of tumor in the CNS for a period of five years are considered cured. Hearing that magic word is every parent's dream.

This chapter covers the emotional and physical aspects of ending a treatment protocol and shifting to a period of observation. It also discusses effective medical follow-up, possible late effects of treatment, and employment and insurance issues for long-term survivors.

## Emotional issues

Treatment for a CNS tumor can span just a few weeks (for those slow-growing tumors completely removed with surgery) to months or years (for fast-growing tumors or slow-growing deep tumors that are not completely removed with surgery or other treatments). Families who have a short treatment process find returning to normal life less stressful than those completing a longer, more complex treatment.

Regardless of the type of tumor, all children eventually reach a point in the treatment process when they move to an observation mode with no immediate plan for surgery, radiation, or chemotherapy. This period of observation may include treatments such as physical, occupational, or speech therapy, medical treatment of seizures or hormonal imbalances, and follow-up scans. It may last for months or go on indefinitely. It is during this inactive period that the family tries to return to normal life.

Parents should anticipate that, after many months or years spent watching their child go through the rigors of active treatment, they may have lost the feeling of a normal life. They may experience relapse scares, and they frequently need to call the doctor to describe the symptoms and be reassured.

> Sam received focal radiation to the tumor bed following surgery as a toddler for an ependymoma. When the radiation treatments were over, it was weird. Suddenly, Sam was no longer under treatment and we didn't have any reason to go to the hospital. No reason to see any doctors or nurses. I had thought that I would be thrilled, and I mostly was, but I was also scared to be on our own. I was filled with thoughts of "what if." What if he gets a fever? What if he has a headache? What if he vomits? I really missed the security of seeing a nurse every day.

> Sam had his first follow-up MRI and lumbar puncture (LP) a week and a half after finishing radiation. They looked good—no signs of cancer! He was done with treatment and cancer-free! All we had to do now was go back to living normally, if that were ever possible, and come back in two months for his next MRI and spinal tap.

> One of the ongoing issues that I still have as a parent is judging what to do in a medical situation. For a long time, I called our pediatrician for every fever or cough. Thankfully, Sam hasn't had many stomach viruses with vomiting. It's hard to go back to being normal about their health. On the one hand, I don't want to panic and make too big a deal out of anything; but on the other hand, what if it's a sign of something serious? I don't want to under-react either.

> Today Sam is cancer-free and a healthy, normal 5-year-old kindergarten student. Sam having cancer is the hardest thing our family has had to deal with. I think the best way to describe it is it's like being on a roller coaster of good news/bad news. The highs and lows were more dramatic in the beginning. Even today, each MRI/LP follow-up puts us back on the ride.

With diagnosis came the awareness that life can be cruel and unpredictable. Many parents feel safe during treatment and feel that therapy is keeping the tumor from growing. The end of treatment leaves many parents and children feeling exposed and vulnerable. When treatment ends, parents must find a way to live with uncertainty, to find a balance between hope and reasonable worry.

> *I had a lot of anticipatory worry—it started about six months before ending treatment. By the last day of treatment I had been worrying for months, so it was just a relief to quit.*

• • • • •

> *We were thrilled when treatment ended. I knew many people who felt that celebrating would jinx them; they just didn't feel safe. Well, I felt that we had won a big battle—getting through treatment—and we were going to celebrate that. If, heaven forbid, in the future we had another battle to fight, we'd deal with it. But on the last day of treatment, we were delighted.*

# Last day of treatment

The last day of treatment usually includes a physical examination, blood work, MRI scan, and a discussion with the oncologist. The treating physician should review the treatment, outline the schedule for MRI scans and blood tests for the future, and sensitively inform the family of the potential for long-term side effects. One group of parents presented to physicians at a major children's hospital the following list of suggestions for the last day of treatment:

- Schedule enough time with the family to have a conversation.
- Bring a sense of closure to the active phase of treatment.
- Express happiness that all has gone well.
- Be realistic but hopeful about the future.
- Praise the child for handling a very difficult time in her life with grace (or courage, or whatever word is appropriate).
- Praise the parents for all of their hard work.
- Allow time for the parents to give the physician feedback and thanks.
- Give a certificate of accomplishment to the child.
- Be aware that families are relieved but fearful of the future.

# Catheter removal

Children and teens usually cannot wait to have the catheter removed, as it symbolizes that treatment has truly ended. Physicians have very different opinions on the best time to remove the catheter. Some remove it on the last day of treatment, while others want to wait until several weeks or months have passed. If your doctor recommends a delay, and you or your child have strong feelings about waiting, take the time to discuss it fully.

Removal of the external catheter is usually an outpatient procedure. The child is given a mild sedative, then the oncologist pulls the catheter out of the child's body by hand. This may also be done under general anesthesia by the surgeon or radiologist who inserted it.

> *Kristin's Broviac removal wasn't too bad. They gave her fentanyl ahead of time, so she was fairly relaxed. I wished that they had offered me a sedative as well! One of the nurses had her hand on Kristin's shoulder and quietly talked to her to try to keep her focused elsewhere. I held her legs, and my wife held her hand. The doctor put one hand on her chest, and pulled on the tubing with the other. It only took about two seconds to come out. There was little blood; they just put a Band-Aid on the site and sent us home.*

Implanted catheters such as the Port-a-cath are removed surgically in the operating room. Children are usually given general anesthesia, and the operation takes less than half an hour. Only one incision is made, usually just above the port at the same place as the scar from the implantation surgery. The sutures holding the port to the underlying muscle are cut, and the port with tubing is pulled out. The small incision is then stitched and bandaged. When the child begins to awaken, he is brought out to the parents. The family then waits until the surgeon has approved their departure. Often, the wait is short, for as soon as the child is awake enough to take a small drink or eat a Popsicle, he is released. If your child becomes nauseated from the anesthesia, the wait can be several hours until he is feeling better.

> *Our docs said that Will's port could come out after the next MRI, which was just after treatment ended. It was a short procedure under general anesthesia, and he actually woke up without thrashing or crying this time. He was so happy to have it gone. He was just barely 5. We talked a little before about the "button" and the tubing coming out, just so he understood it wasn't part of his body that was being taken out.*

# Ceremonies

Some families greatly benefit from having ceremonies to celebrate the end of treatment. Especially for younger children who have spent much of their lives receiving treatment and having procedures, ceremonies can help them grasp that it is truly over. Here are ideas from many families on how to commemorate this important occasion:

- Take good-bye pictures of the hospital and staff.

- Take a picture of your child receiving her last treatment.

- Give trophies to your child and his siblings.

- Ask the clinic to present your child with a certificate.

- Let your child flush all of the leftover oral medications down the toilet.

- Let your child tear or cut up the calendar used to record dates for procedures (not a good idea if any records are on it).

- Throw a big party.

- If your child has been seeing a counselor, schedule a visit to talk about the accomplishment.

- Have friends and family send congratulations cards.

- If consistent with your beliefs, have a religious ceremony of thanksgiving.

- Go on a trip or vacation to celebrate.

Some parents do not feel comfortable celebrating the end of treatment. One mother described her feelings this way:

> Finishing treatment was very difficult. I thought that I would feel like celebrating and cheering—but all I felt was fear. Treatment was over, but cancer was still a part of our lives. I think we will always live with the fear of relapse. It has taken me some time to come to grips with that reality.

As you have read so often in this book, every child, parent, and relative reacts differently to every phase of treatment; what is important is not the differences, but the fact that each family member feels free to express and act on their own feelings, whatever they may be. You may be joyful, relieved, fearful, or terrified, but end of treatment is emotionally charged for every member of the family.

# What is normal?

After the trauma of diagnosis and treatment for a CNS tumor, families grapple with the idea of returning to normal. What is "normal" is variable depending on treatment and circumstances. For instance, for those continuing to monitor a slow-growing tumor deep within the brain, life may return to normal for short periods between follow-up scans and checkups. Other children might require only one surgery, then life becomes predictable again. Many families stay on a roller coaster of being on treatment, then off, then on again for months or years.

It's hard to know what "normal" is after treatment ends. Parents realize that returning to the carefree days before cancer is unrealistic—life has changed. The constant interaction with medical personnel is ending, and support from family and friends recedes. Although it is true that the blissful ignorance of the days prior to CNS tumor are gone forever, many families do enter a period of calm in which routines do not revolve around caring for a sick child, hospital stays, and clinic appointments. Each family needs to carve out a new definition of normal. For some, physical changes or handicaps are a constant reminder of the diagnosis and treatment. This new life often includes physical, occupational, and/or speech therapy and coping with learning issues. For others, there are few reminders of the cancer treatment.

> You can't tell from looking at James, who is 6 now, that he's had brain surgery and chemo. There are no obvious scars or deficits. When he starts to talk or tries to run, then you notice it. He's very friendly and verbal, but his speech is off for his age, his motor skills are slower, he tires easily, and he has partial seizures. He gets services at school, including speech and physical therapy, and we're working on a plan for next year to accommodate schoolwork because of seizures. We've been doing fun things all along, like trips to zoos, walking in the park, and swimming to increase his overall strength. People see us using his wagon to give him a rest when he needs it. Usually someone will look at us strange when they see a big kid using a wagon, and if the moment is right, I've been known to offer some insight. But when you're out having fun, you don't always want to have to explain.

· · · · ·

> These first two months off treatment, I've noticed Kristin steadily gaining in self-confidence and composure.

Many parents and children resolve their complicated feelings by giving back to the cancer community in some way. Helping others, for many people, is a satisfying way to reach out or bring closure to the active phase of cancer treatment. Helping others can create something enormously meaningful out of personal difficulties. Here is what some families have done:

- I requested that the clinic and local pediatricians refer newly diagnosed families to me if the parents wanted someone with a child who experienced the same disease to talk to. I remembered how impossible it was to go to support meetings in the first few months, and how desperately I needed to talk to someone who had already traveled the same road.

- We started a Boy Scout project to keep the toy box full at the clinic.

- My children are counselors at the camp for kids with cancer.

- After my son died, I gave up my parish to be a hospice chaplain.

- We organized a walk to raise funds for the Ronald McDonald House.

- We (a group of parents of children with cancer) requested and were granted a conference with the oncology staff to share our thoughts on ways to improve pain management and communication between parents and staff. It was very well received.

- We circulated a petition among parents to request increased hospital funding for psychosocial support staff. We presented it to the director of the hematology/oncology service.

- I started a Candlelighters group and organized meetings, conferences, and picnics, and I write a quarterly newsletter.

- We held a bone marrow donor drive.

- I give platelets and blood regularly.

- I took all of our leftover Hickman line supplies to camp and gave them to a family who needed them.

The possibilities are endless. Parents use whatever talents they have to help others, from designing head coverings to writing newsletters to going online on their computer to talk with newly diagnosed families.

> I am the administrator of several online support groups for parents
> of children with cancer. We have over 600 participants from sixteen
> countries all over the world. Some of the members' children have been
> cured for years, some are newly diagnosed, and some of the children
> have died. We've become a family. It's important to me to remain

*involved in the fight against childhood cancer. There are so many*
*others that are following behind in our footsteps. Perhaps showing that*
*we've been there, too, yet we're still standing, might help another mom*
*or dad.*

An equally healthy response to ending treatment for cancer is to put it behind you. Many families, after years of struggles, just want to enjoy a newfound sense of normalcy. They don't want constant reminders of cancer, and they feel that it's not good for children to be continually reminded of those hard times. Parents and children need to talk to one another, examine their emotions, decide what course they want to chart, and work together toward a healthy life after cancer.

# Follow-up care

In the past, most survivors of CNS tumors were on their own after treatment ended. With more long-term survivors, it became apparent that these young men and women often faced complex medical and psychosocial effects from their years of treatment. As a result, many institutions began late effects clinics to provide a multidisciplinary team to monitor and support survivors. The nucleus of the team is usually comprised of a nursing coordinator, pediatric oncologist, pediatric nurse practitioner, radiation oncologist, endocrinologist, school liaison, social worker, and psychologist.

The follow-up programs usually include a review of treatments received, counseling regarding potential health risks (or lack thereof), and case-specific diagnostic tests, such as audiograms (to evaluate hearing loss), hormonal studies, or testing for learning disabilities. These follow-up clinics not only provide comprehensive care for long-term survivors, but also participate in research projects that track the effectiveness of and side effects from various clinical trials. In addition, the follow-up clinic acts as an advocate for survivors at schools, insurance agencies, and employers.

As Grace Powers Monaco, one of the founders of Candlelighters Childhood Cancer Foundation, said:

> *Life is a hollow gift unless cancer survivors emerge from treatment as*
> *competent and worthy individuals, able to obtain insurance, equipped to*
> *earn a living, and prepared to participate in a medical surveillance*
> *program to "keep" the life they have won.*

All children with CNS tumors should be followed when off active treatment. If your institution does not provide long-term follow-up care, the following issues should be addressed at the end of treatment

# Follow-up schedule

Protocols for clinical trials require specific follow-up schedules. For instance, your child may require follow-up every three months for a period (usually 1 to 2 years) then every four to six months for a while, and then annually. Follow-up includes:

- Physical exams by primary treating physician
- MRI scans
- Blood tests (CBC and hormonal tests)
- Audiograms
- Neuropsychological testing yearly or biyearly

Find out from the oncologist what the required schedule will be and where the appointments will take place. Make sure your child understands that, after treatment ends, doctor appointments, MRI scans, and blood draws will still be an occasional necessity. In addition to monitoring the tumor status, the follow-up schedule is a mechanism for early identification of late effects of the tumor and treatment.

# Possible late effects

At diagnosis, parents do not know the price their child will ultimately pay for reprieve from the CNS tumor. Short-term effects may be discomfort, seizures, weakness in an arm and/or leg, and school absences. Long-term effects range from none to severe. These can include subtle or pronounced physical disabilities, learning disabilities, an impaired endocrine system, hearing loss, altered bone growth, infertility, and an increased risk of secondary malignancies.

It is important to know the possible risks based on the treatment your child received. You can then store this knowledge in the back of your mind. As one mother said, "I hope for the best and I deal with the rest." For detailed information on possible late effects from childhood cancer, read *Childhood Cancer Survivors: A Practical Guide to the Future*, by Nancy Keene, Wendy Hobbie, and Kathy Ruccione.

> *Our daughter was diagnosed with medulloblastoma when she was 10 months old. She had surgery and two and a half years of chemotherapy. She needed two second look surgeries when MRIs showed a shadow. Both times they found only scar tissue, no tumor. She had minor delays in motor development that a short course of physical therapy resolved. Other than that, she has no late effects. She is a normal, happy, giggling 13-year-old girl. She talks on the phone a lot and likes Backstreet Boys. She is just wonderful and we all feel blessed.*

## Physical disabilities

Permanent weakness of an arm, leg, or entire side of a body can occur from the tumor itself or from swelling related to the treatment. Weakness of the muscles of the eye and face or those involved in swallowing can also occur from the tumor and treatment. Physical, occupational, and speech (swallowing) therapy should continue for months and years to maintain the maximal functioning of the muscles. These services should be provided through the school's IEP (see Chapter 20, *School*). As the child gets older, an exercise program can be established with a physical therapist, occupational therapist, or personal trainer. Insurance companies are reluctant to pay for long-term rehabilitation, so it is helpful for parents to request a case manager or advocate to help them obtain these services.

## Educational issues

School entry and reentry for children who have spent months or years receiving treatment is difficult. Physical changes make it hard for some children with CNS tumors to socially fit in at school. To compound matters, side effects and late effects of the treatments used for CNS tumors often include decline in academic functioning. A decrease in IQ is a side effect for children who receive radiation treatments and sometimes for those who deal with seizures. Difficulty with memory or changes in attention span, verbal fluency, and speed of information processing can also affect many children.

Problems in arithmetic are frequently observed, and reading and spelling difficulties are common. It is imperative that all children receive educational (neuropsychological) testing to identify learning problems. The results of these tests can be incorporated into the individual educational plan (IEP), which is used to plan the school curriculum. A neuropsychologist can also use the results of these tests to help adult survivors identify strategies to cope with learning issues. For further information, refer to Chapter 11, *Radiation Therapy*, and to Chapter 20.

## Hormonal problems

Hormonal problems occur in children with pituitary and hypothalamic tumors and as a late effect of radiation therapy to the brain. The following are types of hormonal problems that your child may develop:

*   Growth hormone deficiency resulting in short stature
*   Deficiency in hormones required to develop normally in puberty
*   Thyroid hormone deficiency

Long-term follow-up should include a visit to an endocrinologist, who can screen for these problems with a blood test. Hormones (pills or injections) can be given to the child to help correct any deficiencies. It is essential that problems with growth and pubertal hormones be identified early, because treatment is only effective when the child is young. Thyroid hormonal replacement (a daily pill) can start at any time. If your child is fatigued or has decreased energy, make sure that the doctor tests thyroid functioning. For more information, refer to Chapter 11.

### Hearing loss

Decrease in hearing (with high-frequency hearing lost first) occurs most often in children treated with cisplatin. The loss is sometimes increased if the child receives radiation therapy as well. Audiograms (hearing tests) are done at frequent intervals while the child is receiving the cisplatin and should be part of the long-term follow-up upon completion of the treatment protocol. A common problem with the loss of high-frequency sounds is the inability to filter out background noise. This presents a problem for these children in the classroom setting, where background noise is common. Your audiologist may be able to recommend devices that will help your child in this situation. Hearing aids are sometimes recommended for children with significant hearing loss.

### Emotional issues

Many children suffer from post-traumatic stress disorder as a result of their experiences with cancer. It is important that you seek proper support for your family members and your child so that these issues can be resolved in a healthy manner.

> There was the time after a long-term EEG that my son had nightmares
> for months. The poor handling of the whole procedure traumatized him.
> For a long time he wouldn't let me touch his head or brush his hair.
> Another time was after treatment ended. Just driving by and seeing clinic
> would make him physically ill. We had to do follow-up visits with another
> doctor for a while, until he was ready to go in there and see everyone
> again. He still won't go into the clinic's infusion room where he got chemo.

## Survivorship

An essential aspect of survivorship is making healthy choices. Good health habits and regular medical care help protect survivors' health as well as reduce the likelihood of late effects from treatment. A sizable number of adult cancers are linked to lifestyle choices. Eating a healthy diet, staying physically active, using sunscreen, avoiding excessive alcohol consumption, maintaining a healthy weight, and not smoking all help to keep survivors healthy and cancer-free. Wearing bike or motorcycle helmets, using seat belts, and calling a cab if the person driving you home has had too much to drink protect survivors from injury. Survivors have little or no control over genetic makeup or the environment in which they live. But making healthy choices on how to live the rest of their lives gives them control over some of their own destiny. For more information on survivor issues, read *Childhood Cancer Survivors: A Practical Guide to the Future,* listed in Appendix B, *Resources.*

## Immunizations

If your child was diagnosed prior to receiving all of his immunizations, ask the oncologist when you should resume the regular schedule for vaccinations. Treatment protocols using high-dose chemotherapy with peripheral stem cell or bone marrow transplant eliminate the effectiveness of previous immunizations. If this is the case, the immunization schedule must be restarted. Ask your oncologist for information regarding this issue.

> My daughter's doctor said to wait a year before beginning to catch up
> on shots. It was nice for her to get a long break before any more pokes.

## Risks of smoking

Teens need continuing counseling on problems associated with smoking (cigarettes or marijuana) or other high-risk behaviors. Any child or teen who received craniospinal radiation is at risk for damage to the lungs or the muscle of the heart. Smoking not only impacts the lungs, but it makes blood vessels hard, further decreasing the heart's ability to pump. The combination of heart and lung damage from radiation therapy and smoking vastly increases the chance of heart disease; heart attack; congestive heart failure; stroke; cancer of the mouth, throat, and lungs; and death from sudden cardiac failure. An article on survivors and smoking contained in the Candlelighters Winter 1994 youth newsletter ends with these words:

> If you've had cancer and your friends haven't, they don't face the same
> risks from smoking that you do. You've fought hard for your life. Don't
> put it out in an ashtray.

## Safe sex

Every teen and young adult who has survived a CNS tumor should be counseled about safe sexual practices. Despite the prevalence of sexual messages in our culture, most teens are woefully under informed about the facts. Many survivors think, erroneously, that if they are infertile, they do not have to be concerned about the use of condoms or other forms of birth control. Many female survivors have found themselves unexpectedly pregnant after not using birth control. In addition, all sorts of diseases, some potentially fatal (hepatitis C, HIV/AIDS) and some not (genital herpes, genital warts, gonorrhea), can be transmitted through sexual intercourse.

One nurse practitioner at a large follow-up clinic stated:

> I tell every teenager who comes through the door, regardless of his or her medical background, that I think that he or she is too young to have sex, and I explain why. But then I say, in the event that you do choose to become sexually active, you ALWAYS need to use a condom, and not just any condom. I tell them to only use a latex condom with a spermicide, which is the most protective barrier. I explain that no sex is the only guarantee to avoid the many diseases out there, but a latex condom with spermicide offers the next best protection. And I really stress that this should be done whoever the partner is, and for whatever type of sex. So many teenagers think that diseases only happen to other kinds of kids.

# Keeping the doctor informed

Once treatment is completed, many children and young adults are no longer cared for by pediatric oncologists who are familiar with their history. A transition back to their community physician occurs. Moreover, many primary care physicians—pediatricians, family practice doctors, internists, gynecologists—are not fully aware of all the different treatments used for the multitude of childhood cancers and of their late effects.

Additionally, when treatment ends, many patients and parents are not adequately informed of the risks of developing physical difficulties months, years, or decades after treatment ends. The risks of such delayed effects are real. It is imperative that survivors be informed advocates for their own healthcare. They need to be educated, in a supportive and responsible way, of the risk for future physical adversities, so that if a problem does arise, it will be recognized early and receive prompt attention. Young adults who have survived childhood CNS tumors need to be fully cognizant of their unique medical history and able to share this information with all future doctors who will care for them.

> Our daughter is a 12-year survivor of medulloblastoma. My husband
> has her entire medical history on the computer. He prints out a booklet for

*each doctor that she sees. We were worried after we moved to another*
*state that if something happened to us, no one would know her history.*
*And she will need to use that info to educate her doctors for the rest of*
*her life.*

A few months before the end of treatment, ask the treating physician to fill out the booklet at the back of this book. This health history will become an indispensable part of your child's medical records for the rest of her life. It should be kept in a safe place, and a copy should be given to each medical caregiver. When your child leaves home to begin her adult life, this booklet should go with her.

If you do not have a copy of the health history booklet, write down the following important information in your child's health history:

• Name of disease

• Date of diagnosis and relapse, if any

• Place of treatment

• Dates of treatment

• Names of attending neurosurgeon, attending oncologist, and primary nurses/nurse practitioners

• Names and total dosages of chemotherapeutic agents used

• Type, areas treated, and amount of radiation used

• Name of radiation center

• Date(s) radiation received

• Dose of radiation and location, e.g., cranial, craniospinal, etc.

• Dates and types of any surgeries

• Date and type of bone marrow or stem cell transplant, if any

• Any major treatment complications

• Any persistent side effects of treatment

• Recommended medical follow-up

• Contact numbers for treating institutions

If your child will not be periodically examined at a long-term follow-up clinic, write down this information and make sure that your child has a copy to give to any future doctor who will be treating him.

# Employment

The population of adults who have survived childhood cancer is growing at a rapid rate. It is estimated that by the year 2010, 1 in every 250 young adults will be a cancer survivor. Thousands of cancer survivors are staying well, growing up, graduating from high school or college, and successfully entering the workforce. As treatment become more successful, more and more brain tumor survivors will be joining these ranks. Survivors of childhood cancer are educators, sports figures, radio announcers, doctors, social workers, dancers, lawyers, and professionals of all types.

Despite their numbers, some survivors still face job discrimination because of fears about cancer and its treatment. Under US federal law and many state laws, an employer cannot treat a survivor differently from other employees because of a history of cancer except in certain circumstances involving health, life, and disability insurance. The Americans with Disabilities Act (ADA) prohibits many types of job discrimination by employers, employment agencies, state and local governments, and labor unions. In addition, most states have laws that prohibit discrimination based on disabilities, although what these laws cover varies widely.

The Americans with Disabilities Act of 1990 (ADA) prohibits discrimination based on actual disability, perceived disability, or history of a disability. Any employer with fifteen or more workers is covered by the ADA.

The ADA requires that:

- Employers may not make medical inquiries of an applicant, unless the applicant has a visible disability, e.g., weakness of arm(s) or leg(s), or the applicant has voluntarily disclosed her tumor history. Such questions must be limited to asking the applicant to describe or demonstrate how she would perform essential job functions. Medical inquiries are allowed after a job offer has been made or during a pre-employment medical exam.

- Employers must provide reasonable accommodations unless it causes undue hardship.

- Employers may not discriminate because of family illness.

- Employers are not required to provide health insurance.

The Equal Employment Opportunity Commission (EEOC) enforces Title 1 (employment) of the ADA. Call (800) 669-4000 for enforcement information and (800) 669-3362 for enforcement publications. Other sections are enforced by or have their enforcement coordinated by the US Department of Justice (Civil Rights Division,

Public Access Section). The Justice Department's ADA web site is at *http://www.usdoj.gov/crt/ada/adahom1.htm*.

The Job Accommodation Network (JAN) is an international consulting service that provides free information about how employers can accommodate people with disabilities. The service also provides information about the Americans with Disabilities Act (ADA). JAN can be reached by calling (800) 526-7234 (USA) or (800) 526-2262 (Canada).

In the United States, JAN is a service of the President's Committee on Employment of People with Disabilities. In Canada (JANCANA), it is a service of Human Resources Development Canada and the Canadian Council on Rehabilitation and Work.

In Canada, the Canadian Human Rights Act provides essentially the same rights as the ADA. The act is administered by the Canadian Human Rights Commission.

If you feel that you have been discriminated against due to your disability or a relative's disability, contact the EEOC or the Canadian Human Rights Commission promptly. In the US, a charge of discrimination generally must be filed within 180 days of the notice of the discriminatory act.

If a survivor of a CNS tumor or a member of the family feels that he has been denied a job, fired, forced from a job, denied reasonable accommodation, or discriminated against for promotions or medical leave because of cancer history, contact the Childhood Cancer Ombudsman (listed in Appendix B) for help. They can provide the following free services:

*   Outside review by experts
*   Citations to medical and legal literature
*   Mediation
*   Analysis of employment contracts
*   Instructions in appeal procedures
*   Assistance with filing complaints
*   Explanations of how to respond to questions on job applications and at interviews

# Insurance for survivors

Job discrimination can spell economic catastrophe for CNS tumor survivors because most health insurance is obtained from employment. As survivors mature, seek employment, and move away from home, many encounter barriers to obtaining health insurance, such as rejection of application based on cancer history, policy reductions, policy cancellation, pre-existing condition exclusions, increased premiums, or extended waiting periods. Current discussions about national healthcare reform are extremely contentious, so it seems unlikely that major reforms of the American health insurance system will occur in the near future. For more on insurance issues for a dependent child in treatment, see Chapter 18, *Record Keeping and Finances*.

> *I realize that I must do whatever is necessary to stay covered on my parent's insurance as long as possible. I don't particularly like that, but it is important. As long as I remain a full-time student, it will be okay.*

Most states offer high-risk individuals, like survivors, access to comprehensive health insurance plans (CHIPS). CHIPS, also called "high-risk pools," are a means for individuals to obtain insurance regardless of their physical condition or medical history. For more information on CHIPS, call your state Office of the Insurance Commissioner. Although neither the US federal nor the state governments mandate a legal right to insurance, there are some legal remedies to insurance discrimination:

- **COBRA.** The Comprehensive Omnibus Budget Reconciliation Act (COBRA) is a federal law that requires public and private companies employing more than twenty workers to provide continuation of group coverage to employees if they quit, are fired, or work reduced hours. Coverage must extend to surviving, divorced, or separated spouses and to dependent children. You must pay for your continued coverage, but it must not exceed by more than 2 percent the rate set for your former co-workers. By allowing you to purchase continued coverage, you have time to seek other long-term coverage.

- **ERISA.** The Employee Retirement and Income Security Act (ERISA) is a federal law that protects workers from being fired because of the cancer history of the employee or beneficiaries (spouse and children). ERISA also prohibits employers from encouraging a person with a cancer history to retire as a "disabled" employee. ERISA does not apply to job discrimination (denial of new job due to cancer history), discrimination that does not affect benefits, and employees whose compensation does not include benefits.

- **Health Insurance Portability and Accountability Act of 1996.** This law allows individuals to change to a new job without losing coverage if they have been insured for at least twelve months. It prevents group health plans from denying coverage based on medical history, genetic information, or claims history, although insurers can still exclude those with specific diseases or conditions. It also increases portability if you change from a group to an individual plan.

ERISA, COBRA, and parts of the Health Insurance Portability and Accountability Act of 1996 are enforced by the Pension and Welfare Benefits Administration in Washington, DC, (202) 219-8776.

For detailed information on the ADA, COBRA, ERISA, and the Health Insurance Portability and Accountability Act of 1996, read *A Cancer Survivor's Almanac: Charting Your Journey*, edited by Barbara Hoffman, JD.

*Well, we finally did it. We took a deep breath, a heavy sigh, and we packed up the medical supplies. While this step may seem insignificant for some, those who have dealt with a chronic/life threatening illness in their family know that the disposal of your arsenal of medical supplies is a symbolic rite of passage. It can only mean two things: your loved one has passed on, or you simply don't need them anymore. We thank God every day that we ended up with the latter reason.*

*Katy's medical "tower" was stored in our hallway, and included various bins and drawers full of central line supplies, a mini IV pump, masks and gloves, hypodermics and sharps containers. It was very conspicuous. You simply couldn't miss it if you walked through the house. It was our constant reminder that we had a sick child, and at times, for me, a crutch. I think I felt that as long as the tower was there and properly stocked and arranged, I was somehow in control of Katy's illness. I feared disposing of, or putting anything away, thinking that if I did, she would most assuredly relapse and I'd need it again. No, of course that's not rational, but rationality has never been one of my strong points.*

*However, as the months passed, the tower gathered its dust, and soon, I couldn't remember the last time we'd even used any of the supplies. A few more months passed, and I began to realize what an eyesore this bunch of junk was! So, after my husband David brought some big boxes home from work, it was time. We did it together. Into the boxes went the tubing and syringes, the masks and dressing change kits for the kids' oncology camp. Into the garbage went all the expired meds, heparin and saline. It was so liberating! I can't imagine why we kept that stuff around for so long. It felt like the end of an era. And in a way it was.*

# CHAPTER 22

# Relapse

PARENTS FREQUENTLY DESCRIBE the recurrence or progression of their child's CNS tumor as more devastating than the original diagnosis. Recurrence refers to the reappearance of a tumor that had previously disappeared with treatment, while progression is defined as an increase in size of an existing tumor. Recurrence or progression may occur while the child is on an active treatment protocol or during an observation phase of treatment.

If recurrence or progression occurs, parents often feel betrayed. They think that they put their child through hell for nothing. They are scared, because they know that any recurrence is serious. The anger is back—they did everything the doctors said, so why did the tumor return? They are afraid that if the first battery of treatments didn't work, what will? And the unspoken but most crushing feeling of all: "If my child dies, how will I survive?"

If your child's tumor has returned or begun to grow, one point is well worth remembering: you are not the same person that you were at diagnosis. You've been through this before, so you know how to get medical and emotional support. You have a relationship with the medical team, and you can speak the language now. You have developed friendships with other families of children with CNS tumors. You know that something that seems insurmountable can be overcome, one day at a time.

This chapter explains how doctors determine if tumor recurrence or progression has occurred, emotional responses of the parents, and how to decide on a treatment plan.

## Signs and symptoms

Recurrence or progression can happen at any time during treatment or after therapy is completed. The signs and symptoms can include many or all of the indicators that were present at diagnosis. For a brain tumor these include:

- Headaches (often with early morning vomiting)
- Dizziness
- Seizures (convulsions)

- Staring spells
- Visual changes: loss of peripheral vision, double vision, jiggling of eyeball, inability to look up, eye turning inward or outward
- Weakness in hands on one or both sides of the body
- Unsteady gait
- Word-finding problems
- Drowsiness
- Facial drooping
- Nausea and vomiting
- Hormonal or growth problems
- Hearing loss
- Changes in appetite or thirst
- Behavior changes
- Change in school performance

For a spinal cord tumor the symptoms may be:

- Back or neck pain that awakens child from sleep
- Scoliosis (curvature of the spine resulting in leaning of shoulders to one side or a hump noticeable in the back)
- Torticollis (tilting of the head and upper spine to one side)
- Weakness or sensory changes in arms or legs
- Changes in bowel and bladder control

Remember that many of these symptoms are also seen with normal childhood illnesses. However, persistent loss of appetite or fatigue or unusually severe symptoms require a call to your treating physician.

> I think our respite is ending. Jen had a scan on Monday and we knew
> when we looked at them it would probably not be good news and that
> was confirmed today when we met with her oncologist. I don't have the
> radiology report yet but the scans will be discussed at tumor board
> Friday. It seems the original area of tumor continues to look stable and
> maybe even a little better but there appears to be an area of new growth
> definitely crossing the midline now to the right side of her brain. Instead
> of starting what would have been her seventh round of Temodar she is on

*hold until Friday. Two possibilities mentioned were CPT-11 and high-dose Tamoxifen.*

*This has been a hard day. I have already made some phone calls as I know from our discussion with the doctor he doesn't think there's much lag time before she needs to be on something. The last four weeks of Procrit shots have moved her blood count from anemia to normal and she is physically active and still feeling good with the exception of some fatigue. She has been having some slight difficulty with her right hand grasping and holding but I am more concerned with her description of losing awareness of what it does. She's getting more memory problems and the beginning of some incontinence. The 29th of this month will be the end of twelve years she has been dealing with this. Enough! But it doesn't look like that is meant to be.*

In some cases, parents have no warning. After bringing their child in for a follow-up scan, they hear the unexpected news. The majority of CNS tumors regrow or progress at the original tumor site. Occasionally, the tumor spreads to another area of the CNS.

# Emotional responses

Parents who have children with a CNS tumor in remission think or speak of relapse with an almost palpable dread. Just the thought can cause the emotions that surged in them at diagnosis to erupt. The depth of the emotions generated by relapse is very hard for parents and survivors to relive and describe. As one survivor said in a shaky voice when being interviewed, "It's been eleven years since I finished treatment, but talking about it shows that you scratch the surface and those overwhelming feelings are still right there."

Parents feel a wide array of emotions at relapse: numbness, guilt, dread, anger, fear, confusion, denial, and grief. Physical symptoms such as dizziness, nausea, fainting, and shortness of breath are common. Parents wonder how they can ask their child to endure it again. They wonder how they will survive it themselves. They oscillate between optimism and panic.

*I found that relapse was far worse than the original diagnosis. At diagnosis, after a certain period of adjustment, you think that treatment has a beginning, a middle, and an end. But relapse creates a bigger burden to accept. You begin to feel that maybe the disease is more powerful than the medicine. I found that for a while I just stopped functioning and thinking rationally. I felt that all the hell of treatment had been just a waste of time. I felt guilt and a tremendous sense of loss of control. I felt like I was on a runaway freight train, hurtling towards an end that didn't look so good anymore. This is the point at which people are willing to use any type of unconventional therapies because they are desperate. I know one mom in our support group who was even willing to try coffee enemas. She looks back on it now and says, "I just went crazy."*

# Deciding on a treatment plan

A rapid response is necessary when faced with a recurrence of childhood CNS tumor. Treatment plans for a first relapse are sometimes specified in your child's protocol, or your physician may suggest a different approach. Suggestions for treatment may include surgery, chemotherapy, a clinical trial, immunotherapy, radiation, or stem cell transplantation.

Physicians make recommendations based on knowledge, experience, and consultations with other experts in the field. Do not hesitate to ask your physician why she has suggested a certain approach to your child's recurrence. Ask your doctor about treatment goals, methods, and possible side effects. Ask your doctor if she has consulted with others in the decision-making process, and if so, whom. Older children and teens need to be involved in decisions regarding their care and treatment choices.

Health Canada's publication, *This Battle Which I Must Fight: Cancer in Canada's Children and Teenagers*, states:

> *This (relapse) is a time of crisis and ambivalence. The decision to be made is whether to continue to try to achieve a remission or to replace this hope with the hope for comfort for the child and a special time together. Each parent, and the child who is old enough to understand, requires differing amounts of time to reach a decision about how to proceed. Careful and frequent discussions with the medical team, as well as with trusted friends and relatives, may help clarify issues and bring some peace-of-mind.*

Just like at diagnosis, time is often a pressing concern. This is especially true for recurrence of tumors.

> *Twenty-five days after surgery for medulloblastoma, Ayla (32 months) started chemo. Six chemo treatments were planned, but we only got*

*through the first three, consisting of vincristine, etoposide (VP-16), cisplatin, and cyclophosphamide. They also collected stem cells for a stem cell transplant, which was never done. During this, the MRIs showed that there was additional spread in ten spots in the midbrain. Chemo was stopped and the last three treatments (thiotepa and carboplatin) weren't used. Exactly one day after Ayla's third birthday, she started radiation, and got the maximum doses for cranial and spinal radiation. Ayla sailed through radiation. She didn't get that sleepy period, although she did add an extra couple hours of nap every day. She had her radiation treatments early in the morning for six weeks. The whole thing took half an hour, and just a few minutes for the actual procedure. The radiation tech would give her the sedative, her special "milkshake" medicine, through her Hickman. Afterwards, we'd go out for the day and play. Most, if not all, of the spots that they were watching are gone now and her original tumor site is showing scar tissue.*

Time is less of a concern for slow-growing tumors that have begun to grow if the child is not yet experiencing symptoms of the progression. In this situation parents have additional time to gather opinions about the next treatment options. Beware rushing into a new treatment plan if you feel uncomfortable. Your child needs to know that you are 100 percent in favor of proceeding, and children have radar for parents' feelings. There is always time for answers to all of your questions and time to get a second opinion.

Refer to Chapter 7, *Forming a Partnership with the Medical Team,* for ways to obtain a second opinion. One excellent resource is the Childhood Cancer Ombudsman Program, an affiliated program of the Childhood Brain Tumor Foundation. Panels of volunteer pediatric oncologists volunteer to give second medical opinions or medical record reviews at the request of families or the treating oncologist. The program is particularly valuable in helping families make well-informed treatment choices, as well as becoming comfortable with the therapeutic approach chosen. For contact information, see Appendix B, *Resources.*

The Physician's Data Query can be reached at (800) 4-CANCER or at *http://cancernet. nci.nih.gov/pdq.htm*. It lists protocols for recurrent disease as well as ongoing clinical trials. The information gleaned from second opinions and/or research may reinforce what your doctor recommended, or it might provide you with some additional treatment options. Either way, it may increase your comfort level during the treatment planning process.

*Our 2-year-old daughter was diagnosed with medulloblastoma in the cerebellum. She was treated with high-dose chemotherapy followed by stem cell transplant. At her two year off treatment MRI, the tumor was back—tiny and at the same site. It was again totally resected and this time we knew she needed radiation. The question was: what kind? We really wanted to avoid as much damage as possible to her developing brain. We did some research and ended up choosing a very new type of radiation called proton beam. The theory, and hope, was that this type of radiation would have less scatter and would do less damage to healthy cells. So, now we wait and hope that it killed the cancer and spared as much of her brain as possible.*

The following are questions that you might want to ask your doctor when discussing the treatment plan:

- What is the goal of this treatment? Is it likely to cure my child, or is it meant to keep him comfortable?

- Why do you think that this treatment is the best option? What are the other choices, and why did you choose this one?

- Have you consulted with other physicians? If so, whom? Did you all agree on this treatment, or was there a range of choices suggested?

- Is there a standard treatment for this type of relapse? What is it?

- What clinical trials are ongoing for this type of relapse?

- Explain the potential benefits and possible side effects of the suggested treatment.

- What are the known or potential risks of the treatment?

- How often will my child need to be hospitalized?

- How long will my child need this treatment?

- If the treatment is investigational, is there scientific evidence that it works for her type of cancer?

- Does insurance cover this type of investigational treatment?

When older children and parents disagree on the details of how to proceed, use the hospital primary nurse/practitioner, social worker, or psychologist to help you negotiate and make compromises. These discussions will help clarify each family member's thoughts and feelings and will allow the child's emotional and physical well-being to be part of the equation.

In the Spring 1995 issue of the Candlelighters newsletter, Arthur Ablin, MD, Director Emeritus of Pediatric Clinical Oncology at the University of California, San Francisco, wrote of the importance of goal setting in the decision-making process after relapse:

> Before determining which treatment is to be chosen, a decision must be made to determine the goal of treatment—in other words, what is it that we are trying to achieve. This crucial first step is the basis upon which any decision concerning treatment must be made. But it is too often omitted from consideration and/or discussion, even by the most experienced. The frustrations accompanying the previous failure of treatment, the fear of the loss of the hope for cure, the pressure of urgency to find solutions, the new awareness of the possibility or probability of death, lead us all to want to consider treatments first rather than these more difficult considerations involved in establishing goals. These also force us to deal with reality earlier, which could mean the almost intolerable confrontation with the death of a very-much-loved child, a tragedy to be avoided at all cost.

After you have set goals, received answers to all of your questions, obtained a second opinion if desired, and decided on a treatment plan, it is time to proceed. Your knowledge and experience may prove to be a double-edged sword. You have no illusions about the difficulties ahead because you've done it before, but you also will be strengthened by your ties with the cancer community, your comfort with your physicians and hospital routines, and your ability to work with the system to get what your child needs. Many parents shared how their child took the lead about relapse treatment. While the parents agonized, their child said simply, "Let's just do it." And they did.

Evan, who had his first surgery shortly after his ninth birthday, in 1992, wrote the following composition. In addition to having a brain tumor, Evan has a diagnosis of high-functioning autism:

> I was 9 when I found out I needed brain surgery. I was nervous then, but I would be scared out of my mind if I was put in that situation now. When I came out of surgery, I couldn't walk, I couldn't even swallow very well or talk much. My first memory after surgery, I was in intensive care. It was bright. I was sound-sensitive, and my head was

throbbing. I found out the type of tumor I had, a pilocytic astrocytoma, is the least malignant, but it was in the brainstem. That meant it was still very serious.

After that surgery, I lost weight. I looked like a Holocaust survivor. I couldn't even stand on the scale, so someone had to hold me. They did a test that I had to swallow food with some chemical thing in it, and then they found out that I had cranial nerve damage so it was hard for me to swallow. I was put on a special diet of soft food, like yogurt or Ensure.

I went to rehab to learn to walk and for physical and occupational therapy. In rehab I could wear regular clothes, and they had a school, too. They had something like periods. At certain times, I'd go to therapy, and then I'd be in school, and so on. Some things were fun, and some things were not.

Some things I enjoyed were seeing movies and playing Uno. Things I did not enjoy were blood tests and the physical therapy, or PT. Every month they had a party. One time there was a magic show, and people dressed up as different people. The first of the parties, I was in a wheelchair and couldn't even sit up straight.

Finally after six weeks, I got to go home. When they sent me home, I could walk and talk, but I had to wear a helmet. That's it for the first time around.

A year later, I made good progress, but then I started to get worse again. I had an MRI, and the tumor had grown, so it was time for another surgery. I was afraid, but I had more of an idea what to expect. After surgery, I didn't lose as much weight, but I had crossed eyes and high blood pressure. I also had this push-button thing for pain. If I was in pain, I would push the button, and it would give me morphine. Besides that, it was pretty much like the previous time.

It felt like a '57 Chevy on my head, as I described the pain then. It was around Halloween, so I didn't go trick-or-treating. I was also eager to get to rehab, because it made me feel so much better the last time.

I wore an eye patch because of the double vision, and I had to switch eyes. A nurse had to take my blood pressure every couple of hours, and I was on medication for high blood pressure.

I had a wheelchair, and I also had to use a walker for several months after getting out of the hospital. Even when I didn't have to use the walker, I still used the wheelchair if I had to go very far, like at Disneyland, or even the mall.

I had a wheelchair costume of an antique car for Halloween. My mom and I made it out of plastic trashcans from the office supply store. I won a costume contest at Knott's Berry Farm with that.

# CHAPTER 23

# Death and Bereavement

THE DEATH OF A CHILD causes almost unendurable pain and anguish for loved ones left behind. Death from a CNS tumor comes after months or years of debilitating treatment, emotional swings, and financial crises. The family begins the years of grief already exhausted from the years of fighting the tumor. It is truly every parent's worst nightmare.

In this chapter, many parents share their innermost thoughts and feelings about their decisions to transition from active treatment, involve hospice, choose death at home or in the hospital, and grief. It made no difference whether parents had recently lost a child or it had happened decades before—tears flowed when talking about their family's experience. Because family members and friends can be strong sources of support, or casualties of the grieving process, parents describe words and actions that help, and they offer suggestions on what to avoid. Grief has as many facets as there are grieving parents; what follows are the experiences of a few.

## Transitioning from active treatment

For children or teenagers whose disease is progressing, medical caregivers and parents at some point need to decide when to end active treatment and begin to work toward making the child comfortable for his remaining days. This is an intensely personal decision.

Some families want to try every available treatment and exhaust all possible remedies. Others reach a point where they feel they have done all they can and they simply do not want their child to suffer any more. They hope for time to share memories, express love, and prepare for death.

> This has been a very difficult weekend with many tears. We have had
> so many wonderful years beyond what we ever thought was possible with
> such a good quality of life for Jen and us. In spite of everything, we have
> no regrets. We selfishly want every moment we can have, but we have

*come to the crossroad where we are asking at what cost to Jen. While we*
*have not made the commitment to hospice yet we are all feeling that we*
*are not far from that place unless there is a dramatic change in Jen soon.*
*She has really fought hard. She made this damn brain tumor work really*
*hard to slow her down. She is very, very tired and while my head*
*understands this, my heart is breaking.*

Dr. Arthur Ablin, Director Emeritus of Pediatric Clinical Oncology at the University of California, San Francisco, wrote in the Spring 1995 Candlelighters newsletter about the difficulties of deciding to end active treatment:

*All too often, the decision to abandon the goal for cure and, reluctantly,*
*accept the reality of inevitable death of a child is too painful and,*
*therefore, never made. This paralyzing pain occurs with equal frequency,*
*perhaps, for the family and the doctor. We of the medical profession have*
*no equal in our ability to prolong dying. We have a powerful array of*
*mechanical, electronic, pharmaceutical, and biotechnical interventions at*
*our command. We can keep people dying for months and even years.*
*Applying or withholding this armamentarium is an awesome*
*responsibility, and it requires infinite wisdom to know how to manage*
*wisely and correctly. We can do great good by applying these tools*
*correctly, but can also do incalculable harm through over-utilization.*
*Physicians and families alike must work together to avoid the possible*
*pitfalls. When cure is beyond all of us, then the challenge is to make the*
*rest of life as worthwhile and rich as possible. There is much to do for*
*the terminally and critically ill child and his or her family. They have*
*that right, we have the privilege, to be of service.*

One of the more difficult tasks that a parent will face is sharing the news with their child that treatments have stopped working. Although no child is a statistic, it is important to look at the probability of tumor control versus the impact of continuing treatment on the child's emotional and physical well-being. Older children and teenagers need to be an integral part in these discussions. Their thoughts and feelings are crucial during the decision-making process. Honest, thorough communication between the ill child or teen, family members, and involved professionals helps everyone work together.

*My niece was diagnosed right after her third birthday and died 2½*
*months short of her fifth birthday. We told her about the "tumor in her*
*head" and she knew that was what was causing all the symptoms she was*

*experiencing. She knew she was sick and wasn't getting better, but we never told her specifically that she would die until after we had stopped all treatment and the outcome was inevitable, probably a month or so before she died.*

*When we told her, we sat down with her and her 2½ year old brother and told them. She acted exactly as though she had already known what was going to happen to her, that we were telling her nothing new.*

*About two months before we told her, the movie "Little Women" came out on video. We had previously taken her to see it in the theatre. We got the video right away, and she watched it probably three times a week or more. She would always tell me, when I watched it with her, that her favorite part was the part where Jo died. It wasn't like she got any pleasure out of that part, but it was like she knew what would happen to her and she could identify very closely with Jo.*

*In retrospect, I think she had known for some time, long before we told her, but she did not speak of it because she had already come to terms with it, and she was not fearful. I think she desperately wanted to live and be cured, but she somehow knew that if a cure could not be found, she would die.*

Often, children take the lead in making the decision to stop treatment.

*When my 6-year-old son Greg was in the hospital in intensive relapse treatment, he would repeat over and over again, "I want to go home." When he was finally well enough to come home for awhile, he kept saying, "I want to go home." In frustration, I said, "Greg, you are home, why do you keep saying that?" He looked up and quietly said, "I want to go to my heavenly home. I want to go to God." I said, "Honey, please don't say that," and, knowing how much we loved him, he replied, "Okay, Mom, I'll fight, I won't go." And he did fight hard for several more months. But he was way ahead of us in acceptance, he was at peace, and he knew it was time to let go.*

When it is clear that death is inevitable, parents struggle with the thought of how to tell the ill child and siblings. All too often in our culture, children are perceived as having to be protected from death, as if this somehow makes their last days better. On the contrary, any pediatric nurse practitioner, oncologist, or social worker can tell you that children, often as young as 4, know that they are dying. If the parents are trying to spare the child, an unhealthy situation develops. The child pretends everything is okay to please the parents, and the parents try to mask their deep grief with false smiles. Everyone loses.

> *Aidan was diagnosed at 4½ and at the time didn't know what the word cancer meant. We kept it that way. A little while later we told him about bad cells, in relation to having radiotherapy. I think this was easier for all of us than with an older child with a better understanding of death. Even so, Aidan now talks about that initial time in hospital as "when you were very worried about me." I think he has some idea about how close he came that week. More recently, now 6, Aidan faced a recurrence from the medulloblastoma. When he was having a lumbar puncture I told him the doctor would put a needle in his back. He asked why and I answered that he needed to see if there were any bad cells there.*
>
> *After a bit of thinking he asked, "What happens if there are?" I put on my brave face and said we hoped there weren't but we just have to wait and see. Then he said, "They'll go everywhere won't they?" My brave face was certainly tested then and so was his. He was very quiet that afternoon.*

Denial can keep children and parents alike from finishing up business—distributing belongings, telling each other how much they love one another, and saying good-bye. It also strips parents of their ability to prepare their child for the journey from life to death. Children need to know what to expect. They need to know that they will be surrounded by those they love, that their parents will be holding them, and they need to know the family's beliefs about what happens after death.

> *Jennifer contracted a respiratory fungal infection that resulted in her being hospitalized on a ventilator. She was given lots of morphine so that she wouldn't feel air hungry. She was alert off and on for a few days. We read to her and played tapes. After one week on the respirator, she took a turn for the worse. She didn't respond to me after that. Her kidneys were ceasing to function, and she started to get puffy. Her liver was deteriorating, and her painful pancreatitis had come back. After ten days on the respirator, I couldn't bear it any longer. I lay down in her bed, took her in my arms, and kissed her at least 200 times. I talked to her for a long time, and told her that we would take care of her cats, and that I was sorry that she had to suffer so much, and how beautiful Heaven is. I told her to go be with Jesus, her Grandpa, and her dog. I also told her how much we all loved her and how proud we were of her. I got off the bed to*

*change positions, and the nurse rushed in. Her heart had suddenly stopped the second I got up. I believe she heard me and just needed to know it was okay to go. She didn't want to leave until she knew her mommy was ready.*

*Jennifer had told me that she wasn't afraid to die, and this has been a great source of comfort to us. I believe that she was preparing for her death, even as we hoped for her remission. Before she went to the hospital, she spent all her money, gave away some of her possessions to her sisters, and said a final good-bye to her home, cats, teachers, and friends.*

One father shares how his family faced his daughter's terminal prognosis:

*When Stacia was diagnosed with glioblastoma in April, 1997, the prognosis was given as nine to twelve months. With experimental treatments, I guessed that I might be able to extend her life another year. But the bottom line was that our child, our beautiful Stacia, was going to die. The recognition of this truth is a paralyzing event. Simply said, it breaks your heart in half, and leaves you weeping uncontrollably. When the crying subsided, the questions came flooding. Whatever in the world am I going to do? Two ideas came to mind. The first was absolutely normal: I will scour the world for treatments and try to save my child's life. This thought occurs to every parent in this situation. Understandably, most parents become completely absorbed by this single idea.*

*My second thought was: How can I give Stacia the best possible life in the time that she (and we) have left? The concept I came up with was LIVING BIG. And live big we did. I set about with my wife Linda, our children, Jodi and David, Stacia's extended family, and all of her good friends, to create a network of love and support that would always be there to help her live life to the fullest, no matter what happened. In practical terms, what this meant was creating a schedule of "living" to compliment her schedule of "treatments."*

*We did not play it safe. We took Stacia everywhere: Canada, Yosemite, Shasta Lake, Tahoe, Pinecrest, Cayucos, Monterey, San Francisco, even Mexico. That was one of the greatest weeks of our lives. Pure fun, pure memories. You see, Stacia was the life of the party. All we had to do was treat her that way.*

*There is another element of living big, other than just taking big trips. That's the intimate part. Setting aside a night, when you take your child out for dinner—just you and her. I asked Stacia if it would be okay to make Thursday nights our father-daughter night. She readily agreed. We went to our favorite pizza parlor, every Thursday, even if she did not eat. At the beginning, she could walk in on her own. Later she used a cane, still later we did a Texas two-step, where we walked in hand in hand, still later a 4-point walker, and still later her wheelchair. We never missed a night. And she often did not eat or drink much. She didn't really care. Because we were together. We made small talk, most of the time. Other times, we spoke about life and death. Mostly about life.*

*The rest of the family set about making their own special days or weekends with Stacia. We threw parties and had her friends over. Her friends threw parties, and we brought her over, even when I had to carry her inside, in my arms. We never left her out.*

*We tried to enjoy life to the fullest, even when we knew the situation was terminal. We packed a lifetime of living into two years. Stacia lived 26 months from her initial diagnosis. Cut down in her prime by a disease that the medical community doesn't understand all that well. An orphan disease that could have made orphans of my whole family, except that we did not let it.*

*We miss Stacia terribly, and our hearts are still broken over losing her. But our spirits are not broken, because we lived big, with the life of the party. God bless you Stacia Jennifer.*

# Supportive care

In the US and Canada, there are very active and effective hospice systems. Hospices ease the transition from hospital to home and provide support for the entire family. Hospice personnel ensure adequate pain control, allow the patient to control the last days or weeks of her life and provide active bereavement support after death.

Usually, if the family wishes the child to die at home, a smooth transition occurs from the oncology ward to hospice care. Unfortunately, sometimes pediatric patients are not referred to hospice, and the parents are left to deal with their child's last days at home with no experienced help and no clear idea of what is to come. Your nurse practitioner, case manager, or hospital social worker can refer you to or help you find a pediatric hospice in your area. Before you leave the hospital, it is wise to find out the name of a contact person at the agency that will be taking over the home care of your child.

*Yesterday we got a visit from the hospice nurse. We had been putting it off but felt that we should have it in place for when we really need it for Ryan. Everyone keeps telling me what a great thing it is, and maybe that's how they feel, but personally, I think birthday parties are great, Disneyland is great, even Chuck E. Cheese is great. Hospice is not great.*

• • • • •

*When our children were babies and learning, I always used the principle of reinforcing things I wanted them to learn or understand with all their senses: hearing, seeing, touch, smell, and taste. During Jen's last days, we kept her room filled with light the way she liked it, and even a soft low light at night so whenever her eyes opened so she knew one of us was right there. We played her favorite music continuously, more upbeat during the day and softer choices at night, and we talked with her and then to her when she could no longer respond with her voice, although the squeeze of her hand and her big blue eyes spoke volumes.*

*We touched her constantly, sometimes just sitting next to her holding her hand and not moving, other times stroking her head, rubbing "udder" cream on her elbows and heels so she didn't get bedsores. She had lost quite a bit of her sense of smell, but we kept everything very fresh and all the flowers that came to the house were all around her because she visually could remember their wonderful scent. We learned to use the great swabs that hospice provided with very cool water and a bit of mint Listerine so her mouth felt clean and fresh, especially as she became less able to take care of herself and even more so when she was no longer able to take in water and then food. One of the nurses told us to take ice chips and put them in a very worn piece of cloth and make it tiny so she wouldn't gag and let in rest in her mouth for a few minutes at a time so she had some moisture, and when that became impossible because she could hardly open her mouth, we swabbed her lips and the gums outside of her closed teeth. All this was meant to convey the message you are loved and cared for and we will be right here for you every step of the way.*

Hospice not only provides assistance in physically caring for your child, it can also provide emotional support for your child, you and your spouse, and any other children in your home.

*We were very fortunate in our hospice experience, which lasted a mere eight days. On the first day, a nurse arrived to meet all of us. She came in with a big smile and introduced herself. The nurse began by taking a very complete medical history, and I remember being surprised by the depth of information she wanted. It was like she wanted to fully understand the entire brain tumor journey and what he had been through, while I suppose I had expected her to laugh off with disinterest everything that had happened before "the end," as if it wouldn't matter anymore. She listened intently, reacted appropriately at incidents that had been a bit unusual, and wrote down a great deal. Then she did a brief exam, just BP, pulse, and general appearance, and assured him that she wouldn't bother him anymore. He relaxed when he realized that she wouldn't be poking him as so many others had already done. We had been apprehensive before her arrival, but afterward, it felt like the night crew had arrived after a very long day shift.*

If you have questions about hospice or what support is available, you can contact Children's Hospice International at (800) 24-CHILD.

# Dying in the hospital

Some children die in the hospital suddenly, while others slowly decline for weeks or months. If your child is slowly dying, you may have choices about where he will spend his last days. There are no right or wrong choices. Much depends on the number of people available to provide care at home, and how comfortable they are doing so. Many parents ask their child where he prefers to be. Some children and teens like to be with the nurses in a hospital environment, but others want to stay at home with brothers, sisters, friends, and pets.

Parents, children, and staff should talk honestly to decide on the appropriate place for the child and then obtain the support (hospice, private nurses in the hospital, family members) needed to make the choice a comfortable reality. Remain flexible so that as the situation changes, options remain open.

Parents of children who died in the hospital stressed the importance of clear communication. Parents need to be strong advocates for adequate pain control, and they need to clearly tell the staff how they would like things to be.

In most hospitals, patients are routinely resuscitated using CPR and electric shocks to the heart (this is called a "code"). Parents need to discuss their wishes with the oncologist and ensure that an order of "NO CODE" is put in the chart and on the child's door. Family members should understand that a DNR (Do Not Resuscitate) order does not mean "do not care" for my child. On the contrary, it allows the medical team to provide comfort measures, such as:

- Allowing the child to sleep during the night without interruptions for temperature and blood pressure

- Providing adequate pain medications

- Allowing family and friends open visitation without restrictions as to length and time of stay and number of people in the room

- A private room

> *Alannah was medicated at any indication of discomfort, and after a week of semi-consciousness followed by a week of coma, we finally got up the guts to have her taken off the respirator, to let her go. She opened her mouth a couple of times, as if trying to breathe, and that was it. With her mother and I holding her, the staff just left us alone. Fifteen minutes later, the attending doc came back and declared time of death. Alannah left very peacefully. We were told to expect that she might seem to be struggling or gasping, and that it would just be reflex, that she wouldn't really be struggling. It didn't happen.*

Parents also should discuss whether they want nurses or doctors present when their child dies. Many families feel very close to the hospital staff and feel supported by their presence, while others prefer to have only family and close friends at the bedside. Advance planning helps to ensure that, as death approaches, the family's wishes are understood and respected.

# Dying at home

A child's death at home and the time just before can be a peaceful experience, depending on the extent of preparation and the quality of support available to the family. Unlike other childhood cancers, pain is rarely associated with CNS tumors, although families should keep their doctor or hospice team apprised if their child is experiencing any discomfort. For this reason, many families of children with CNS tumors choose for their children to die at home.

> *Four weeks before Stacia died, she called us into her room. One by one, she proclaimed her love for each of us, and thanked us for being the best family a girl could ever have. She told us not to worry, that she was going to be all right, and that one day, we would all be together again. On*

*Memorial Day, 1999, Stacia died in her mother Linda's arms, with all of us at her side.*

. . . . .

*Just before Thanksgiving, 1998, ten days before Jay's 15th birthday, my worst fear was realized—the tumor was back, an anaplastic ependymoma, and this time, in the brainstem. Because of location, surgery was not possible. And this time, radiation wasn't possible either. We faced the decision of attempting an aggressive and not usually very successful chemotherapy or calling it quits and letting him go. Choosing hospice was the hardest decision of our lives.*

*Jay wanted to die at home, it was important to him. Towards the end, we sat near Jay's bed talking softly. A few minutes later, I leaned over to check on our son. He seemed to be slipping away.*

*"Squeeze my finger if you can hear me," I pleaded. Jay gave my finger a light squeeze, so weightless I could barely feel it. He slept in a classic fetal position, knees beneath his chest, occupying as small a space as possible. A few minutes later, I spoke to him again, this time no response. Gently, I grasped his wrist with my thumb and forefinger and counted a pulse. We called hospice and they offered to send a nurse over, but we refused, preferring to receive their support by telephone.*

*We sat at Jay's bedside. At nine o'clock, our daughter Vanessa came home. She spoke to her brother, his eyebrows arched, but he didn't respond in any other way. We felt positive he could hear her. At first, I thought I must have given my son too much morphine. Gary called the doctor and the doctor insisted that I hadn't. Deep down I knew I hadn't done anything wrong. There wasn't anything I could have done differently to help my son become fully alert again.*

*Throughout the night, we all stayed with Jay. We folded ourselves onto the bed with him, surrounding him. In the center, Jay lay between the three of us, small, quiet, immobile, with his dog at his side. All night, his breathing stopped and then started again.*

*"Maybe we need to tell him that it's okay to die," Vanessa offered. "Jay, I love you," she said. "Don't worry, I'll do your chores and help Mom. Time is different in heaven; we'll be there with you before you know it," she cooed.*

*I kissed Jay on his forehead. "It's okay," I whispered. "Don't wait for anything, it's time for you to go." At that moment, Jay smiled the*

*sweetest smile, and a peaceful feeling as wide as the sky settled over us,*
*something warm and cozy fell across my heart, and then he was gone.*

Whether your child is dying at home or in the hospital, any siblings should be included in the family response. Being part of things and having jobs to do helps brothers and sisters remain involved, contributing members of the family. Young children can answer the doorbell, go on errands, or make tapes to play for the sibling. Older children can help with meals, stay with the ill child to give parents a break, answer the phones, or help make funeral arrangements. These jobs should not be "make-work"—children should truly be helping. This not only allows them to clarify their role in the family, but helps them to prepare for the death as well as have an opportunity to say good-bye. These jobs help siblings feel that they are a useful part of the family rather than a forgotten and perhaps less loved brother or sister.

*We gave our children free rein to pick out the clothes that Jesse would*
*be buried in. They made very thoughtful choices: her favorite, very*
*comfortable pajamas with little tea cups on them, and her teddy bear.*

## The funeral

Funerals and related rituals (memorial services, wakes, burial, shiva) are important not only as a time to say good-bye and to begin to accept the reality of death, but also to provide an opportunity to recognize the relationships and impact that the child or teen has had on others. Funerals allow friends and family to gather together to share memories and to show support for the remaining family members. A funeral is a tangible demonstration of love.

*As the car drove us to Guildford Cathedral, the rain started to come*
*down in torrents, even the angels were crying. It got darker and darker*
*and I felt lower and lower.*

*As we walked around the corner into the Nave, we were absolutely*
*amazed. There were 700 people in the Cathedral. 700. I could not*
*believe my eyes. Michael obviously touched a lot of hearts.*

*When the service started, the singing was just out of this world.*
*And right next to me our son Christopher shut his eyes and sang along*
*with his friends from St. George's who had come along to bolster the*
*Guildford Choir. And that was quite something, to see the boys from*
*the two choirs sitting side by side in the choir stalls, together with the*
*men of two choirs. Michael had always wanted to sing with his brother*

*when he was still a chorister. He finally got the two Choral Foundations together.*

*The tribute from his godfather was perfect: funny, witty, poignant, and included a wonderful tribute to Christopher as well. The sermon from Canon Maureen told everyone what a strong faith Michael had and how he was so sanguine in living and in dying. "Here was someone who was alive from top to toe!" she said. And he WAS.*

*The anthem was moving, the prayers touching, and then the undertakers moved in to pick up the coffin, and Graham, Christopher, and I moved behind it to take that long, long walk down the Nave. By now I was in tears—and walking past 700 people, most of whom were also in tears, was not easy. As we got to the Great West Door, the pallbearers turned round so that Michael was facing the altar, and everything was so quiet you could hear a pin drop. Suddenly, over the speakers, came the sound of Michael singing, "In the morning when I rise ..."*

*Christopher and I stood with our arms round each other and tears pouring down our cheeks. As it finished, the organ swung into action and Michael's body was turned around and carried out for the last time of his beloved Cathedral, just as the sun came out.*

Children of all ages should be allowed to attend the funeral if they wish, but only after they have been prepared about what to expect. They need an explanation of where they will be going (funeral, shiva, wake, memorial service, burial) and what it means. They need to know what type of room they are going to, if the casket will be there, if it will be open, if there will be flowers, who will be there, how the mourners will be acting, who will stay with the them, what they will be expected to say, and how long they will be there. All questions should be answered honestly and children's feelings respected.

*We celebrated our 3-year-old son's Kevin's life today. The past week has been a whirlwind. All of Kevin's favorite women worked nonstop for 48 hours leading up to last night. The funeral home was beautiful. There were pictures everywhere—on pedestals, in photo albums, collages, and frames.*

*There were children's books throughout the funeral home as well as red balloons, Kev's favorite color. We had patchwork squares out to create a memorial quilt for his younger sisters, Courtney and Katie.*

*People wrote special messages and drawings on them to capture their feelings: "Kevin, Sending you love and kisses and one BIG scoop of mashed potatoes!"*

*We also had sheets of paper to write stories and memories of Kevin to make a memorial book for the girls. Kevin's favorite things were on a memorial table: his green blankie with the hole in it, his books, his Buzz Lightyear, his green bike, his catcher's mitt, his baseball and yellow bat, golf clubs, and more.*

*We rented a 6' projector screen and a big screen TV to display a 20 minute video in both rooms at the funeral home. It showed Kevin's life over the past year. And it was a pretty good life too: putting candles on Grammy's cake with Matthew, gymnastics with Grampie, wrestling with Courtney, reading with Daddy, playing football with Nana, kissing Auntie JoJo and Auntie Karin, playing golf in the yard, laying on the floor laughing, telling knock knock jokes, riding bikes in the house, at the beach at the Cape.*

*What does a mom do? She loves, cherishes, teaches, protects, and lets go. For one brief, shining moment, we had Kevin. For happily ever after we have our memories of him.*

Many siblings benefit from giving one last gift to the departed, such as writing a private note and dropping it in the casket, or bringing some of their sister's favorite flowers to put in her hands. If you have any questions or concerns about what to tell your children or whether they should attend the services or burial, read *How Do We Tell the Children? A Parent's Guide to Helping Children Understand and Cope when Someone Dies*, by Dan Schaefer and Christine Lyons.

Ministers, priests, and rabbis have a unique opportunity to provide support, love, and comfort to the grieving family and friends. They usually know the family well and can evoke poignant memories of the deceased child or teen during the service. Members of the clergy often have excellent counseling skills and can visit the family after the funeral to provide ongoing help during mourning.

# The role of family and friends

Family members and friends can be a wellspring of deep comfort and solace during grieving. Some people seem to know just when a hug is necessary or when silence is most welcome. Unfortunately, in our society there are few guidelines for handling the social aspects of grief. Many well-meaning people voice opinions concerning the time it is taking to "get over it" or question the parents' decision to not give away their child's clothing. Others do not know what to say, so they are silent, pretending that life's greatest catastrophe has not occurred. Many friends never again mention the deceased child's name, not knowing that this silence, as if the cherished child never existed, only adds to parents' pain. Holidays can become uncomfortable, because they bring sadness as well as joy.

In an attempt to alleviate these difficulties, bereaved parents helped compile the following lists of what helps and what does not, in the hope that it may guide those family members and friends who deeply care, but just don't know how to help. These suggestions are offered with the understanding that what works for one person may not work for another. Try to use your knowledge of the bereaved family to choose options that you think will make them comfortable. If in doubt, ask them. As Mother Teresa said, "Kind words can be short and easy to say, but their echoes are truly endless."

## Things that help

The long lists of things that help from Chapter 6, *Family and Friends* (e.g., keeping the household running, feeding the family, and helping with bills), are still appropriate here. The following lists are specific suggestions for grief.

Helpful things to say:

- I am so sorry.
- I cannot imagine the pain you are feeling, but I am thinking about you.
- I really care about you.
- You and your family are in my thoughts and prayers.
- We would like to hold a memorial service at the school for your son if you think that it would be appropriate.
- I will never forget John's sunny smile.
- I will never forget Jane's gentle way with children and animals.

Parents also offer a list of helpful things to do:

- Go to the funeral or memorial service.

> We were overwhelmed and touched by all of the people who came to the funeral. Even people that I had not seen in years—like some of my college professors—attended. Her oncologist and nurse drove 100 miles to be there.

- Show genuine concern and caring by listening.

    *What has helped me the most is for people to just listen. Finding time to remember and reminisce is sometimes very difficult and painful, yet other times I feel much pride and happiness. Friends whose children also have cancer have been the greatest help to me during my daughter's illness and after her death.*

- Help the siblings.

    *We had friends just call and say, "We will pick up Nick on Saturday and take him to Water World, then to our house for dinner. We were hoping he could spend the night. Will that be all right?" They did this many times, and it not only was fun for him, but gave us a chance to be alone with each other and our grief.*

- Write the parents a note instead of sending just a preprinted sympathy card with your signature. Include special things you remember about their child or your feelings about their child. Letters, poems, or drawings from classmates and friends allow children to share their feelings with the family of the deceased, as well as provide poignant testimonials that the family will cherish.

- Talk about the child who has died. Parents forever carry cherished memories of their child and enjoy hearing others' favorite recollections.

    *Months after the funeral, we gathered family members and some close friends to share memories on tape. We did a lot of laughing as well as shed a few tears. But I will always cherish those tapes.*

    · · · · ·

    *I think most of all parents want their child to be remembered. It really comforts me to go to Greg's grave and find flowers, notes, or toys left by others.*

- When parents express guilt over what they did or did not do, reassure them that they did everything they could. Remind them that they provided their child with the best medicine had to offer.

- Remember anniversaries. Call or send a card or flowers on the anniversary of the child's death.

- Respect the family's method of grieving.

- Give donations in the child's name to a favorite charity of the child or parents, for instance, the child's school library, Candlelighters, the local children's camp, a brain tumor organization, or US Children's Hospice International.

> *Every year we still get a card saying that Caitlin's occupational therapist donated money to Camp Goodtimes. It makes me feel good that she is remembered so fondly and that the money will help other kids with cancer and their brothers and sisters.*

- Commemorate the child's life in some tangible way. Examples of this are: planting trees, shrubs, or flowers, erecting a memorial or plaque, or displaying a picture of the child.

> *The spring after Matthew's death, his school contacted me and said they wanted to do something special in his honor. They planted a little leaf linden tree in front of the building and built a wonderful seat around its base. They picked this particular tree because of its wonderful fragrance, and because the leaves were shaped like little hearts. A plaque beside the tree proclaims that this is Matthew's Friendship Tree. In addition to his name and the date of his birth and death, it reads: "When you remember me, please have a smile and cherish the good times we shared. And in these memories I will live with you forever."*

- Be patient. Acute grief from the loss of a child lasts a long, long time. Expectations of a rapid recovery are unrealistic and hurtful to parents.
- Encourage follow-up from medical personnel.

> *Caitlin had a very kind, very gentle radiation oncologist. I went back to see her after Caitlin died; she said, "We were so happy when we saw the progress that Caitlin made, from a stretcher to sitting to talking and walking again; and then our hearts broke when she relapsed. I wept." It was so human and so wonderful for her to let me know that she cared.*

## Things that do not help

Please do not say the following to the parents:

- I know exactly how you feel.
- It's a blessing her suffering has ended.
- Thank goodness you are young enough to have another child.
- At least you have your other children.
- Be brave.
- Time will heal.
- God doesn't give anyone more than they can bear.

- It was God's will.
- He's in a better place now.

> *Every time someone approached me at the funeral home with the words, "He's gone to a better place," I felt as if I would scream. Matthew's place was with me, his mother. Seven-year-old boys need their mother. It also really angered me when people repeatedly said, "Oh, with all he suffered, you wouldn't wish him back if you could." Well, yes, I would wish my child back! I would wish him back healthy and well. To this very day I would wish my child back, even if I could hold him for just a moment or hear the sound of his laughter one more time.*

- God must have needed another angel.
- It's lucky this happened to someone as strong as you.
- Don't worry, in time you'll get over it.
- Why did you decide to cremate him?
- How is your marriage holding up?
- You need to be strong for your other children.

The following are not helpful things to say to the siblings:

- You need to be strong for your mom and dad.
- Don't cry, it upsets your parents.
- You're the man of the house now.
- How does it feel to be the big sister?

Even if a bereaved parent has deep religious faith, it is often tested by their child's death. Parents are not comforted by well-meaning friends who assume faith is making the grief bearable; indeed, many parents find it to be infuriating. It's better to just say "I'm sorry."

In the months and years following the child's death, any of the following might not be appreciated:

- Don't you think it's time to get over it?
- It's been six months; it's time to put the past behind you.
- Life goes on.
- You need to get on with your life.

- You shouldn't be feeling that way.

- Don't you think you should give away all of her clothes?

- Don't cry.

- Doesn't it bother you to have his pictures around?

- Please don't talk about Johnnie, it just stirs up all those memories.

- It's not good to just sit around, you need to get out and have some fun.

Don't let your own sense of helplessness keep you from reaching out. Pretending that nothing is wrong or being afraid to talk about the child who has died hurts grieving parents.

The following are suggestions from parents on what not to do:

- Don't remove anything that belonged to the child who died, unless specifically asked to by the parents.

    > One family member took my son's toothbrush out of the bathroom and threw it away. I missed it immediately. She probably felt that she was doing me a favor, but it made me so angry. I needed to keep things. I have his hair from the second time it fell out, because he wanted to save it, and I've kept his teeth which had to be pulled during treatment. I just need to have those things, and I resent people who insist you must clear out a child's things. Parents should be able to keep things or get rid of them— whichever is comfortable—regardless of others' opinions.

- Don't offer advice.

    > Christie's room is still her room. We still refer to it as Christie's room. People just don't have the right to say you shouldn't leave that room empty: it's not empty, it's full of her life. I know that they are not trying to hurt us. It just bothers them to see that room. Sometimes it is just a reminder of death; yet, there are times when being in there and surrounded by all her things brings us closer to her and her time with us.

- Don't say anything that in any way suggests that the child's medical care was inadequate. Parents already feel intense guilt over what should have been or could have been.

    > I can't tell you how many people said things like "If only you had gone to a different treatment facility," or "If only you had used this or that treatment." What people need most is support for what they are doing or did do.

- Don't look on the bright side or find silver linings.

  *I became unexpectedly pregnant the month after my daughter died. I can't tell you how many people said things like "The circle of life is complete," or "God is taking one and giving you another," or "God is replacing her." She can never be replaced. It was horrible to hear those things, and I felt it was unfair to both the unborn baby and to my daughter who died.*

- Don't drop bereaved parents from the support group. Talk about your options; grief-stricken parents have enough silence in their lives.

  *When my daughter was terminal, in really bad shape, I went to the support group. We had all bonded and were very close. I felt guilty because I really wanted to cry and was trying to hold it back because I didn't want to upset everybody else. All of the sudden, I felt like I was the alien, like you feel when your child is diagnosed. Here I was in a room full of people I loved, where I had felt safe. Now I was alone again, this time with no hopes of Christie's recovery. It was truly the end. I never felt more scared or alone.*

- Don't make comments about the parents' strength.

  *People would say things to me like "You're so strong," or "I just couldn't live through what you have." It makes me want to scream. Do they mean I loved my child less than they love theirs because I have physically survived?*

# Sibling grief

Siblings are sometimes called the "forgotten grievers" because attention is typically focused on the parents. Children and teens hesitate to express their own strong feelings in an attempt to prevent causing their parents additional distress. Indeed, adult family members and friends may advise the brothers and sisters to "be strong" for their parents or to "help your parents by being good." These requests place a terribly unfair burden on children who have already endured months or years of stress and family disruption. Siblings need continual reinforcement that each of them is an irreplaceable member of the family and that the entire family has suffered a loss. They have a right to mourn openly, in their own way, and in their own time (which may be delayed or intermittent).

> *The family requires such reorganization after a child's death, and there is nowhere to look for an example. Each person in the family constellation*

*has different feelings and different ways of grieving; there is just no way to reconcile all of this when the supposed leaders of the group are totally out of it. Not to mention the fact that both my husband and I wanted more understanding and compassion from each other than we were possibly able to give.*

Children express grief in many ways, including physically (changes in eating habits, toileting, sleeping, stomachaches); emotionally (regression to earlier behaviors, risk taking); fear (of the dark, being away from parents); guilt (once said "I wish you would die," to the sibling, and the sibling died); and emotional changes (tantrums, crying, sadness, anxiety, withdrawal, depression). Older children and teens may appear nonchalant, angry, or withdrawn or take risks involving alcohol and drugs.

In families with siblings of different ages, parents need to engage them at their developmental level. Sometimes private times together or individual outings with the parent can be very helpful for siblings.

Many families pull apart because it is too painful to share their deep, but different, feelings of grief. Some parents worry that if they start talking, they will "break down" in front of the children. But children who are excluded from the family's mourning may begin to feel alienated from the family. Here are suggestions from families about how to help pull together while mourning:

- Let the siblings go to the funeral. They have suffered a loss; they need to say good-bye; they need support for their grief just as much as adults.

- Children and teens experience the same feelings as adults. By sharing your own feelings, you can encourage them to identify their own. (For example, "I'm really feeling sad today. How do you feel?")

- Some families establish a regular meeting time to talk about their feelings. Both tears and laughter erupt when family members talk about funny or touching memories of the departed child.

- Jointly discuss how holidays and anniversaries should be observed. Some families hang a Christmas stocking every year for the departed child, others merely mention her name during the blessing. Each family devises different ways to handle the child's birthday and the anniversary of her death.

> *Last year we marked our first Christmas since Matthew's death. It was so incredibly hard for me to open the boxes of decorations knowing that inside I would find treasures he had made for me over the years with his own two little hands. I cried when I found his stocking, because I didn't*

*know what to do with it. Somehow it didn't seem right to not hang it as usual.*

*I decided that I would continue to place Matthew's stocking beside David's and Kristina's. Instead of Santa filling it with treats, I asked my family to fill it for me. A few weeks before Christmas, I ask members of my family to write a memory of Matthew on a piece of paper. The only stipulation is that it must be a happy memory. On Christmas morning I look forward most of all to the gifts my children have made for me in school, and the memories that fill Matthew's stocking. Matthew will always be included in our Christmas. That's because he will always be an important member of our family.*

# Parental grief

There are as many ways to grieve as there are bereaved parents. There is no timetable, no appropriate progression from one stage to the next, no time when parents should "be over it." Losing a child is one of life's most horrific and painful events. Therese A. Rando, in her book *Grieving: How to Go On Living When Someone You Love Dies,* writes:

> *Parental grief is particularly intense. It is unusually complicated and has extraordinary up-and-down periods. It appears to be the most long lasting grief of all.*

The death of a child shatters the very order of the universe—children are not supposed to die before their parents. It seems unnatural, incomprehensible. Losing a child entails mourning not only the child himself, but all of the hopes, dreams, wishes, fantasies, and needs relating to him. When you lose a child, you lose part of yourself, part of your future.

This book will not go through psychological descriptions of the grieving process. There are excellent reference books available, several of which are listed in Appendix B, *Resources.* Here, the parents themselves tell you about grief.

> *I truly think that it is the worst thing in the entire world. Nothing worse can happen than losing your child. There is no reprieve. None.*

> • • • • •

> *I was having a very hard time grieving when a wonderful therapist that I was seeing said to me, "You are beating yourself up about grieving. Think about it. When you enter marriage, what are you called? A wife. When your spouse dies, what are you called? A widow. When you don't*

have a home and you are living on the street, what is the name for that? A homeless person. When you lose a child, what's it called, what's the name?" I said, "I don't know." She said, "Exactly. There is not even a word in our vocabulary. That's how terrible it is. It doesn't even have a name."

• • • • •

Every day when I walk out of my house I tell myself to grab the mask. I feel like I walk different than everybody and talk different than everybody and look different than everybody. It's the worst part of bereavement, the isolation caused by people who just don't know how to talk to you, when really all they need to do is listen and remember with you.

• • • • •

I found myself getting busier and busier, thinking that I could outrun the pain. I realized that I couldn't avoid the hurt; I just had to grit my teeth, cry, and live through it.

• • • • •

I felt like our sick daughter was the center of our universe for so long, that now I need to start feeling some responsibility for my other kids whom I've been away from for so long, both physically and emotionally. I told my husband the other night that I didn't even know if I loved the three kids anymore. I cannot feel a thing. Pinch me, I don't feel it. Hug me, I don't feel it. I'm numb.

• • • • •

It's hard to admit, but there was an element of relief when my daughter died. Not relief for myself, but for her. I was almost glad that she wouldn't face a life full of disabilities, that she wouldn't face the numerous surgeries that would have been required to repair the damage from treatment, that she wouldn't face the pain of not having children of her own. I just felt relief that she would no longer feel any pain.

• • • • •

At first we didn't feel like a family anymore. Now it's better, but it's still not the family that I was used to, that I want. I still feel like the mother of four children, not three. I find it very hard to answer when someone asks me how many children I have. I also can't sign cards like I used to, with all of our names, so now I just write "from the gang." I guess that's not fair to the boys, but I just can't bear to leave her name off.

• • • • •

Birthdays are hard for us. Greg's birthday was June 10, and his brother's is June 9. So it's pretty hard to ignore. On Greg's birthday and *the anniversary of his death, we blow up balloons, one for every year he would have been alive, write messages on them with markers, and release them at his grave.*

• • • • •

*It seems like just about every holiday has some difficult memory attached to it now. He was diagnosed on Easter, and then relapsed the next year on Valentine's Day. I hate them both now. Christmas is always hard. And Halloween is tough because he so loved to dress up. I see all those little ones in their costumes and I'm just flooded with pain.*

• • • • •

*This evening my heart was so saddened. I paced up and down in front of the mantel pausing to look at each picture of my daughter. Something that I cannot describe catches in my chest, and I can't breathe right. I look at her face and try to will it to life for a kiss and a touch, for softly spoken endearments at night. How we love all of our children, yet one missing leaves such a stabbing pain.*

• • • • •

*The past few weeks have been tough. Everything is a reminder of Kevin, a spoon with his name on it, toys throughout the house, syringes in the drawer, the dozens of books on the shelf. I can hear his 3-year-old singsong voice with the things he used to say at least a thousand times, "Momma, you shut the TV off?" "Momma, where are ya?" "Momma, I want my blankie" "Momma, how come Courtney's not cooperating" "Momma, you read me a book" "Momma, you lay down and scratch my back" "Momma, you sing hush baby."*

*The "firsts" are going to be the hardest, going to the park, going food shopping, going to the Maine house, going to Target, driving by the library and not popping in to pick up a book for Kev. I find that I don't want to spend time with anyone who didn't know Kevin. I'm not sure if it's because they won't know of how big the loss is or because I need to have people around who can talk about him and the things he used to say and do. So when people say, "How are you doing?" I say, "We're doing." We're doing a lot of thinking, a lot of laughing, and a lot of crying.*

• • • • •

*It's hard when people I have just met ask, "How many children do you have?" In the beginning I always felt that I had to explain that I had two but one died. Now, I just say one. I don't want their sympathy, I don't want their pity, but most of all I just don't want to have to explain. After*

*two years or so, I started to feel uncomfortable giving out my life history
and then having to deal with other people's discomfort. So now I just say
one, and yet it still feels like I'm betraying him every time I do it.*

Bereaved parents are frequently reassured that "time will ease the pain." Most find that this is not the case. Time helps them understand the pain; the passage of time reassures them that they can adjust and they will survive. The acute pain becomes more quiescent, but still erupts when parents go to what would have been their child's graduation, hear their child's favorite song, or just go to the grocery store. Grief is a long, difficult journey, with many ups and downs. But, with time, parents report that laughter and joy do return. They acknowledge that life will never be the same, but it can be good again.

Judith Barrington wrote in her book *Grief Postponed*:

> *Certain smells, certain moments when I feel unloved, certain aspects of
> the Christmas rituals, and hundreds of other ordinary details of life, will
> reopen the wound. But at least now I can let it bleed for a while and go
> on. At least now I can be open, not only to those painful moments, but
> also to the many joys of my life.*

*I just wish I had armfuls of time*

—Four-year-old with cancer
*Armfuls of Time*

# CHAPTER 24

# Toward the Future

IT IS HARD TO BELIEVE that when the first astronaut stepped out onto the moon in 1969, the technology available to diagnose and treat children with CNS tumors was primitive at best. Many children were placed on medication for seizure disorders without ever knowing that the cause of the seizures was a tumor. If diagnosed, most children died from their tumor.

The first CT scanner became available in the late 1970s, and the MRI (the gold standard for diagnosis of a CNS tumor) was not widely used until the late 1980s. Surgery, when performed, utilized extremely unsophisticated equipment until the 1980s. The risks of surgical procedures were quite high. Radiation treatments provided some temporary relief of symptoms and occasionally a cure. Children who survived after high-dose radiation almost always developed devastating late effects. Chemotherapy was not used, because it was thought that the drugs would not penetrate the blood/brain barrier and get to the tumor.

It is clear that treatments have come a long way in the past two decades. Technology is now available to successfully diagnose, treat, and cure many children with brain and spinal cord tumors. Diagnostic tools, especially the MRI, allow for earlier diagnosis and treatment. The MRI helps surgeons plan delicate surgeries and is also used to give surgeons a three-dimensional picture of the tumor during surgery. MRI is also used to plan radiation treatments and allows the newer radiation therapy machines to deliver more focused doses of radiation, thus sparing nearby healthy brain cells. Chemotherapy has been shown to penetrate the blood/brain barrier, and many drugs have been found to be effective in destroying CNS tumor cells.

The enrollment and participation in national clinical trials has fueled the success in understanding and treating CNS tumors. Approximately 75 percent of children with tumors enroll in clinical trials. This has enabled researchers of the past three decades to learn about the many different subgroups of tumors and how each should be treated. Research has also shown that:

- Each tumor is an individual. Children with the same diagnosis have incredibly variable responses to treatment. Therefore, some children with grim prognoses are cured, but others with a tumor considered to be very treatable relapse.

- Children with tumors that are totally removed with surgery have a much better prognosis than do those whose tumors cannot be totally removed.

- Slow-growing tumors may remain dormant for months or years without any treatment.

- Some slow-growing tumors shrink in size in response to chemotherapy.

- Chemotherapy when used alone or in conjunction with radiation therapy is effective in treating some CNS tumors (especially medulloblastoma, PNET, and germ cell tumors)

- Radiation therapy, which used to be the gold standard, is now withheld for slow-growing tumors until other treatment methods have been tried.

- Radiation therapy treatments are delayed in young children with fast-growing tumors because of the adverse effects on the developing brain.

> When you have an aggressive malignant tumor growing in your child's brain, the choice to wait for newer, superior treatments to come along may not be an option. In the case of our daughter Morgan, who was first diagnosed with a malignant medulloblastoma a few days before her second birthday, the decision to wait on having her undergo radiation therapy was a hard and complicated one. After a successful resection of her tumor, Morgan went on to receive six rounds of intense chemotherapy followed by a stem cell transplant. Afterward, her doctors requested that we follow her therapy with radiation treatments. Because of her age, not yet 3, we opted to not expose her to the powerful tool of radiation, which may have increased her chance of long-term survival but at the same time may have left her cognitive abilities severely handicapped. Our decision was not a hasty one. We also had well-respected doctors telling us not to do any other therapy, including radiation, because Morgan's chemo treatment was the most powerful of its day and some kids were actually achieving long-term survival without radiation.
>
> Morgan stayed cancer free for two years. It was at Morgan's two year MRI scan that a small tumor was found—she had relapsed at the original tumor site. Now we had no choice but to treat Morgan with radiation therapy. What we immediately realized was that by waiting, we bought Morgan some time. Now almost 5, Morgan's cognitive development would fare better after radiation than if she were 3. What we didn't know was that technology in radiotherapy had improved greatly with the introduction of a sophisticated treatment called proton

*beam radiation. Different from the traditional method, proton beam*
*causes less damage to the good brain cells and delivers a more direct hit*
*to the tumor bed. The result, many doctors believe, is less damage to the*
*good brain tissue (sparing cognitive impairment) and similar results for*
*long-term survival as traditional radiation treatments.*

*Morgan received proton beam radiation for six weeks to her head and*
*spine. Today she is a happy, well-adjusted 6-year-old who goes to school,*
*dance classes, and gymnastics. Although it is still too early for us to know*
*just how much proton beam radiation therapy may have helped Morgan,*
*we feel fortunate that she had the opportunity to undergo this new and*
*improved treatment.*

There is good reason to believe that the technological advances on the horizon will result in a more positive outlook for those diagnosed in the future. This, combined with continued enrollment of children with CNS tumors on national clinical trials, will expedite the identification of effective treatments.

It is hoped that the following areas of current research will provide a greater understanding of CNS tumors:

- Improvements in MRI technology/MR spectroscopy will help physicians better understand rate of tumor cell growth at any specific time.

- Intraoperative MRI scans will be widely available and will further increase the amount of tumor that the surgeons can remove safely.

- New surgical instruments and improved intraoperative monitoring will provide valuable information to the surgeons during the operation.

- Radiation therapy technology will continue to fine-tune the delivery of ultra-focused radiation treatments while sparing normal tissues.

- New chemotherapy agents will be developed and tested for efficacy against CNS tumors.

- Biologists will study genetic mutations and environmental factors that may cause CNS tumors.

- Research in the areas of immunotherapy and gene therapy will create brand new treatments that are more effective and less damaging.

The increased numbers of long-term survivors have raised awareness of late effects of the disease and treatments. The expansion of rehabilitative medicine has allowed for physical, occupational, and speech therapy to be available at home, at school, and in the community. Special education and the mandate for individual educational plans provide education for children with CNS tumors who have cognitive problems. Such programs have expanded to include career and college counseling.

As researchers, doctors, and nurses forge ahead in the fight to improve diagnosing and treating children with CNS tumors, they share the same dreams of the patients and their families:

> During the twenty years that I have spent as a nurse and a nurse practitioner, I have worked only with children with cancer. Fifteen of those years were spent working with children who have CNS tumors. I have witnessed countless families coping with the diagnosis and treatment of their children. In the early days there were no MRI scans, no broviacs or mediports, and children who had brain tumors mostly died. As clinicians, we would sigh to ourselves with each new diagnosis thinking in the back of our minds, "How many months or years will this child live?"
>
> The MRI scanner and advances in surgery have completely changed the pessimism associated with CNS tumors. We now know that many tumors can be cured or controlled with surgery and observation with MRI scans. Chemotherapy and radiation can cure or control those that will grow back or can't be removed with surgery. We have learned that to do nothing but watching often buys us time for a newer treatment that may come along. Aggressive research continues with the support of many groups organized by families of children with CNS tumors to find a cure for each and every type of tumor.
>
> In the bigger picture, it isn't the diseases or the treatments that I remember, it is the children:
>
> Kristen who had four surgeries and two years of chemotherapy for her medulloblastoma which was diagnosed when she was 9 months of age. She is now 15, a normal adolescent.
>
> Ryan at age 2 had a brainstem and spinal cord tumor diagnosed and underwent several surgeries and radiation. He couldn't move a muscle, was dependent on a respirator, and had a feeding tube because he could not swallow. I cried four years later when I got a holiday card with Ryan riding a bicycle. He is now 16.

*Brian, diagnosed at 15, underwent surgery, chemotherapy, and radiation. Ten years later I went to his wedding.*

*Charlie was operated on at ages 4 and 8 for a brainstem tumor. He invited me to his Bar Mitzvah this year...he is 13.*

*There is reason to hope.*

# Blood Counts and What They Mean

KEEPING TRACK OF THEIR CHILD'S BLOOD COUNTS becomes a way of life for parents of children with cancer. Unfortunately, misunderstandings about the implications of certain changes in blood values can cause unnecessary worry and fear. To help prevent these concerns and to better enable parents to help spot trends in the blood values of their child, this appendix explains the blood counts of healthy children, the blood counts of children being treated for cancer, and what each blood value means.

## Values for healthy children

Each laboratory and lab handbook has slightly different reference values for each blood cell, so your lab sheets may differ slightly from those that appear later in this appendix. There is also variation in values for children of different ages. For instance, in newborn to 4-year-old children, granulocytes are lower and lymphocytes higher than the numbers listed below. Geographic location affects reference ranges as well. The following table lists blood count values for healthy children:

| Blood count type | Values for healthy children |
| --- | --- |
| Hemoglobin (Hgb.) | 11.5–13.5 g/100 ml |
| Hematocrit | 34–40% |
| Red blood count | 3.9–5.3 m/cm or 3.9-5.3 x $10^{12}$/L |
| Platelets | 160,000–500,000 mm$^3$ |
| White blood count | 5,000–10,000 mm$^3$ or 5–10 K/ul |
| WBC differential: | |
|     Segmented neutrophils | 50–70% |
|     Band neutrophils | 1–3% |
|     Basophils | 0.5–1% |
|     Eosinophils | 1–4% |
|     Lymphocytes | 12–46% |
|     Monocytes | 2–10% |
| Direct (conjugated) | 0.1–0.4 mg/dl |
| Indirect (unconjugated) | 0.2–0.18 mg/dl |
| AST (SGOT) | 0–36 IU/l |
| ALT (SGPT) | 0–48 IU/l |
| BUN | 10–20 mg/dl |
| Creatinine | 0.3–1.1 mg/dl |

## Values for children on chemotherapy

Blood counts of children being treated for cancer fluctuate wildly. White blood cell counts can go down to zero or be above normal. Red cell counts decrease periodically during treatment, necessitating transfusions of packed red cells. Platelet levels also decrease, requiring platelet transfusions. Absolute neutrophil counts (ANC) are closely watched, because they give the physician an idea of the child's ability to fight infection. ANCs vary from zero to in the thousands.

Oncologists consider all of the blood values to get the total picture of the child's reaction to illness, chemotherapy, radiation, or infection. Trends are more important than any single value. For instance, if the values of three tests were 5.0, 4.7, 4.9, then the second result was insignificant. If, on the other hand, the values were 5.0, 4.7, 4.2, then there is a decrease in the cell line.

The explanations below will describe each blood value. If you have any questions about your child's blood counts, ask your child's doctor for a clear explanation. Especially in the beginning, many parents agonize over whether the rapid changes in blood counts (often requiring transfusions, changes in chemo dosages, and changes in whether the child can have visitors) are normal or expected. The only way to address your worries and prevent them from escalating is to ask what the changes mean.

## What do these blood values mean?

The following sections explain each line of the table of blood values shown earlier. See Figure A-1 to get an idea of the different ways these values might be displayed on the actual lab reports prepared for your child.

### Hemoglobin (Hgb)

Red cells contain hemoglobin, the molecules that carry oxygen and carbon dioxide in the blood. Measuring hemoglobin gives an exact picture of the ability of the blood to carry oxygen. Children may have low hemoglobin levels at diagnosis and during the intensive parts of treatment. This is because both cancer and chemotherapy decrease the bone marrow's ability to produce new red cells. Signs and symptoms of anemia—pallor, shortness of breath, fatigue— may start to show if the hemoglobin gets very low.

### Hematocrit (HCT), also called packed cell volume (PCV)

The purpose of this test is to determine the ratio of plasma (clear liquid part of blood) to red cells in the blood. Blood is drawn from a vein, finger prick, or Hickman or Port-a-cath and is spun in a centrifuge to separate the red cells from the plasma. The hematocrit is the percentage of cells in the blood. For instance, if the child has a hematocrit of 30 percent, it means that 30 percent of the amount of blood drawn was cells and the rest was plasma. When the child is on chemotherapy, the bone marrow does not make many red cells, and the hematocrit will go down. This results in less oxygen being carried in the blood, and your child may have less energy. The child may be given a transfusion of packed red cells when the hematocrit goes below 18 to 19 percent.

| TEST | RESULTS | | UNITS | REFERENCE RANGE | | | |
|------|---------|---|-------|-----------------|---|---|---|
| Collection Cmt. - | | | | | | | |
| | | | | | | | |
| *CBC** | | | | | | | |
| White Blood Count | 1.7 | L | x10-3 | 3.8 | - | 12.5 | JK |
| Red Blood Cnt | 3.02 | L | x10-6 | 3.90 | - | 5.30 | JK |
| Hemoglobin | 8.9 | L | g/d1 | 11.5 | - | 13.5 | JK |
| Hematocrit | 26.1 | L | % | 34.0 | - | 40.0 | JK |
| MCV | 86.0 | | um3 | 75.0 | - | 87.0 | JK |
| MCH | 29.4 | | uug | 24.0 | - | 30.0 | JK |
| MCHC | 34.1 | | % | 32.0 | - | 36.0 | JK |
| Segs | 33 | | % | 30 | - | 70 | JK |
| Bands | 1 | | % | 0 | - | 5 | JK |
| Lymphocytes | 19 | L | % | 20 | - | 70 | JK |
| Monocytes | 42 | H | % | 0 | - | 8 | JK |
| Eosinophiles | 5 | H | % | 0 | - | 3 | JK |
| Morphology Cmt 1 Anisocytosis | | | 2+ | | | | |
| Platelets | 34 | L | x10-3 | 250 | - | 550 | JK |

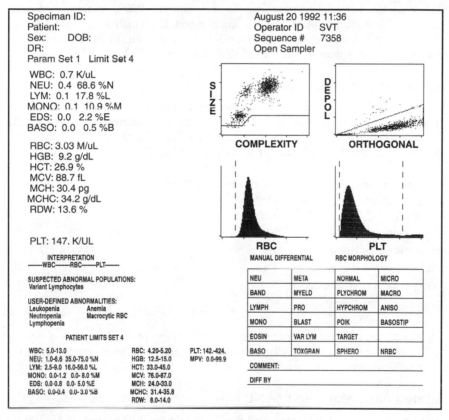

Speciman ID:
Patient:
Sex:        DOB:
DR:
Param Set 1   Limit Set 4

WBC: 0.7 K/uL
NEU: 0.4 68.6 %N
LYM: 0.1 17.8 %L
MONO: 0.1 10.9 %M
EDS: 0.0 2.2 %E
BASO: 0.0 0.5 %B

RBC: 3.03 M/uL
HGB: 9.2 g/dL
HCT: 26.9 %
MCV: 88.7 fL
MCH: 30.4 pg
MCHC: 34.2 g/dL
RDW: 13.6 %

PLT: 147. K/UL

August 20 1992 11:36
Operator ID    SVT
Sequence #    7358
Open Sampler

SIZE / COMPLEXITY

D EPOL / ORTHOGONAL

RBC

PLT

INTERPRETATION
------WBC------RBC------PLT------

SUSPECTED ABNORMAL POPULATIONS:
Variant Lymphocytes

USER-DEFINED ABNORMALITIES:
Leukopenia        Anemia
Neutropenia       Macrocytic RBC
Lymphopenia

PATIENT LIMITS SET 4

WBC: 5.0-13.0
NEU: 1.0-6.6 35.0-75.0 %N
LYM: 2.5-9.0 16.0-56.0 %L
MONO: 0.0-1.2 0.0- 8.0 %M
EDS: 0.0-0.8 0.0- 5.0 %E
BASO: 0.0-0.4 0.0- 3.0 %B

RBC: 4.20-5.20
HGB: 12.5-15.0
HCT: 33.0-45.0
MCV: 76.0-87.0
MCH: 24.0-33.0
MCHC: 31.4-35.8
RDW: 8.0-14.0

PLT: 142.-424,
MPV: 0.0-99.9

MANUAL DIFFERENTIAL

RBC MORPHOLOGY

| NEU | META | NORMAL | MICRO |
|-----|------|--------|-------|
| BAND | MYELD | PLYCHROM | MACRO |
| LYMPH | PRO | HYPCHROM | ANISO |
| MONO | BLAST | POIK | BASOSTIP |
| EOSIN | VAR LYM | TARGET | |
| BASO | TOXGRAN | SPHERO | NRBC |

COMMENT:

DIFF BY

Figure A-1. Two sample lab data sheets

# Red blood cell count (RBC)

Red blood cells are produced by the bone marrow continuously in healthy children and adults. These cells contain hemoglobin, which carries oxygen and carbon dioxide throughout the body. To determine the RBC, an automated electronic device is used to count the number of red cells in a sample of blood.

Red cell indices (MCV, MCH, MCHC) are mathematical relationships of hematocrit to red cell count, hemoglobin to red cell count, and hemoglobin to hematocrit. They give a mathematical expression of the degree of change in shape found in red cells and the concentration of hemoglobin within each cell. The higher the number (low teens are fine), the more distorted the red cell population is.

# White blood cell count (WBC)

The total white blood cell count determines the body's ability to fight infection. Treatment for cancer kills healthy white cells as well as diseased ones. Parents need to expect prolonged periods of low white counts during treatment. To determine the WBC, an automated electronic device counts the number of white cells in a liter of blood. If your lab sheet uses K/ul instead of $mm^3$, multiply by 1,000 to get the value in $mm^3$. For example, on the lab sheet in Figure A-1, the total WBC on the bottom lab sheet is 0.7 K/ul. Therefore, $0.7 \times 1,000 = 700$ $mm^3$.

# White blood cell differential

When a child has blood drawn for a complete blood count (CBC), one section of the lab report will state the total white blood cell (WBC) count and a differential, in which each type of white blood cell is listed as a percentage of the total. For example, if the total WBC count is 1,500 $mm^3$, the differential might appear as in the following table:

| White blood cell type | Percentage of total WBCs |
|---|---|
| Segmented neutrophils (also called polys or segs) | 49% |
| Band neutrophils (also called bands) | 1% |
| Basophils (also called basos) | 1% |
| Eosinophils (also called eos) | 1% |
| Lymphocytes (also called lymphs) | 38% |
| Monocytes (also called monos) | 10% |

You might also see cells called metamyelocytes, myelocytes, promyelocytes, and myeloblasts listed. These are immature white cells usually only found in the bone marrow. They may be seen in the blood during recovery from low counts.

# Absolute neutrophil count (ANC)

The absolute neutrophil count (also called the absolute granulocyte count or AGC) is a measure of the body's ability to withstand infection. Generally, an ANC above 1,000 means that the child's infection fighting ability is near normal.

To calculate the ANC, add the percentages of neutrophils (both segmented and band) and multiply by the total WBC. Using the example above, the ANC is 49% + 1% = 50%. 50% of 1,500 (.50×1,500) = 750. The ANC is 750.

## Platelet count

Platelets are necessary to repair the body and stop bleeding, through the formation of clots. Because platelets are produced by the bone marrow, platelet counts decrease when a child is on chemotherapy. Signs of lowering platelet counts are small vessel bleeding, such as bruises, bleeding gums, or nosebleeds. Platelet transfusions may be given when the count is very low or when there is bleeding. Platelets are counted by passing a blood sample through an electronic device.

Approximately one-third of all platelets spend a great deal of time in the spleen. Any splenic dysfunction, such as enlargement, may cause the counts to drop precipitously. If the spleen is removed, platelet counts may skyrocket. This transient thrombocytosis (elevated platelet count) will abate within a month.

## ALT (alanine aminotransferase), also called SGPT (serum glutamic pyruvic transaminase)

When doctors talk about liver functions, they are usually referring to tests on blood samples that measure liver damage. If the chemotherapy is toxic to your child's liver, the damaged liver cells release an enzyme called ALT into the blood serum. ALT levels can go up in the hundreds or even thousands in some children on chemotherapy. Each institution and protocol has different points at which they decrease dosages or stop chemotherapy to allow the child's liver to recover. If you notice a change in your child's ALT, ask for an explanation and plan of action (for example, "John's ALT is now 450—what are your thoughts about reducing or stopping the chemotherapy to allow his liver to recover?").

## AST (aspartate aminotransferase), also called SGOT (serum glutamic oxaloacetic transaminase)

SGOT is an enzyme present in high concentrations in tissues with high metabolic activity, including the liver. Severely damaged or killed cells release SGOT into the blood. The amount of SGOT in the blood is directly related to the amount of tissue damage. Therefore, if your child's liver is being damaged by the chemotherapy, the SGOT can rise into the thousands. In addition, there are other causes for an elevated SGOT, such as viral infections, reaction to an anesthetic, and many others. If your child's level jumps unexpectedly, ask the physician for an explanation and a plan of action.

## Blood urea nitrogen (BUN)

Blood urea nitrogen (BUN) is a blood test used to assess kidney function. It is also used to detect liver disease, dehydration, congestive heart failure, gastrointestinal bleeding, starvation, shock, or urinary tract obstruction by a tumor. The test measures the amount of an end product of protein metabolism, called urea nitrogen, in the blood. For children with kidney or liver disease, BUN is often found in abnormal levels.

| Blood Counts | | | | | | | | | |
|---|---|---|---|---|---|---|---|---|---|
| **Date:** | | | | | | | | | |
| **WBC**<br>*ref. range_____* | | | | | | | | | |
| **Neutrophils**<br>*(polys or segs)* | | | | | | | | | |
| **Neutrophils**<br>*(bands)* | | | | | | | | | |
| **ANC**<br>*(polys + bands,<br>multiplied by WBC)* | | | | | | | | | |
| **Hematocrit**<br>*ref. range_____* | | | | | | | | | |
| **Platelets**<br>*ref. range_____* | | | | | | | | | |
| **Chemistries** | | | | | | | | | |
| | | | | | | | | | |
| | | | | | | | | | |
| | | | | | | | | | |
| **Chemotherapy** | | | | | | | | | |
| | | | | | | | | | |
| | | | | | | | | | |
| | | | | | | | | | |
| **Side Effects** | | | | | | | | | |
| | | | | | | | | | |
| | | | | | | | | | |
| | | | | | | | | | |

*Figure A-2. **Example of a record-keeping sheet***

## Creatinine

Creatinine is the breakdown product of protein metabolism found in the urine and the blood. Creatinine is measured to assess kidney function and to determine the presence and severity of suspected kidney disease. An elevated blood creatinine level is often seen in children with kidney insufficiency and renal failure. Doctors use a creatinine clearance test to assess kidney function, particularly to see how efficiently the kidney filters and excretes creatinine.

## Your child's pattern

Each child develops a unique pattern of blood counts during treatment, and observant parents can help track these changes. This appendix contains a record-keeping sheet (see Figure A-2) that you can use to record your child's blood values. If there is a change in the pattern, show it to your child's doctor and ask for an explanation. Doctors consider all of the laboratory results to decide how to proceed, but they should be willing to explain their plan of action to you so that you better understand what is happening and worry less.

If your child is participating in a clinical trial and you have obtained the entire clinical trial protocol, it will contain a section that clearly outlines the actions that should be taken by the oncologist if certain changes in blood counts occur.

# Resources

THE RESOURCES LISTED BELOW are starting points for finding the help you need. Each may supply you with additional ideas and services beyond those listed here.

## List of pediatric neurosurgeons

Appendix D, *List of Pediatric Neurosurgeons,* contains a list of pediatric neurosurgeons organized by state. It was accurate for the fall of 2001, but because physicians move and phone numbers change, some listings may not remain correct. The American Society of Pediatric Neurosurgeons maintains an updated list at *http://www.aspn.org.*

## Service and disability organizations

**The Academy for Guided Imagery**
PO Box 2070
Mill Valley, CA 94942
(800) 726-2070
*http://www.interactiveimagery.com*

This organization can assist in locating a professional in your area to help your child learn visualization.

**American Brain Tumor Association**
2720 River Road, Suite 146
Des Plaines, IL 60018
(800) 886-2282
*http://www.abta.org*

Provides publications about brain tumors, holds patient conferences, offers support by telephone, publishes newsletters three times yearly, and funds research.

**American Cancer Society**
1599 Clifton Road NE
Atlanta, GA 30329-4251
(800) ACS-2345
*http://www.cancer.org*

Its programs include patient-to-patient visitation, transportation to appointments, housing near treatment centers, equipment and supplies, support groups, educational literature, and summer camps for children with cancer.

**The American Society of Clinical Hypnosis**
33 West Grand Avenue, Suite 402
Chicago, IL 60610
*http://www.asch.net*

A membership organization for doctors, psychologists, and dentists who use hypnosis in their practices. Will provide referrals to local members.

**American Speech-Language-Hearing Association (ASHA)**
10801 Rockville Pike
Rockville, MD 20852
(800) 638-8255
*http://www.asha.org*

Provides referrals to local speech/language/hearing specialists.

**Brain Tumor Foundation for Children, Inc.**
1835 Savoy Drive, Suite 316
Atlanta, GA 30341
(770) 458-5554
*http://www.btfcgainc.org*

Provides patient conferences, educational information, and some financial assistance to families in Georgia (hopes to expand this service to other states). Also funds research.

**Brain Tumor Foundation of Canada**
650 Waterloo Street, Suite 100
London, Ontario N6B 2R4 Canada
(519) 642-7755
*http://www.btfc.org/*

Provides patient and family support, publications, quarterly newsletter, and funds for research.

**The Brain Tumor Society**
124 Watertown Street, Suite 3-H
Watertown, MA 02472
(800) 770-8287
*http://www.tbts.org*

Provides resource guides and educational materials, public education and patient conferences, telephone support, and funds for research. Publishes six newsletters yearly and a brain tumor booklist (bibliography of helpful books).

**Canadian Cancer Society**
565 W. 10th Avenue
Vancouver, BC V5Z 4J4 Canada
(888) 939-3333
*http://www.bc.cancer.ca*

Provides same services as the US Cancer Society.

**Candlelighters Childhood Cancer Foundation**
3910 Warner Street
Kensington, MD 20895
(800) 366-CCCF
*http://www.candlelighters.org*

Founded in 1970, Candlelighters has more than 40,000 members worldwide. It provides yearly bibliography and resource guides, quarterly newsletters, referrals, information, and various handbooks to help families of children with cancer.

**Candlelighters Childhood Cancer Foundation Canada**
55 Eglinton Avenue E., Suite 401
Toronto, Ontario M4P 1G8 Canada
(800) 363-1062 (Canada only)
*http://www.candlelighters.ca*

Provides resource guides, newsletters, and information.

**Childhood Brain Tumor Foundation**
20312 Watkins Meadow Drive
Germantown, MD 20876
(301) 515-2900
*http://www.childhoodbraintumor.org*

Provides information and advocacy for children and families, funds research, and publishes three annual newsletters.

**Childhood Cancer Ombudsman Program**
27 Witch Duck Lane
Heathsville, VA 22473
Fax: (804) 580-2502
Email: *gpmonaco@rivnet.net*

This free service helps children with cancer and their families who are experiencing difficulties getting access to appropriate education, medical care, healthcare cost coverage, and meaningful employment.

**Children's Brain Tumor Foundation**
274 Madison Avenue, Suite 1301
New York, NY 10016
(888) 228-4673
*http://www.cbtf.org*

Provides support for families and children, resource guides, and funds for research.

**The Charles A. Dana Foundation**
745 Fifth Avenue, Suite 700
New York, NY 10151
(202) 223-4040
*http://www.dana.org*

The Dana Press publishes a quarterly journal, *Cerebrum,* which presents articles, debates, and book excerpts from leading neuroscientists. The *Brain in the News* is a compilation of news stories from major papers concerning brain research and treatment news.

**Epilepsy Foundation of America**
4351 Garden City Drive
Landover, MD 20785
(800) 332-1000
*http://www.epilepsyfoundation.org*

Provides support nationally and locally on issues regarding seizure management at home and school, sponsors self-help groups and summer camps, provides information on laws and legal rights, and hosts forums for discussion. Publishes Epilepsy USA magazine six times a year.

**Federation for Children with Special Needs**
1135 Tremont Street, Suite 420
Boston, MA 02120
(617) 236-7210
*http://www.fcsn.org*

Federally funded organization with representation in every state. Provides information on special education rights and laws, conferences, referrals for services, parent training workshops, publications, and advocacy information.

**Hydrocephalus Association**
870 Market Street, Suite 705
San Francisco, CA 94102
(888) 598-3789
*http://www.hydroassoc.org*

Provides support, education, and advocacy through conferences, newsletters, and informational pamphlets. *About Hydrocephalus: A Book for Families* is available in English and Spanish and is an excellent booklet describing hydrocephalus and its treatment.

**Making Headway Foundation, Inc.**
115 King Street
Chappaqua, NY 10514
(914) 238-8384
*http://www.makingheadway.org*

Provides supportive services for families of children with brain and spinal cord tumors. Offers a variety of services in the New York-New Jersey area including counseling with trained specialists and educational programs.

**National Association for Parents of Children with Visual Impairments**
PO Box 317
Watertown, MA 02471
(800) 562-6265
*http://www.spedex.com/NAPVI/*

NAPVI maintains a national support network via telephone and mail correspondence; provides publications, information, referrals, conferences, outreach programs, and a quarterly newsletter with membership.

**The National Brain Tumor Foundation**
414 Thirteenth Street, Suite 700
Oakland, CA 94612
(800) 934-2873
*http://www.braintumor.org*

Provides telephone support, national and regional patient conferences, publications, free quarterly newsletter, caregiver programs, patient support network, support groups, and funds for research.

**National Cancer Institute (NCI)**
Cancer Information Service
Building 31, Room 10A03
31 Center Drive
Bethesda, MD 20892
(800) 4-CANCER
*http://www.cancernet.nci.nih.gov*

Provides a nationwide telephone service for people with cancer, their families, friends, and the professionals who treat them. It provides answers and sends out informational booklets on a variety of cancer-related topics.

The NCI and the National Institute of Neurological Disorders and Stroke (NINDS) published The Report of the Brain Tumor Progress Review Group, in November, 2000. It is available online at *http://osp.nci.nih.gov/Prg_assess/PRG/BTPRG/*.

**National Center for Complementary and Alternative Medicine**
PO Box 8218
Silver Spring, MD 20907
(888) 644-6226
*http://nccam.nih.gov*

Dedicated to exploring complementary and alternative healing practices in the context of rigorous science, training researchers, and disseminating authoritative information.

**National Center for Learning Disabilities**
381 Park Avenue South, Suite 1401
New York, NY 10016
(888) 575-7373
http://www.ncld.org

Offers extensive resources, referral services, and educational programs regarding learning disabilities. Promotes public awareness and advocates for effective legislation to help people with learning disabilities.

**National Childhood Cancer Foundation**
440 E. Huntington Drive
PO Box 60012
Arcadia, CA 91066-6012
(800) 458-NCCF
http://www.nccf.org

Supports pediatric cancer treatment and research in more than 350 hospitals in North America and Australia. Their newsletter, *Childhood Cancerline,* provides information on new treatments and psychosocial support.

**National Coalition for Cancer Survivorship**
1010 Wayne Avenue Suite 770
Silver Spring, MD 20910
(877) 622-7937
http://www.cansearch.org/

Organization that addresses the needs of long-term cancer survivors and advocates for changes in healthcare to maximize survivors' access to optimal treatment and support. Extensive publications list, awareness events, support services, Cancer Survival Toolbox.

**National Hydrocephalus Foundation**
12413 Centralia Road
Lakewood, CA 90715
(562) 402-3523
http://www.nhfonline.org

Membership entitles families to quarterly newsletter, publications, access to reference library, referrals, and video rentals.

**National Information Center for Children and Youth with Disabilities**
PO Box 1492
Washington, DC 20013-1492
(800) 695-0285
http://www.nichcy.org

A clearinghouse that provides free pamphlets and information on disabilities and the rights of disabled children and their parents.

**National Neurofibromatosis Foundation**
95 Pine Street, 16th Floor
New York, NY 10005
(800) 323-7938
*http://www.nf.org*

NNFF funds research to find effective treatments and a cure for neurofibromatosis. It provides direct services to children and adults with NF, as well as information and resources to the public and medical professionals.

**National Spinal Cord Injury Association**
6701 Democracy Blvd. Suite 300-9
Bethesda, MD 20817
(800) 962-9629
*http://www.spinalcord.org*

Educates and empowers survivors of spinal cord injury and disease through toll-free help line and local support groups to achieve and maintain higher levels of independence.

**Pediatric Brain Tumor Foundation of the United States**
302 Ridgefield Court
Asheville, NC 28806
(800) 253-6530

Promotes awareness of pediatric brain tumors, provides patient support and teleconferences, and publishes educational materials and a quarterly newsletter, *The Helping Hand.* Scholarships are available for pediatric brain tumor survivors who wish to extend their education past the high school level.

**The Sensory Integration Resource Center**
The KID Foundation
1901 West Littleton Blvd.
Littleton, CO 80120
*http://www.sinetwork.org/*

This organization provides information for both families and professionals. It supplies a FAQ (frequently asked questions) list, explanations of sensory integration disorders, treatment information, a bibliography, ways to contact a therapist, resources, and links to related sites.

**Sensory Integration International: The Ayres Clinic**
1514 Cabrillo Avenue
Torrance, CA 90501
(310) 320-2335
*http://home.earthlink.net/~sensoryint/*

Provides courses in sensory integration, information for families, a newsletter, and online database for therapists.

**US Department of Justice**
ADA Information Line
Civil Rights Division
PO Box 66738
Washington, D.C. 20035
(800) 514-0301
TDD: (800) 514-0383
*http://www.usdoj.gov/crt/ada/adahom1.htm*

Answers questions about the Americans with Disabilities Act, explains how to file a complaint, and provides dispute resolution.

**We Can, Pediatric Brain Tumor Network**
PO Box 614
Manhattan Beach, CA 90266
*http://www.wecan.cc*
*info@wecan.cc*

This Los Angeles-based network sponsors lectures, social events, support groups, phone and e-mail network, "veteran parent" programs (organized mentoring at participating hospitals), and parent advisory councils (national and local).

# Organizations that provide emotional support

**Cancer Care, Inc.**
275 7th Ave.
New York, NY 10001
(800) 813-4673
*http://www.cancercare.org*

A national, nonprofit organization that provides referrals, one-on-one counseling, specialized support groups, educational and teleconference programs, and direct financial assistance.

**Center for Attitudinal Healing**
33 Buchanan Drive
Sausalito, CA 94965
(415) 331-6161

A nonprofit, nonsectarian group that sponsors local and national workshops for children with chronic or life-threatening diseases, their siblings and their parents. It sponsors support groups for children, teens, and parents and provides home and hospital visit. It has published several excellent books.

## Chai Lifeline/Camp Simcha
National Office
48 West 25th Street, 6th Floor
New York, NY 10010
(212) 255-1160 or (800) 343-2527

A national, nonprofit Jewish organization that provides support service programs to children and their families in crisis, including medical referrals, support groups, visits to hospitalized and housebound children, financial aid, transportation, a kosher camp for kids with cancer, and more.

## Children's Hopes and Dreams Foundation
280 Route 46
Dover, NJ 07801
(973) 361-7348

This organization operates a free, worldwide pen-pal program for children ages 5 to 17 with disabilities, chronic illnesses, or life-threatening illnesses. Also provides wishes.

## Friends Network
PO Box 4545
Santa Barbara CA 93140
(805) 693-1017
*http://www.kidscancernetwork.org*

A national, nonprofit organization that distributes *The Funletter,* a full-color activities newsletter, to children with cancer.

## National Children's Cancer Society
1015 Locust, Suite 600
St. Louis, MO 63101
(800) 532-6459
*http://www.children-cancer.org*

Advocates for children affected by childhood cancer and their families by providing financial assistance, educational materials, and emotional support.

## Parents Caring and Sharing
c/o Chumie Bodek
109 Rutledge Street
Brooklyn, NY 11211
(718) 596-1542 or 596-9002 (call during business hours, Eastern time)

Provides outreach, a support network, and newsletter for Jewish Orthodox families with children with cancer. Holds monthly meetings and links families of children with similar diseases.

**Songs of Love Foundation**
PO Box 750809
Forest Hills, NY 11375
(800) 960-7664
*http://www.songsoflove.org*

A nonprofit organization that has a volunteer group of more than 350 artists who produce personalized musical portraits for children and teens with chronic or life-threatening diseases.

# Bone marrow and stem cell transplantation

**BMT Infonet**
2900 Skokie Valley Road, Suite B
Highland Park, IL 60035
(888) 597-7674
*http://www.bmtnews.org/*

Nonprofit organization with the best site on the Internet for people who need a transplant. Provides newsletters, books, helpful services, a list of transplant centers, drug database, extensive resource list, and more.

**The National Transplant Assistance Fund**
3475 West Chester Pike Suite 230
Newtown Square, PA 19073
(800) 642-8399
*http://www.transplantfund.org*

Provides fundraising assistance and donor awareness material to transplant patients and catastrophically injured patients nationwide.

# Financial help

**Cancer Fund of America**
2901 Breezewood Lane
Knoxville, TN 37921
(800) 578-5284
*http://www.cfoa.org*

Helps defray cancer-related expenses not covered by insurance.

**The Sparrow Foundation**
4192 NW 61st
Redmond, OR 97756
(541) 549-1144, ext. 8307
*http://www.sparrow-fdn.org/*

Promotes youth-compassion by establishing and supporting Sparrow Clubs to help local children in medical crisis.

# Free air services

**AirLifeLine**
(877) AIRLIFE
*http://www.airlifeline.org*

AirLifeLine is a national nonprofit charitable organization of over 1,500 private pilots who fly ambulatory patients who cannot afford the cost of travel to medical facilities for diagnosis and treatment.

**Corporate Angel Network, Inc. (CAN)**
Westchester County Airport, Building 1
White Plains, NY 10604
(914) 328-1313

A nationwide, nonprofit program designed to give patients with cancer the use of available seats on corporate aircraft to get to and from recognized cancer treatment centers.

**Hope Air Transportation Network**
Proctor & Gamble Building
4711 Young Street
North York, Ontario M2N 6K8 Canada
(416) 222-6335

Provides free air transport to Canadians in financial need who must travel from their own communities to recognized facilities for medical care.

**National Patient Air Transport Hotline**
24-hour hotline: (800) 296-1217

Specialists refer callers to the most appropriate, cost-effective charitable or commercial services, including volunteer pilot organizations and airline transport programs.

# Wish fulfillment organizations

In addition to the two large organizations listed below, there are many other organizations that grant wishes to seriously ill children. A comprehensive list of wish fulfillment organizations is available on the Web at *http://www.patientcenters.com/childcancer.*

**Make-A-Wish Foundation of America**
3550 N. Central Ave. Suite 300
Phoenix, AZ 85012
(800) 722-WISH
*http://www.wish.org*

Grants wishes to children under the age of 18 with life-threatening illnesses. US and international chapters and affiliates exist.

**The Starlight Children's Foundation**
5900 Wilshire Boulevard, Suite 2530
Los Angeles, CA 90036
(323) 634-0080

Fulfills wishes for seriously ill children ages 4 to 18. There are chapters in the United States, Canada, Australia, and the United Kingdom.

# Rehabilitation centers and organizations

**The Alex Center and The Alex Foundation For Brain Injury**
165 North Myrtle Avenue
Tustin, CA 92780
(714) 734-6062
*http://www.alexfoundation.com*

The Alex Center is a school serving the educational and rehabilitative needs of children and adolescents with brain injury. The Alex Foundation is a nonprofit organization, started by the family of a child with a brain tumor, that raises the money to support the school.

**Bancroft NeuroHealth**
Hopkins Lane, PO Box 20
Haddonfield, NJ 08033-0018
(800) 492-8249
*http://www.bancroft.org/*

Bancroft NeuroHealth provides services for children, adolescents, and adults with brain injuries. These include early intervention programs, special education and vocational services, residential and in-home services, a neurobehavioral stabilization program and more. They have programs in New Jersey, Maine, and Louisiana.

**Brain Injury Association, Inc.**
105 North Alfred Street
Alexandria, VA 22314
(800) 444-6443
*http://www.biausa.org*

The Brain Injury Association's affiliated state offices offer detailed information about regional resources and refers families to physicians, therapists, and other professionals as well as peer and family support groups.

**The Easter Seals Society, USA**
230 West Monroe Street, Suite 1800
Chicago, IL 60606
(800) 221-6827
*http://www.easter-seals.org*

**The Easter Seal Society, Ontario**
1185 Eglinton Avenue East, Suite 800
Toronto, Ontario M3C 3C6 Canada
(800) 668-6252
*http://www.easterseals.org*

Easter Seals' primary services include medical rehabilitation, job training, employment, inclusive childcare, adult day services, summer camp, recreation, research, advocacy, and education.

**Lash and Associates Publishing/Training**
*http://www.lapublishing.com*

This organization publishes an array of books on brain injury issues in children and provides links ranging from brain injury associations in Canada and the United States to state programs and resources regarding special education.

**The May Center for Education and Neurorehabilitation**
35 Pacella Park
Randolph, MA 02368
(800) 778-7601
*http://www.mayinstitute.org*

A nationally recognized center for children, adolescents, and young adults with cognitive, behavioral, or emotional challenges related to acquired brain injury or neurological disease.

**Melmark**
Locations in Pennsylvania, Massachusetts, and Maryland
(888) MELMARK
*http://www.melmark.org*

Melmark provides educational, residential, medical, nursing, and rehabilitation services to children and adults with a wide range of cognitive, emotional, and medical disabilities, including autism, acquired brain injury, and neurological impairments.

## Sports organizations

**National Disability Sports Alliance**
25 West Independence Way
Kingston, RI 02881
(401) 792-7130
*http://www.ndsaonline.org*

The NDSA offers a variety of sports for athletes who have cerebral palsy, traumatic brain injuries, and related conditions.

**North American Riding for the Handicapped Association (NARHA)**
PO Box 33150
Denver, CO 80233
(800) 369-RIDE
*http://www.narha.org*

Accrediting organization for therapeutic riding programs. Their Web site maintains regional listings of accredited centers in the United States and Canada. Therapeutic riding programs are covered by some insurance plans under physical therapy, and some have sliding scale fees.

**Special Olympics, Inc.**
1325 G Street, NW, Suite 500
Washington, DC 20005
(202) 628-3630
*http://www.specialolympics.org*

Special Olympics is an international program of year-round sports training and athletic competition for more than one million children and adults with cognitive challenges.

# Bereavement

**The Centering Corporation**
7230 Maple Street
Omaha, NE 68134
(402) 553-1200
*http://www.centering.org*

Publishes a free catalog that contains an extensive listing of books, cards, and audio and videotapes on death and grieving.

**Children's Hospice International**
901 North Pitt Street, Suite 230
Alexandria, VA 22314
(703) 684-0330
(800) 24-CHILD
*http://www.chionline.org/*

Provides a network of support and care for children with life-threatening conditions and their families. Will provide referrals to nearest hospice.

**The Compassionate Friends National Office**
PO Box 3696
Oak Brook, IL 60522-3696
(877) 969-0010
*http://www.compassionatefriends.org*

A self-help organization that offers understanding and friendship to bereaved families through support meetings at local chapters and telephone support (they match persons with similar losses). It publishes a national magazine called "We Need Not Walk Alone" and local chapters offer free newsletters, lending libraries, and support.

## APPENDIX C

# Books and Online Sites

A WEALTH OF INFORMATION is available through libraries and computers. Brain tumor organizations provide extensive listings of books and Internet resources as well. This appendix briefly describes how to get the most from your library and computer and lists specific books and online sites that you might find helpful when researching your child's medical condition or treatment.

## How to get information from your library or computer

Most libraries now have a computerized database of all materials available in their various branches. Some libraries may still use a manual card catalog system. Ask a librarian if you need help learning to use these systems. A librarian can also tell you how to request a book from another branch and how to put a book on hold if it is currently checked out.

If a book is not in your library's collection, ask the librarian if she can obtain it from another library by requesting an inter-library loan. This is a common practice, and you might be able to get medical texts from university or medical school libraries.

In addition to books, you can find relevant magazine and medical journal articles at the library. The librarian can show you how to use the database to search for articles and where to find the periodicals.

Public libraries usually subscribe to only the most popular medical journals, such as the *New England Journal of Medicine*. If you are able to visit a university or medical school library, you will find many more medical journals available. To find the nearest medical library open to the public, call the National Network of Libraries of Medicine at (800) 338-7657. If you do not live close to one of these libraries, ask your local librarian if he can help you obtain copies of the articles you want.

There is an astonishing amount of information available through the Internet. Libraries from all over the world can be accessed, and you can download information in minutes from huge databases like MEDLINE or Cancerlit. Obtaining information from large medical databases, established journals, or large libraries is exceedingly helpful for parents at home with sick children. However, the huge numbers of people using the Internet have spawned chat rooms, bulletin boards, and thousands of FAQs (frequently asked questions) that may or may not contain accurate information. You may want to adopt the motto "Let the buyer beware."

If you do not have a home computer, many libraries provide Internet access. Ask the librarian to help you connect to MEDLINE, Physician's Data Query (PDQ), or other databases you wish to search. Don't hesitate to ask for assistance in finding web sites or whatever else you need on the Internet. For a step-by-step tutorial that explains how you can best use all the options of

PubMed (the National Library of Medicine's search program), see *http://www.nlm.nih.gov/bsd/ pubmed_tutorial/m1001.html.*

## Brain anatomy

*A Primer of Brain Tumors, Seventh Edition.* American Brain Tumor Association. Available online at: *http://www.abta.org/primer.* In addition, the ABTA publishes many informational pamphlets about specific types of brain and spinal cord tumors and individual treatments. These books include *About Ependymoma, About Glioblastoma Multiforme and Malignant Astrocytoma, About Medulloblastoma/PNET,* and *About Oligodendroglioma and Mixed Glioma.* Treatment books include *Chemotherapy of Brain Tumors, Radiation Therapies,* and *Sterotactic Radiosurgery.*

*About Hydrocephalus: A Guide for Patients and Families.* Hydrocephalus Association: (415 ) 732-7040 or go to *http://www.hydroassoc.org.*

Diamond, M.C., et al. *The Human Brain Coloring Book.* New York: HarperCollins Publishers, 1985. Provides detailed black-and-white illustrations of the brain and its structure. Intended for informal learners through students in the field of neuroscience.

### Neuroscience for Kids
*http://faculty.washington.edu/chudler/neurok.html*

Thorough web site for children and adults. Covers full range of topics regarding anatomy, seizures, and more.

## Online dictionaries

A number of online medical dictionaries are listed on the National Library of Medicine's web site at *http://www.nlm.nih.gov/medlineplus/dictionaries.html.*

CancerWEB (*http://www.graylab.ac.uk/omd/index.html*) is a good medical online dictionary.

Merriam-Webster, Inc. (*http://www.Merriam-Webster.com*) provides free access to the complete text and audio pronunciations of *Merriam-Webster's Collegiate Dictionary, Tenth Edition.*

## General reading

*Alex's Journey: The Story of a Child with a Brain Tumor.* American Brain Tumor Association. Contact ABTA at (800) 886-2282 or go to *http://www.abta.org.*

Armstrong, Lance, with Sally Jenkins. *It's Not About the Bike: My Journey Back to Life.* Penguin Putnam, Inc., 2000. True story of world-renowned bicycling champion who overcame metastatic testicular cancer and won the 1999 Tour de France.

Candlelighters Childhood Cancer Foundation. *Bibliography and Resource Guide.* 1998. (800) 366-CCCF, or for CCCF-Canada, (800) 363-1062. Extensive listing of books and articles on childhood cancer, coping skills, death and bereavement, effects on family, long-term side effects, medical support, and terminal home care. Excellent resource.

Johnson, Joy, and S. M. Johnson. *Why Mine?: A Book for Parents Whose Child Is Seriously Ill.* Omaha, NE: Centering Corporation, 1981. To order, call (402) 553-1200. Quotes from parents about fears, feelings, marriages, siblings, and the ill child.

Kushner, Harold. *When Bad Things Happen to Good People*. Boston: G.K. Hall, rev. ed., 1997. A rabbi wrote this comforting book on how people of faith deal with catastrophic events.

Lerner, Michael. *Choices in Healing: Integrating the Best of Conventional and Complementary Approaches to Medicine*. Cambridge, MA: The MIT Press, 1996. A comprehensive overview of both conventional and complementary approaches to cancer treatment. Available online at *http://www.commonweal.org/choicescontents.html*.

National Cancer Institute. *Young People With Cancer: A Handbook for Parents*. This booklet describes the different types of childhood cancer, medical procedures, coping skills, and family issues, and gives sources of information. (800) 4-CANCER.

*PDR for Herbal Medicines, Second Edition*. Medical Economics Company, 2000. Guide to herbal therapies. Profiles 700 medicinal herbs, including actions, adverse effects, and contraindications.

White Smith, Gregory and Steven Naifeh. *Making Miracles Happen*. Boston: Little, Brown, 1997. Empowering personal account from a Pulitzer Prize-winning author about his search for treatment for an inoperable brain tumor, plus useful insights into dealings with the medical community.

## Reading for children/teens/siblings

### Children

Crary, Elizabeth. *Dealing with Feelings*. I'm Frustrated; I'm Mad; I'm Furious Series. Seattle: Parenting Press, 1992. Fun, game-like books to teach preschool and early elementary children how to handle feelings and solve problems.

Foss, Karen. *The Problem with Hair: A Story for Children Learning about Cancer*. Centering Corporation, 1996. A poem about a group of friends and what happens when one of them loses her hair from chemotherapy.

Hautzig, Deborah. *A Visit to the Sesame Street Hospital*. New York: Random House, 1985. Grover, his mother, Ernie, and Bert visit the Sesame Street Hospital in preparation for Grover's upcoming operation.

Krishner, Trudy. *Kathy's Hats*. Concept Books, 1992. Written by a mother of a 9-year-old with Ewing's sarcoma, this attractively illustrated book explains how Kathy used different hats to cope with her treatments.

Rogers, Fred. *Going to the Hospital*. New York: Putnam's Sons, 1997. With pictures and words, TV's beloved Mr. Rogers helps children ages 3 to 8 learn about hospitals.

Rogers, Fred. *Some Things Change and Some Things Stay the Same*. American Cancer Society. Order by calling (800) ACS-2345. Very comforting book for preschool-age children with cancer and their siblings.

*Mr. Rogers Talks About Childhood Cancer*. 1990. Videotapes (2), guidebook, storybook. VHS, 45 minutes. Available from American Cancer Society, (800) ACS-2345. Mr. Rogers talks to children and uses characters from the land of make believe to stress the importance of talking about feelings.

Saltzman, David. *The Jester Has Lost His Jingle*. Jester Co., Inc., 1995. With glossy color pictures and lyrical writing, this story gently teaches children and adults about the importance of love, laughter, and overcoming adversity.

## Teens

Gravelle, Karen, and Bertram A. John. *Teenagers Face to Face with Cancer.* New York: Julian Messner, 2000. Seventeen teenagers talk openly about their cancer.

## Siblings

American Cancer Society. *When Your Brother or Sister Has Cancer.* For a free copy, call (800) ACS-2345. Sixteen-page booklet that describes the emotions felt by siblings of a child with cancer.

O'Toole, Donna. *Aarvy Aardvark Finds Hope: A Read Aloud Story for People of All Ages About Loving and Losing, Friendship and Hope.* Compassion Books, 1988. Aarvy Aardvark and his friend Ralphie Rabbit show how a family member or friend can help another in distress.

Peterkin, Allan. *What About Me? When Brothers and Sisters Get Sick.* Magination Press, 1992. Describes the conflicted feelings of siblings when their brother or sister is hospitalized.

# Medical Treatment

## Coping with procedures

Benson, Herbert, MD. *The Relaxation Response.* New York: Avon Books, 2000. This is an excellent resource for the relaxation method of pain relief.

Kuttner, Leora, PhD. *No Fears, No Tears.* Videotape, 27 minutes. Available through the Canadian Cancer Society, (604) 872-4400 or *http://www.bc.cancer.ca/ccs.* Documentary of eight young children and their parents as they learn how to manage the pain of cancer treatment.

Kuttner, Leora, PhD. *No Fears, No Tears—13 Years Later.* Videotape, 46 minutes. To order, fax request to: (604) 294-9986, or email: *leora_kuttner@sfu.ca.* Thirteen years after learning how to manage their painful cancer treatments, seven survivors of childhood cancer make sense of their early traumatic experiences, and demonstrate the power of mind-body pain relief.

## Partnership with medical team

Center for Attitudinal Healing. *Advice to Doctors and Other Big People from Kids.* Berkeley, CA: Celestial Arts, 1991. Written by children with catastrophic illnesses; offers suggestions and expresses feelings about healthcare workers. Wise and poignant.

Keene, Nancy. *Working with Your Doctor: Getting the Healthcare You Deserve.* Sebastopol, CA: O'Reilly & Associates, Inc., 1998. Practical guidance to help patients take an active role in maintaining health, and steps to help improve the doctor/patient relationship.

## Hospitalization

Keene, Nancy. *Your Child in the Hospital: A Practical Guide for Parents,* rev. ed. Sebastopol, CA: O'Reilly & Associates, 1999. A pocket guide full of parent stories to help others prepare their children physically and emotionally for hospitalizations.

Kellerman, Johnathan. *Helping the Fearful Child.* New York: W.W. Norton, 1981. Although this book was written as a guide for everyday and problem anxieties, it is full of excellent advice for parents of children undergoing traumatic procedures. This book is out of print, but may be available in your local library.

## Clinical trials

Finn, Robert. *Cancer Clinical Trials: Experimental Treatments and How They Can Help You.* Sebastopol, CA: O'Reilly & Associates, 1999. Excellent guide that explains the structure, ethics, and types of clinical trials. Also covers how to evaluate a trial and deal with financial issues.

National Cancer Institute. *What Are Clinical Trials All About?* For a free copy, call (800) 4-CANCER. 22-page booklet covers basic information about clinical trials.

## Chemotherapy

Dodd, Marylin J., RN, PhD. *Managing the Side Effects of Chemotherapy & Radiation Therapy: A Guide for Patients and Their Families.* UCSF Nursing, 1996. This book contains thorough explanations of possible side effects of chemotherapy and radiation and suggestions for managing them.

National Cancer Institute. *Chemotherapy & You: A Guide to Self-Help During Treatment.* For a free copy, call (800) 4-CANCER. 56-page booklet includes answers to commonly asked questions about chemotherapy, its side effects, emotions while on chemotherapy, and nutrition.

*Physicians Desk Reference.* Oradell, New Jersey: Medical Economics Data, 2001. Issued yearly, lists authoritative information on all FDA approved drugs. Technical language. Available at reference desk in most libraries.

USP DI, Volume II, *Advice for the Patient: Drug Information in Lay Language.* United States Pharmacopeial Convention, Inc., 2001. Contains detailed drug information in non-medical language. Available in most libraries.

## Radiation

McKay, Judith, and Nancee Hirano. *The Chemotherapy and Radiation Survival Guide.* Oakland, CA: New Harbinger, 1998. Basic, understandable guide to chemotherapy and radiation and their side effects.

National Cancer Institute. *Radiation Therapy and You: A Guide to Self-Help During Treatment.* For a free copy, call (800) 4-CANCER. 52-page booklet clearly defines radiation, explains what to expect, describes possible side effects, and discusses follow-up care.

O'Connell, Avice, MD, and Norma Leone. *Your Child and X-Rays: A Parents' Guide to Radiation, X-Rays and Other Imaging Procedures.* Rochester, NY: Lion Press, 1988. 89-page book explains x-ray treatments in easy-to-understand language.

## Surgery

Epstein, Fred, and Elaine Fantle Shumberg. *Gifts of Time.* New York: William Morrow and Company, Inc., 1993. Out-of-print title, but worth the search at your local library. Compelling stories from a pioneering pediatric neurosurgeon.

McClone, David, MD, Arthur Marlin, MD, and R. Michael Scott, MD, eds. *Pediatric Neurosurgery: Surgery of the Developing Nervous System.* Philadelphia: W.B. Saunders, 2001. Extremely technical.

O'Neill, James A., ed. *Pediatric Surgery.* St. Louis: Mosby-Year Book, 1998. Extremely technical.

## Bone marrow and stem cell transplantation

Stewart, Susan, and Jan Sugar. *Autologous Stem Cell Transplants: A Handbook for Patients.* BMT Infonet, *http://www.bmtinfonet.org/basics.html.* This book walks readers through a transplant, clearly explaining each step of the procedure. Included is information about preparing for a transplant, managing complications and side effects, coping with psychological stress, pediatric transplants, and much more.

## Terminal illness

Callanan, Maggie, and Patricia Kelley. *Final Gifts: Understanding the Special Awareness, Needs, and Communications of the Dying.* New York: Poseidon Press, 1997. Written by two hospice nurses with decades of experience, this book helps families understand and communicate with terminally ill patients. Highly recommended.

# Online medical resources

See additional web sites listed in Appendix B, *Resources.*

**American Cancer Society**
*http://www.cancer.org*

**BMT InfoNet**
*http://www.bmtnews.org*

**Canadian Cancer Society**
*http://www.cancer.ca/*

**CANSearch**
*http://www.cansearch.org/canserch/canserch.htm*

This guide to cancer resources is produced by the National Coalition for Cancer Survivorship.

**Centerwatch**
*http://www.centerwatch.com*

The Centerwatch Clinical Trials Listing Service contains a searchable database of 7,500 current clinical trials in all areas of medicine, including cancer.

**Clinical Trials and Noteworthy Treatments for Brain Tumors**
Musella Foundation for Brain Tumor Research and Information
*http://www.virtualtrials.com*

A patient-friendly web site dedicated to providing current brain tumor information to families and patients. Maintains a database of clinical trials and a variety of Internet support mailing lists.

**Clinical Trials**
*http://www.clinicaltrials.gov*

The US National Institutes of Health, through its National Library of Medicine, has developed ClinicalTrials.gov to provide patients, family members, and members of the public current information about clinical research studies.

**Medicine Online**
*http://www.meds.com/*

Provides patients and professionals with in-depth educational information on specific diseases. Also includes information on reimbursement and a treatment guide.

**Med help International**
*http://medhlp.netusa.net*

A nonprofit organization that provides medical information written in nontechnical language. The all-volunteer staff is comprised of physicians and other healthcare professionals.

**The Multimedia Medical Reference Library**
*http://www.med-library.com/medlibrary/*

**Oncolink**
*http://cancer.med.upenn.edu*

A text and multimedia service available through the Internet. Oncolink offers a wide variety of cancer-related information, including articles, handbooks, case studies, writings by patients and their families, and visual images, including a children's art gallery.

**Patient Advocacy Numbers**
*http://infonet.welch.jhu.edu/advocacy.html*

**Patient Support.com**
*http://www.patientsupport.com*

**Pediatric Oncology Resource Center**
*http://www.acor.org/ped-onc*

Site provides useful information on diseases, treatments, signs of childhood cancer, family issues, and activism. Also includes information on bereavement. Numerous links to helpful support and medical resources.

**Rx List—The Internet Drug Index**
*http://www.rxlist.com/*

# Emotional Support

*Family Portrait: Coping with Childhood Cancer.* Videotape. VHS, 25 minutes. Purchase from Films for the Humanities and Sciences, (800) 257-5126. Five family portraits cover such issues as guilt, sibling rivalry, divorce, the adopted child, and involvement of other family members.

*Mr. Rogers Talks with Parents About Childhood Cancer.* 1990. Videotapes (2), guidebook, and pamphlet. VHS, 47 minutes. Available from American Cancer Society, (800) ACS-2345. Interviews with parents. The first tape illustrates ways to deal with emotions during diagnosis and treatment. The second tape sensitively deals with bereavement.

Sourkes, Barbara M., PhD. *Armfuls of Time: The Psychological Experience of the Child with a Life-Threatening Illness.* University of Pittsburgh Press, 1995. Features the voices and artwork of children with cancer. Highly recommended.

# Support groups

American Psychological Association. *Finding Help: How to Choose a Psychologist.* To obtain free brochure, send self-addressed stamped envelope to *Finding Help,* APA Public Affairs Office, 750 First St., NE, Washington, DC 20002-4242. Covers psychotherapy, the types of problems people discuss, and how to choose a therapist.

Bogue, Erna-Lynne, ACSW, and Barbara K. Chesney, MPH. *Making Contact: A Parent-to-parent Visitation Manual.* Bethesda, MD: The Candlelighters Childhood Cancer Foundation, 1987. (800) 366-CCCF. For parents of children with cancer. Includes guidelines for selection of parent visitors, training to improve parent-visitor contact, developing referral systems, and support resources.

Chesler, Mark A., PhD, and Barbara K. Chesney. *Cancer and Self-Help: Bridging the Troubled Waters of Childhood Illness.* Madison, WI: The University of Wisconsin Press, 1995. Explains how self-help groups are formed, how they function and recruit, and why they are effective.

National Cancer Institute. *Taking Time: Support for People with Cancer and the People Who Care About Them.* NIH Publication No. 88-2059. (800) 4-CANCER. 61-page booklet includes sections on sharing feelings, coping within the family, and when you need assistance.

**ACOR, The Association of Cancer Online Resources, Inc.**
*http://www.acor.org*

ACOR has information and electronic support groups for young patients, caregivers, and anyone affected by cancer.

**The Healing Exchange**
P.O. Box 425743
Cambridge, MA 02142
(617) 623-0066
*http://www.braintrust.org*

Host to a number of Internet support e-lists, including the large Braintmr list.

**SpeciaLove**
*http://www.speciallove.org*

A resource devoted to parents and children with cancer to facilitate networking. This resource is oriented to the family aspects of childhood cancer. SpeciaLove, Inc., was started in 1983 by Tom and Sheila Baker, who lost their 13 year-old daughter to leukemia.

**Touchstone Support Network**
*http://www.php.com/touchstone.htm*

A nonprofit, nonsectarian, volunteer organization that provides emotional and practical support services for families and their children with chronic and life-threatening illnesses.

## Siblings

Faber, Adele, and Elaine Mazlish. *Siblings Without Rivalry: How to Help Your Children Live Together So You Can Live Too.* New York: Avon Books, 1998. Required reading for parents with fighting siblings. Offers dozens of simple yet effective methods to reduce conflict and foster a cooperative spirit.

Murray, Gloria, and Gerald Jamplosky, eds. *Straight from the Siblings: Another Look at the Rainbow.* Millbrae, CA: Celestial Arts, 1982. Written by sixteen children who have brothers and sisters with a life-threatening illness who met at the Center for Attitudinal Healing. A must-read for both parents and siblings.

### Feelings, communication, and behavior

Faber, Adele, and Elaine Mazlish. *How to Talk So Kids Will Listen...and Listen So Kids Will Talk.* New York: Rawson, Wade Publishers, 1999. The classic book on developing new, more effective ways to communicate with your children, based on respect and understanding. Highly recommended.

Kurcinka, Mary Sheedy. *Raising Your Spirited Child: A Guide for Parents Whose Child Is More Intense, Sensitive, Perceptive and Energetic.* New York: HarperCollins, 1992. Many of the strategies in this reassuring guide are very effective for children stressed by cancer treatment.

Nelsen, Jane. *Positive Discipline.* rev. ed. New York: Ballantine Books, 1999. Written by a psychologist, educator, and mother of seven, this book teaches parents how to promote self-discipline and personal responsibility.

Rich, Dorothy. *MegaSkills: Building Children's Achievement for the Information Age,* expanded edition. Boston, New York: Houghton Mifflin, 1998. Innovative school program in text form aimed at developing friendships and social skills.

## Practical support

### Finances

Tolley, Diane. *Finding the Money: A Guide to Paying Your Medical Bills.* *http://www.bmtinfonet.org/cgi-bin/orderform_infonet.pl.* Drawing from her experience as an insurance salesperson, a fundraiser, and the mother of a BMT patient, Tolley offers a host of practical suggestions on how to assess what your transplant and after-care will cost and how to track and pay for your bills.

Leeland, Jeff. *One Small Sparrow: The Remarkable Real-Life Drama of One Community's Compassionate Response to a Little Boy's Life*. Sisters, OR: Multnomah Books, 1995. Contains numerous ideas for methods to raise funds. Christian perspective.

## Nutrition

Freeman, John M., MD, Jennifer B. Freeman, et al. *The Ketogenic Diet: A Treatment for Epilepsy.* Demos Medical Publishing: 2000. Practical guidance from leading expert on using the ketogenic diet to help control seizures.

National Cancer Institute. *Managing Your Child's Eating Problems During Cancer Treatment* and *Eating Hints for Cancer Patients.* (800) 4-CANCER. These booklets cover how cancer treatments affect eating, how to cope with side effects, special diets, family resources, and recipes.

Wilson, J. Randy. *The Non-Chew Cookbook.* Glenwood Springs, CO: Wilson Publishing, Inc., 1986. P.O. Box 2190, 81602. (303) 945-5600. Contains recipes for patients unable to chew due to the side effects of chemotherapy and/or radiation.

## School

American Brain Tumor Association. *When Your Child is Ready to Return to School.* (800) 886-2282 or go to *http://www.abta.org.*

American Cancer Society. *Back to School: A Handbook for Parents of Children with Cancer.* (800) ACS-1234. 16-page introductory booklet covers school re-entry, classroom presentations, the importance of advocates, legal issues, IEPs, and special needs.

Anderson, Winifred, Stephen Chitwood, and Deidre Hayden. *Negotiating the Special Education Maze: A Guide for Parents and Teachers,* 3rd ed. Bethesda, MD: Woodbine House, 1997. Step-by-step guide to obtaining help for your child. If you only read one book on this subject, this should be the one.

Baron, Ida Sue, et al. *Pediatric Neuropsychology in the Medical Setting.* New York: Oxford University Press, 1995. Text (written primarily for clinicians) that details neuropsychological evaluations, brain development, and medical conditions that can affect the brain, including epilepsy and cancer.

Bateman, Barbara D., and Mary Anne Linden. *Better IEPs: How to Develop Legally Correct and Educationally Useful Programs.* Sopris Press, Inc., 1998. One of the better resources for writing specific test-measured goals and objectives.

Candlelighters Childhood Cancer Foundation Canada. *School Reentry Resource Manual.* 1992. (416) 489-6440. For parents, educators, and healthcare professionals, addresses siblings, adolescence, survivor's quality of life, programs, bereavement, and grief.

Chai Lifeline. *Back to School: A Handbook for Educators of Children with Life-threatening Diseases in the Yeshiva/Day School System.* 1995. (212) 465-1300. Covers diagnosis, planning for school reentry, infection control, needs of junior and senior high school students, children with special educational needs, and saying good-bye when a child dies.

The Compassionate Friends. *Suggestions for Teachers and School Counselors.* P.O. Box 3696, Oak Brook, IL 60522. (630) 990-0010.

Diamond, Marian, and Janet L. Hopson. *Magic Trees of the Mind.* New York: Plume Press, 1999. Discusses how to enrich brain development from birth through adolescence.

Gliko-Braden, Majel. *Grief Comes to Class: A Teacher's Guide.* 1992. Centering Corporation, 1531 N. Saddle Creek Rd., Omaha, NE 68104. (402) 553-1200. Comprehensive guide to grief in the classroom.

Peterson's Guides. *Peterson's Guides to Colleges with Programs for Learning Disabled Students or Attention Deficit Disorders,* 5th ed. Princeton, NJ: Peterson's Guides, 2000. Excellent reference. Online search services are available at *http://www.petersons.com.*

Siegel, Lawrence M. *The Complete IEP Guide: How to Advocate for Your Special Ed Child.* Nolo Press, 2001. An easy-to-read and helpful guide to the entire IEP process.

**Wrightslaw**
*http://www.wrightslaw.com*

Wrightslaw is one of the better privately operated web sites on special education law. *Wrightslaw: Special Education Law* is one of their own books on the subject. They also provide hundreds of articles and cases online, strategies for advocacy, free publications, and a free monthly email newsletter.

## After treatment ends

Harpham, Wendy Schlessel. *After Cancer: A Guide to Your New Life.* Harperperennial, 1995. Written in a question and answer format, doctor/cancer survivor Harpham addresses the medical, psychological, and practical issues of recovery.

Hoffman, Barbara, JD, ed. *A Cancer Survivor's Almanac: Charting Your Journey.* National Coalition for Cancer Survivorship, 1998. Comprehensive guide to the issues of cancer survivorship.

Keene, Nancy, Wendy Hobbie, and Kathy Ruccione. *Childhood Cancer Survivors: A Practical Guide to Your Future.* Sebastopol, CA: O'Reilly & Associates, 2000. A user-friendly, comprehensive guide on late effects after treatment for childhood cancer.

# Bereavement

## Parental grief

*Bereavement: A Magazine of Hope and Healing.* Provides support for the grieving, allows for feedback from professionals, and teaches nonbereaved how to help. (719) 282-1948. Other grief-related publications are also available.

Centering Corporation. *Creative Care Package.* (402) 553-1200. Lists more than 300 books and videos on coping with serious illness, loss, and grief.

Compassionate Friends. *Resource Guide.* (630) 990-0010. Contains hundreds of books, pamphlets, videos, and audiotapes on all aspects of grief.

Gilbert, Laynee. *I Remember You: A Grief Journal.* San Francisco: HarperCollins, 2001. A journal for written and photographic memories during the first year of mourning. Beautiful book filled with quotes and comfort.

Kubler-Ross, Elisabeth, MD. *On Children and Death.* New York: Macmillan, 1983. This comforting book offers practical help in living through the terminal period of a child's life with love and understanding.

Morse, Melvin, MD. *Closer to the Light: Learning from Near Death Experiences of Children.* New York: Villard Books, 1990. About startlingly similar spiritual experiences of children who almost die.

Rando, Therese, PhD, ed. *Parental Loss of a Child.* Champaign, IL: Research Press, 1986. Addresses death from a serious illness; guilt and grief; advice to physicians, clergy, and funeral directors; professional help; and support organizations.

## Sibling grief (adult reading)

Doka, Kenneth, ed. *Children Mourning, Mourning Children.* Hemisphere Publications, 1995. Topics include children's understanding of death, answering grieving children's questions, and the role of the schools. Write to Taylor and Francis, 1900 Frost Road, Suite 101, Bristol, PA, 19007. Include $14.95 plus $2.50 for shipping and handling.

Grollman, Earl. *Talking About Death: A Dialogue Between Parent and Child.* Boston: Beacon Press, 1990. This very comforting book teaches parents how to explain death, understand how children react to specific types of death, and when to seek professional help. Highly recommended.

Schaefer, Dan, and Christine Lyons. *How Do We Tell the Children?: A Step-by-Step Guide for Helping Children Two to Teen Cope When Someone Dies,* updated edition. New York: Newmarket Press, 1993. If your terminally ill child has siblings, read this book.

## Sibling grief (young child reading)

Buscaglia, Leo. *The Fall of Freddy the Leaf: A Story of Life for All Ages.* New York: Holt, Rinehart and Winston, 1982. This wise yet simple story about a leaf named Freddy explains death as a necessary part of the cycle of life. This book is out of print, but may be available in your local library.

Mellonie, Bryan, and Robert Ingpen. *Lifetimes: The Beautiful Way to Explain Death to Children.* New York: Bantam Books, 1987. Paintings and simple text explain that dying is as much a part of life as being born.

## Sibling grief (school-aged children)

*Drying Their Tears.* Produced by CARTI, Communication Division, Markham University, P.O. Box 55050, Little Rock, AR 72215. (800) 482-8561. Video and manual to help counselors, teachers, and other professionals help children deal with the grief, fear, confusion, and anger that occur after the death of a loved one.

Temes, Roberta, PhD. *The Empty Place: A Child's Guide Through Grief.* Far Hills, NJ: New Horizon Press, 1992. (402) 553-1200. Explains and describes feelings after the death of a sibling, such as the empty place in the house, at the table, in a brother's heart.

White, E.B. *Charlotte's Web.* New York: Harper, 1952. Classic tale of friendship and death as a part of life. (The videotape is widely available to rent.)

## Sibling grief (teenagers)

Gravelle, Karen, and Charles Haskins. *Teenagers Face to Face with Bereavement.* Englewood Cliffs, NJ: J. Messner, 2000. The perspectives and experiences of seventeen teenagers coping with grief.

Grollman, Earl. *Straight Talk About Death for Teenagers: How to Cope with Losing Someone You Love.* Boston, MA: Beacon Press, 1993. Wonderful book that talks to teens, not at them. Discusses denial, pain, anger, sadness, physical symptoms, and depression.

*The Healing Path.* The Compassionate Friends' sibling video addresses concerns of surviving siblings, such as sadness, pain, anger, and fear. Call (630) 990-0010 or fax (630) 990-0246.

# List of Pediatric Neurosurgeons

THE FOLLOWING LIST is based on updated information from The American Society of Pediatric Neurosurgeons (*http://www.aspn.org*). Each institution was called by phone, and any changes to personnel or contact information was made. Because doctors retire, move to different institutions, and switch from clinical practice to research, and area codes occasionally change, the following information may not remain current over time. The following is not an endorsement of any physician or institution.

## ALABAMA

**Jeffrey P. Blount, MD**
**Paul A. Grabb, MD**
**W. Jerry Oakes, MD**
Children's Hospital of Alabama
Birmingham, AL 35233
Phone: (205) 939-6914

## ARIZONA

**Kim H. Manwaring, MD**
**S. David Moss, MD**
Phoenix Children's Hospital
Phoenix, AZ 85006
Phone: (602) 239-4880

**Harold L. Rekate, MD**
Barrow Neurological Institute
Phoenix, AZ 85013
Phone: (602) 406-3632

## CALIFORNIA

**James Boggan, MD**
University of California, Davis
Sacramento, CA 95817
Phone: (916) 734-3658

**Clarence Greene, MD**
Kid's Neurosurgery
Long Beach, CA 90806
Phone: (562) 426-4121

**Michael S. B. Edwards, MD**
Sutter Memorial Hospital
Sacramento, CA 95816
Phone: (916) 454-6850

**Nalin Gupta, MD**
University of California
San Francisco, CA 94143
Phone: (415) 353-7500

**Michael L. Levy, MD**
**J. Gordon McComb, MD**
Los Angeles Children's Hospital
Los Angeles, CA 90027
Phone: (323) 663-8128

**Hector E. James, MD**
San Diego, CA 92123
Phone: (858) 560-4791

**Michael G. Muhonen, MD**
Children's Hospital of Orange County
Mission Hospital
Orange, CA 92868
Phone: (714) 289-4151

**Daniel Won, MD**
Pediatric Neurosurgical Associates
San Bernardino, CA 92408
Phone: (909) 384-1210

**Meredith V. Woodward, MD**
Valley Children's Hospital
Madera, CA 93638
Phone: (559) 353-6277

## COLORADO

**Michael II. Handler, MD**
**Lori McBride, MD**
**Ken R. Winston, MD**
The Children's Hospital
Denver, CO 80218
Phone: (303) 861-6000

## CONNECTICUT

**Charles C. Duncan, MD**
Yale University School of Medicine
New Haven, CT 06520
Phone: (203) 785-2809

## DISTRICT OF COLUMBIA

**Philip H. Cogen, MD, PhD**
Children's National Medical Center
Washington, DC 20010
Phone: (202) 884-3020

## FLORIDA

**Carolyn Marie Carey, MD**
**Gerald F. Tuite, MD**
Pediatric Neurosurgery
St. Petersburg, FL 33701
Phone: (727) 892-4143

**Glenn Morrison, MD**
**Jogi V. Pattisapu, MD**
Pediatric Neurosurgery
Orlando, FL 32806
Phone: (407) 649-7686

**David Pincus, MD**
University of Florida
Gainesville, FL 32510
Phone: (352) 392-4335

**John Ragheb, MD**
Miami Children's Hospital
Miami, FL 33155
Phone: (305) 662-8386

## GEORGIA

**William R. Boydston, MD**
**Roger J. Hudgins, MD**
Pediatric Neurosurgery Associates
Atlanta, GA 30342
Phone: (404) 255-6509

**Ann Marie Flannery, MD**
**Mark Lee, MD**
Medical College of Georgia
Augusta, GA 30912-0004
Phone: (706) 721-5568

**Timothy B. Mapstone, MD**
Emory University
Atlanta, GA 30322
Phone: (404) 778-4489

**Mark S. O'Brien, MD**
Children's Healthcare of Atlanta
Atlanta, GA 30345
Phone: (404) 321-9234

## ILLINOIS

**David M. Frim, MD**
The University of Chicago Hospitals
Chicago, IL 60637
Phone: (773) 702-2475

John A. Grant, MD
David G. McLone, MD
Tadanori Tomita, MD
Children's Memorial Hospital
Chicago, IL 60614
Phone: (773) 880-4373

Francisco Gutierrez, MD
Chicago, IL 60611
Phone: (312) 926-3490

Yoon Hahn, MD
Christ Hospital & Medical Center
Oak Lawn, IL 60453
Phone: (708) 346-1013

## INDIANA

Joel C. Boaz, MD
Thomas G. Luerssen, MD
James W. Riley Hospital For Children
Indianapolis, IN 46202-5200
Phone: (317) 274-8852

Michael S. Turner, MD
Indianapolis Neurosurgical Group
Indianapolis, IN 46202
Phone: (317) 926-5411

## IOWA

Arnold H. Menezes, MD
University of Iowa Hospital
Iowa City, IA 52242
Phone: (319) 356-2768

## LOUISIANA

Richard A. Coulon Jr., MD
Ochsner Clinic
New Orleans, LA 70121
Phone: (504) 842-4033

Joseph Nadell, MD
Children's Hospital
New Orleans, LA 70118
Phone: (504) 899-0575

John W. Walsh, MD
Tulane University Medical Center
New Orleans, LA 70112
Phone: (504) 588-5565

## MARYLAND

Benjamin S. Carson, MD
Johns Hopkins Hospital
Baltimore, MD 21287-8811
Phone: (410) 955-5000

## MASSACHUSETTS

Peter M. Black, MD, PhD
Dana-Farber Cancer Institute
Boston, MA 02115
Phone: (617) 355-6008

William Butler, MD
Paul H. Chapman, MD
Michael Medlock, MD
Massachusetts General Hospital
Boston, MA 02114
Phone: (617) 726-3887

Liliana Goumnerova, MD
Joseph R. Madsen, MD
Mark R. Proctor, MD
R. Michael Scott, MD
Children's Hospital
Boston, MA 02115
Phone: (617) 355-6011

## MICHIGAN

Holly Gilmer-Hill, MD
Steven Ham, MD
Monica Loke, MD
Sandeep Sood, MD
Children's Hospital of Michigan
Detroit, MI 48201
Phone: (313) 833-4490

Karin M. Muraszko, MD
University of Michigan
Ann Arbor, MI 48109-0338
Phone: (734) 936-5016

**Mark Watts, MD**
Henry Ford Hospital
Detroit, MI 48202
Phone: (313) 916-3528

## MINNESOTA

**Michael McCue, MD**
**Mahmoud G. Nagib, MD**
Minneapolis, MN 55407-3799
Phone: (612) 871-7278

**Michael D. Partington, MD**
Neurosurgery Associates
St. Paul, MN 55102-2481
Phone: (651) 227-7088

**Corey Raffel, MD**
Mayo Clinic
Rochester, MN 55905
Phone: (507) 284-8167

## MISSOURI

**David F. Jimenez, MD**
Univ. Of Missouri Hospital & Clinic
Columbia, MO 65212
Phone: (573) 882-4908

**Jeffrey G. Ojemann, MD**
**T. S. Park, MD**
St. Louis Children's Hospital
St. Louis, MO 63110
Phone: (314) 454-2810

## MISSISSIPPI

**Andrew D. Parent, MD**
Univ. of Mississippi Medical Center
Jackson, MS 29216
Phone: (601) 984-5703

## NORTH CAROLINA

**William O. Bell, MD**
Carolina Neurosurgical Associates
Winston-Salem, NC 27103
Phone: (336) 768-1811

**Herbert E. Fuchs, MD, Ph.D.**
**Timothy George MD**
Duke Medical Center
Durham, NC 27710
Phone: (919) 684-5013

**C. Scott McLanahan, MD**
Carolinas Medical Center
Charlotte, NC 28207
Phone: (704) 376-1605

## NEBRASKA

**Leslie C. Hellbusch, MD**
University of Nebraska
Omaha, NE 68114
Phone: (402) 398-9243

## NEW JERSEY

**Arno H. Fried, MD**
Hackensack University Medical Center
Hackensack, NJ 07601
Phone: (201) 996-5251

**Gary Magram, MD**
N.J. Neuroscience Institute
Edison, NJ 08818
Phone: (732) 321-7950

## NEW YORK

**Rick Abbott, MD**
**Fred J. Epstein, MD**
**George Jallo, MD**
**Karl Kothbauer, MD**
Beth Israel North Medical Center
New York, NY 10128
Phone: (212) 870-9600

**Michael R. Egnor, MD**
Stony Brook University
Stony Brook, NY 11794
Phone: (631) 444-1210

**Neil A. Feldstein, MD**
Babies and Children's Hospital of New York
New York, NY 10032
Phone: (212) 305-1396

**James Goodrich, MD**
Montefiore Medical Center
The Bronx, NY 10467
Phone: (718) 920-4197

**Veetai Li, MD**
Children's Hospital of Buffalo
Buffalo, NY 14222
Phone: (716) 878-7386

**John Miller, MD**
Rego Park, NY 11374
Phone: (718) 459-7700

**Steven J. Schneider, MD**
Long Island Neuro. Associates
New Hyde Park, NY 11042
Phone: (516) 354-3401

**John B. Waldman, MD**
Albany Medical College
Albany, NY 12208
Phone: (518) 262-5088

**Jeffrey H. Wisoff, MD**
New York University Medical Center
New York, NY 10016
Phone: (212) 263-6419

## OHIO

**Alan R. Cohen, MD**
**Shenandoah Robinson, MD**
Rainbow Babies and Children's Hospital
Cleveland, OH 44106
Phone: (216) 844-5741

**Kerry R. Crone, MD**
Children's Hospital Medical Center
Cincinnati, OH 45229-3039
Phone: (513) 636-4726

**Edward J. Kosnik, MD**
Neurological Associates
Columbus, OH 43221
Phone: (614) 457-4880

## PENNSYLVANIA

**P. David Adelson, MD**
**A. Leland Albright, MD**
**Ian F. Pollack, MD**
Children's Hospital of Pittsburgh
Pittsburgh, PA 15213
Phone: (412) 692-8142

**Karin S. Bierbrauer, MD**
**Joseph H. Piatt, Jr., MD**
St Christopher's Hospital for Children
Philadelphia, PA 19134-1095
Phone: (215) 707-7200

**Mark S. Dias, MD**
**Paul M. Kanev, MD**
Hershey Medical Center
Hershey, PA 17033
Phone: (717) 531-8807

**Leslie N. Sutton, MD**
Children's Hospital of Philadelphia
Philadelphia, PA 19104
Phone: (215) 590-2780

## SOUTH CAROLINA

**Lenwood Smith, Jr., MD**
Columbia, SC 29203-6873
Phone: (803) 434-8323

## TENNESSEE

Frederick A. Boop, MD
Stephanie Einhaus, MD
Michael S. Mulbauer, MD
R. Alexander Sanford, MD
Simms-Murphy Clinic
Memphis, TN 38103
Phone: (901) 522-7762

Noel Tulipan, MD
Vanderbilt University
Nashville, TN 37221
Phone: (615) 322-6875

## TEXAS

Patricia Anne Aronin, MD
Children's Hospital of Austin
Austin, TX 78756
Phone: (512) 479-3843

Derek A. Bruce, MD
Kenneth N. Shapiro, MD
Frederick H. Sklar, MD
Center for Pediatric Neurosurgery
Dallas, TX 75235
Phone: (214) 456-6660

Michael J. Burke, MD
Neurosurgery Institute of South Texas
Corpus Christi, TX 78411
Phone: (361) 561-1387

Robert C. Dauser, MD
John P. Laurent, MD
Texas Children's Hospital
Houston, TX 77030
Phone: (832) 824-3950

David J. Donahue, MD
S.W. Neurosurgery Assoc.
Fort Worth, TX 76104
Phone: (817) 336-1300

Sarah J. Gaskill, MD
Arthur E. Marlin, MD
Pediatric Neurosurgery of South Texas
San Antonio, TX 78229
Phone: (210) 615-1218

Ronald J. Wilson, MD
Austin, TX 78746
Phone: (512) 306-1323

## UTAH

Douglas L. Brockmeyer, MD
John R. Kestle, MD
Marion L. Walker, MD
Primary Children's Medical Center
Salt Lake City, UT 84113-1100
Phone: (801) 588-3400

## VIRGINIA

John D. Ward, MD
Medical College of Virginia
Richmond, VA 23298-0631
Phone: (804) 828-9165

## WASHINGTON

Richard G. Ellenbogen, MD
Saddi Ghatan, MD
John Loeser, MD
Children's Hospital
Seattle, WA 98105
Phone: (206) 526-2544

## WISCONSIN

Bruce A. Kaufman, MD
Cheryl A. Muszynski, MD
Children's Hospital of Wisconsin
Milwaukee, WI 53201
Phone: (414) 266-6435

# CANADA

**Keith E. Aronyk, MD**
Edmonton, Alberta, T6G 2B7 Canada
Phone: (780) 407-6870

**D. D. Cochrane, MD**
**Paul Steinbok, MD**
British Columbia Children's Hospital
Vancouver, BC, V6H 3V4 Canada
Phone: (604) 875-2094

**James M. Drake, MD**
**Robin P. Humphreys, MD**
**James T. Rutka, MD**
The Hospital for Sick Children
Toronto, ON, M5G 1X8 Canada
Phone: (416) 813-6125

**Jean-Pierre Farmer, MD**
**Jose L. Montes, MD**
The Montreal Children's Hospital
Montreal, Quebec, H3H 1P3 Canada
Phone: (514) 412-4400

**Enrique C. G. Ventureyra, MD**
Children's Hospital of Eastern Ontario
Ottawa, ON, K1H 8L1 Canada
Phone: (613) 737-2316

# Index

## A

## B

Baby talk, 275

Backpacks for school, 400

Back pain
    spinal cord tumors, 29
    as symptom, 2

Bactrim, 77, 267

Bag Balm, 271–272

Balanced diet, 345–347

Baldness. *See* Hair loss

Balloons, 82–83
    hospital policies, 97

Bancroft NeuroHealth, 501

Barrington, Judith, 477

Basic soap, 279–280

Bathing/showering with catheters, 178

BCNU, 219–220
    lung infections, 267

Bed wetting, 275–276

Behavioral changes
    of children, 308–314
    of parents, 314–320
    in siblings, 327
    as symptom, 2

Benadryl, 245
    for platelet transfusions, 71

Benign tumors, 34, 35
    debulking procedures, 143
    time issues, 449

Bereavement, 471–472

Beta HCG marker, 40

BiCNU, 219–220

Biofeedback, 253
    and procedures, 53

Biologic modifiers, 46

Biopsies, 142–143
    bone marrow aspiration/biopsy, 61
    needle aspiration biopsy, 70

Birth control, 439

Birthdays, 475–476

Bis-chloronitrosurea, 219–220

Bladder control
    postoperative complications, 155
    as relapse symptom, 446
    spinal cord tumors, 29
    as symptom, 2

Blaming by siblings, 328–329

Bleeding, bone marrow transplants and, 296–297

Blended families, 117–118

Blenoxane, *See* Bleomycin

Bleomycin, 217–218
    lung infections, 267

Blindness. *See* Vision

BLM. *See* Bleomycin

Blood chemistries, 59

Blood counts. *See also* Low blood counts;
                Recordkeeping
    charts, 363
    complete blood cell counts (CBCx), 59
    meanings of, 483–489
    red blood cell count (RBC), 486
    white blood cells count (WBC), 263, 486

Blood cultures, 59

Blood donations, 98

Blood draws, 59–60

Blood patch, 73

Blood transfusions, 60–61

Blood urea nitrogen (BUN), 487

BMT Infonet, 288, 499

Board certified doctors, 123

Body surface area (BSA), 215

Bone growth x-rays, 61

Bone marrow aspiration/biopsy, 61

Bone marrow registry, joining, 99

Bone marrow transplants, 44, 283, 284–285
    allogenic transplants, 288
    appetite loss, 298
    bleeding, 296–297
    complications of, 292–293
    conditioning regimens, 291–292
    costs of, 290–291
    emotional responses to, 293–294
    external catheters for, 178
    facility, choosing a, 288–290
    financial assistance for, 291
    growth problems, 299
    hemorrhagic cystitis, 297
    infection complications, 294–296
    long term side effects, 299–300
    mouth sores, 277
    mucositis, 297
    necessity for, 283–284
    neurological complications, 298
    organizational resources, 499
    procedure for, 291–293
    puberty/sterility problems, 299–300
    pulmonary edema, 298
    questions to ask, 283
    recovery times, 285
    recurrence after, 299
    secondary cancers after, 300
    thyroid function and, 299
    tooth development and, 299
    venoocclusive disease (VOD), 296

Bone scans, 62

Books
    as resources, 504–515
    for siblings, 331

Cereals, servings of, 346
Cerebellar mutism, 157–158
Cerebellum, 20–21
Cerebral fissure, 15
Cerebrospinal fluid, 20, 26
Cerebrum, 15–20
    frontal lobes, 16–17
    lobes of, 16
    occipital lobes, 20
    parietal lobes, 18–20
    symptoms of tumors in, 16
    temporal lobes, 18
Ceremonies. *See also* Funerals
    at end of treatment, 431
Chai Lifeline/Camp Simcha, 498
Chaplains. *See* Clergy
Charge nurses, 124
Charitable donations in name of child, 468
The Charles A. Dana Foundation, 492–493
Chat rooms, 383
Chemical modifiers, 195
Chemo Angels, 332
Chemotherapy, 43–44, 213. *See also* Bone marrow
        transplants; Nutrition
    adjunctive treatments, 253
    anemia from, 60
    for astrocytomas, fast-growing, 38
    bed wetting during, 275–276
    blood count values, 484
    chicken pox during, 268
    clinical trial information, 479
    colony-stimulating factors, 243–244
    current research, learning about, 385
    debulking prior to, 143
    dosages, 215
    effectiveness of, 213–214
    free medicine programs, 375–376
    giving drugs, 214
    guidelines for calling doctor, 216
    list of drugs, 217–243
    for medulloblastoma, 36
    myelosuppressive high-dose chemotherapy, 287
    neuropsychological testing after, 414–415
    platelet transfusions and, 70
    pulmonary function tests, 71
    questions to ask, 216
    spinal taps and, 72
    urine specimens for, 79
    vitamin supplements and, 347–348
    window study, 43
Chest x-rays, 63
Chicken pox, 216
    bone marrow transplants and, 296
    low blood counts and, 267–268
    school, avoidance at, 401

Childhood Brain Tumor Foundation, 492
Childhood Cancer Ombudsman Program, 291
    contact information, 492
    employment issues, 442
    insurance claim denials, challenging, 373
    for relapses, 449
*Childhood Cancer Survivors: A Practical Guide to the*
        *Future* (Keene, Hobbie & Ruccione),
        208, 435, 438
Child life therapists, 48, 81
    surgery, preparation for, 152
Children's Brain Tumor Foundation, 492
Children's Cancer Group (CCG), 164
Children's Hopes and Dreams Foundation, 498
Children's Hospice International, 461
    contact information, 503
Children's Inn, 381
Children's Oncology Group
    chemical modifiers, studies of, 195
Children's Oncology Group (COG), 41, 127, 164
Children's Special Health Care Services (CSHCS)
        (Michigan), 376
Chloral hydrate for MRIs, 68
Choroid plexus carcinomas, 40–41
Choroid plexus papillomas, 40–41
Choroid plexus tumors, 35, 40–41
Christmas stockings, 474
Churches. *See* Religious community
Cigarette smoking, risks of, 438
Cisplatin, 43, 221–223, 449
    hearing loss from, 58, 437
Citrotein, 356
Citrucel, 272
Civil Rights Division, Justice Department, 441–442
Classmates
    help from, 106–107
    involvement of, 396
    of terminally ill children, 423–424
Claustrophobia, MRIs and, 69
Clear fluids, serving, 348
Clergy
    counseling by, 389
    support from, 386–387
Clinical nurse managers, 124
Clinical nurse specialists, 124
Clinical trials, 151–172
    designers of, 164
    entire documentation, parents receiving, 169–170
    finding out about, 46
    information from, 478–480
    informed consent to, 166–167
    Institutional Review Board (IRB), 165
    Phase II studies, 162, 163–164
    pros and cons of, 171–172

# D

Dacarbazine, 225–226
Dairy products
    intolerance, 344
    nutrition in, 346
Dana Press, 493
Dance classes, 407–408
Deafness. *See* Hearing/hearing loss
Death of child, 454–477
    active treatment, transition from, 454–459
    anniversary of, 468
    classmates and, 424
    communicating with child, 455–457
    family and friends, role of, 466–474
    at home, 462–464
    hospice care, 459–461
    in hospital, 461–642
    organizations helping with, 503
    school for terminally ill children, 423–424
    siblings understanding, 327
    talking to children, 312–313
Debulking, 143–144
    for non-germinoma tumors, 40
Decadron. *See* Dexamethasone
Dehydration
    diarrhea and, 271
    nausea and, 261
Demerol, 249–250
Denial, 6
    by parents, 314–315
    with terminally ill child, 456–457
Dental care. *See also* Tooth development
    chemotherapy and, 276–277
    low blood counts and, 277
Depression
    adolescents and, 305
    of parents, 315
    withdrawal and, 310–311
Depth EEG, 65–66
Depth perception, 18
Designated Disabled Program (DDP) (Canada), 413
Desitin, 271–272
Destructive children, 310
Detachol, 178, 185, 186
Dexamethasone, 234–235, 245
    appetite changes, 343
    for hydrocephalus, 148
    lung infections, 267
    side effects, 205, 281
    taste of, 76
    temper tantrums and, 321
Diabetes insipidus, 25
Diagnosis, 326–327

Diamond, Marian C., 26
Diarrhea
    with chemotherapy, 216, 270–272
    with irinotecan, 231
    lactose intolerance, 344
    from topotecan, 241
Diencephalon, 24–25
Diet. *See* Nutrition
*Diet and Nutrition Eating Hints* booklets, 344
Digital thermometers, 78
Dilantin
    calcium supplements and, 344
    with irinotecan, 231
Dilaudid, 250–251
Diphenhydramine, 245
    with prochlorperazine, 247
Directory of Pharmaceutical Patient Assistance, 375
Discipline
    household rules, application of, 316–317
    improving, 320–324
    overindulgence of child, 317
Dishonesty of parents, 314–315
Distraction from procedures, 53
Diuretics, 343
Dizziness
    cerebellum tumors, 20–21
    as relapse symptom, 445
    as symptom, 1
DNA, 213
DNR (Do Not Resuscitate) orders, 461–462
Dogs, 269
Dolophine, 251
Dominance of brain, 16
Donations in name of child, 468
Dosages for chemotherapy, 215
Double lumen access, 178
Double vision, 2
    intracranial pressure and, 28
    as postoperative complication, 157
Drain for hydrocephalus, 147
Dressings
    changes, 159
    for PICC lines, 184
    on subcutaneous ports, 181–182
Drowsiness
    intracranial pressure and, 28
    as relapse symptom, 446
    somnolence syndrome, 207
    as symptom, 2
Droxia, 227–228
Drug abuse, 319
DTIC-Dome, 225–226
Ducosate, 272
Dull affect, 18

# E

Early intervention services, 402–403
Earobics, 425
Easter Seals programs, 408, 502
Easter Seals Society, Ontario, 502
Easter Seals Society, USA, 502
Easy Listener, 425
Echinacea, 255
Echocardiogram/EKG, 64
Education. *See* School
Education for all Handicapped Children Act, 412
Elected representatives and insurance issues, 373
Electroencephalogram/EEG, 64–66
Electromagnetic radiation, 34
Electromyogram/EMG, 66
Electronic mailing list services, 383
Elks Club, 376
Embarrassment, parents feeling, 11
Embryonal CNS tumors, 283
EMLA cream, 54, 250
   for bone marrow aspiration/biopsy, 61
   for finger pokes, 66–67
   for gallium scans, 67
   for IVs, 73–74
   for spinal taps, 72
   for subcutaneous injections, 75
   for subcutaneous port access, 181
Emotional responses, 5, 304–306
   to bone marrow transplants, 293–294
   comfort objects, 311–312
   to end of treatment, 427–429
   late effects and, 437
   regression, 311
   to relapse, 447–448
   of siblings, 327–333
   withdrawal, 310–311
Employment Insurance Act, Canada, 114
Employment issues, 441–442
Encephalitis, 267
Endocrine function, 210
Endocrinologists, 122
End of treatment, 427–444
   catheter removal, 430
   ceremonies at, 431
   emotional issues, 427–429
   last day, 429
   normal, returning to, 432–434
Enemas, 254
Ensure products, 356, 357, 359
Enteral access, 150
Enteral nutrition, 358–359
Environmental factors, 34
Enzymes, chemotherapy with, 214

Ependymomas, 24, 35, 39–40
   internal radiation for, 194
   posterior fossa syndrome, 157–158
   radiation therapy for, 195, 200
   spinal taps for monitoring, 72
Epilepsy Foundation of America, 282, 493
Epogen, 243–244
Equal Employment Opportunity Commission
   (EEOC), 441
ERISA (Employment Retirement and Income Security
   Act), 443–444
Erthropoietin, 243–244
Estrogen, 300
Ethyl chloride
   spray, 54
   for subcutaneous port access, 181
Etopophos, 43, 226–227, 449
Etoposide, 43, 226–227, 449
Exercise in hospitals, 91
Expectations, 323
Experimental treatments. *See also* Clinical trials
   with radiation, 195
Explanation of benefits (EOBs), 368
Extended family, 95–99
   keeping in touch, 96–97
   suggestions for, 97–99
External catheters
   blockages, 176
   breakage, 177
   clamps for, 177
   costs of, 187–188
   Dacron cuff on, 174
   daily care of, 174–175
   infections from, 175–176
   kinks in, 176–177
   liquid adhesive removers for tape, 178
   risks of, 175–177
External radiation, 191–193
   description of treatment, 203–204
Eye movement, 2
   brainstem tumors, 22
   cranial nerves controlling, 22
   posterior fossa tumors, 20

# F

Facial drooping, 2
   brainstem tumors, 22
   cranial nerves controlling, 22
   posterior fossa tumors, 20
   as postoperative complication, 157
   as relapse symptom, 446
Family. *See also* Extended family; Siblings
   anger at, 9–10
   billing problems, dealing with, 368

## K

Kaopectate, 270
Keene, Nancy, 435
Ketamine, 55
Kimo Bear Project, 180
Kinks
    in external catheters, 176–177
    in subcutaneous ports, 183
Kiwanis Club, 376
Knights of Columbus, 376
Kytril, 245, 262

## L

Lactose intolerance, 344
Lash and Associates Publishing/Training, 502
*The Last Day of April* (Roach), 8
Last day of treatment, 429
Late effects
    educational issues, 436
    physical disabilities, 436
    types of, 435–437
Laundry, hospital stays and, 84
LCSW (Licensed Clinical Social Worker), 389
Learning disabilities. *See* Cognitive problems
Least restrictive environment (LRE), 412
Leave-sharing, 104–105
Left cerebral hemisphere of brain, 15
Leg pain, spinal cord tumors, 29
Leucovorin, 233
Leukapheresis, 286
Leukemia, 34, 287
Lidocaine
    for bone marrow aspiration/biopsy, 61
    in EMLA cream, 250
    in Numby Stuff, 252
    in procedures, 54
Life-threatening emergencies, 196
Light sensitivity, 18
Lions Club, 376
Lip glosses, 280
Liquid adhesive removers, 178
Liquid medicines, 77
Listening to children, 307
*Little Women,* 456
Liver, bone marrow transplants and, 296
LMFCC (Licensed Marriage and Family Child Counselor), 389
LMFT (Licensed Marriage and Family Therapist), 389
Lomotil, 270
Lomustine, 43, 231–232
    lung infections, 267
Lorazepam, 246
Loss of appetite. *See* Appetite changes

Loss of control, 10
Low blood counts, 263–270
    dental care and, 277
    pneumonia, 266–267
LPC (Licensed Professional Counselor), 389
LPNs (licensed practical nurses), 124
LSW (Licensed Social Worker), 389
Lumbar puncture. *See* Spinal taps
Luteinizing hormone, 209
Lyons, Christine, 466

## M

McDonnall, Sara, 334–335
Magnesium citrate, 272
Magnetic resonance imaging. *See* MRIs
Make-A-Wish Foundation of America, 500
*Making Contact* booklet, 385
Making Headway Foundation, 493
Malignant tumors, 34, 35
Mannitol
    with carboplatin, 220–221
    with cisplatin, 222
Marijuana smoking, risks of, 438
Marriage
    coping styles in, 115–116
    counseling, 388–392
    pressures on, 114–117
Masks in radiation therapy, 198–199
Masons, 376
Massage, 253
    and procedures, 53
Mathematics problems, 410, 436
Matulane, 236–237
Maximal surgical resection, 144–146
Maximum tolerated doses (MTDs), 162, 163
The May Center for Education and
        Neurorehabilitation, 502
Mealtimes, suggestions for, 349
Measles
    exposure to, 216
    school and, 401
Meat/meat substitutes, 346
Medicaid, 375
    fund raising and, 377
Medical charts, parents reading, 131
Medical records
    blood count charts, 363
    calendar system, 362–363
    computers for maintaining, 364
    information needed in, 360–361
    journals for, 361–362
    tape recorders for, 363–364
Medical students, 123

Medical supplies, 444
Medical team, 120
    anger at, 9
    appreciation for, 133–134
    changing doctors, 138–139
    communication with, 129–134
    conferences with, 133
    conflict resolution, 136–138
    cooperation with, 130–131
    hierarchy of doctors, 123–124
    in hospital, 121–125
    multidisciplinary team, 4, 121–122
    relationships with, 128–129
    second opinions, 134–135
    sensitivity and, 136
    siblings, educating, 326
    surgeons, locating, 125–127
Medications. *See also* specific medications
    Canada, assistance programs in, 375–376
    for emotional difficulties, 323
    errors, checking for, 90
    experimental drugs, 163–164
    free medicine programs, 375–376
    hospitalizations and, 87–88
    insurance covering, 370
    recognition of problems from, 321
    school performance and, 399
Medi-port, 173
Meditation, 253
    for nausea, 261
Medline, 385, 504
Medulla, 22
Medulloblastomas, 21, 34, 108, 148
    autologous stem cell rescue and, 283
    death, talking about, 312–313
    description of, 35–37
    high-risk tumors, 36–37
    posterior fossa syndrome, 157–158
    radiation therapy, 195
        side effects, 207
    speech problems, 83
    spinal taps for monitoring, 72
    standard-risk/high-risk tumors, 36–37
Megase, 205
Melmark, 502
Memorial services, 464–466
Memory problems
    cerebrum tumors, symptoms of, 16
    diencephalon tumors, 24
    intracranial pressure and, 28
    parietal lobe tumors, 19
    postoperative complications, 156
    relapse and, 447
    temporal lobe tumors, 18

Meninges, 26
Meningitis, aseptic, 156
Meperidine, 249–250
Mesna
    with cyclophosphamide, 223
    hemorrhagic cystitis and, 297
Metamucil, 272
Methadone, 251
Methotrex. *See* Methotrexate
Methotrexate, 232–233
    folic acid with, 254
    sun sensitivity, 265
Midbrain, 21
Milk of magnesia, 272
Milk products. *See* Dairy products
Ministers. *See* Clergy
Mini transplants, 283–284
Miralex, 272
*The Misunderstood Child* (Silver), 310
Mixed gliomas, 37
Moi-Stir, 206
Monaco, Grace Powers, 434
Moodie, Amanda, 333–334
Mood swings, 281
Moon face, 343
More children, decision for, 117
Morphine, 54, 251–252
Motor area, 17
Mouth/throat sores, 277–279
    glutamine for, 278
    as radiation side effect, 206
    rinses for, 278
MRIs, 3–4, 68–69, 478
    biopsies with, 143
    with computer-guided surgery, 147
    with depth EEG, 65
    nitrous oxide and, 56
    observation with, 45
MTX. *See* Methotrexate
Mucositis, 297
MUGA scans, 69–70
Multidisciplinary second opinions, 135
Multidisciplinary teams, 4, 121–122
Multi-lumen subcutaneous ports, 180
Multiple-gated acquisition (MUGA) scans, 69–70
Music in hospital rooms, 83
Myeloablative chemotherapy, 287
Myelosuppressive high-dose chemotherapy, 287
Myleran, 218–219
Myoplex Lite, 356

# N

Nail problems and chemotherapy, 279–280
Nasogastric tubes, 150, 343
   for enteral nutrition, 358–359
   post-surgical, 155
National Association for Parents of Children with Visual Impairments, 494
The National Brain Tumor Foundation, 494
National Cancer Institute (NCI)
   clinical trials, information on, 162
   contact information, 494
   designing clinical trials, 164
   *Diet and Nutrition Eating Hints* booklets, 344
   hospitals, choosing, 127
National Center for Complementary and Alternative Medicine, 494
National Center for Learning Disabilities, 495
National Childhood Cancer Foundation, 495
National Children's Cancer Society, 498
National Coalition for Cancer Survivorship (NCCS), 134, 495
National Disability Sports Alliance, 502
National Hydrocephalus Foundation, 495
National Information Center for Children and Youth with Disabilities, 495
National Institutes of Health, National Center for Complementary and Alternative Medicine, 254
National Neurofibromatosis Foundation, 496
National Organization for Social Security Claimants' Representatives (NOSSCR), 375
National Patient Air Transport Hotline, 500
National Spinal Cord Injury Association, 496
The National Transplant Assistance Fund, 499
National Wilms Tumor Study Group (NWTSG), 164
Natulanar, 236–237
Nausea. *See also* Antinausea drugs; Vomiting
   acupuncture for, 261–262
   from chemotherapy, 260–262
   as radiation side effect, 206
   as relapse symptom, 446
   Relief Band, 262
   as symptom, 2
Neck
   cranial nerves controlling, 22
   symptom, pain as, 2
Needle aspiration biopsy, 70
Nembutol for MRIs, 68
Nestle NuBasic, 280, 359
Neumega, 244
Neupogen, 75, 286, 295, 298
Neuroblastoma, 287
Neurofibromatosis (NF1), 38, 426
   learning disabilities and, 208
   National Neurofibromatosis Foundation, 496

Neurological complications. *See also* Cognitive problems
   bone marrow/stem cell transplants, 298
   late effects, 409
Neuro-oncologists, 125
   second opinions sought by, 135
Neuropsychological testing, 70
   insurance coverage of, 370
Neuropsychologists/psychologists, 122
*Neuroscience for Kids* Web site, 26
New treatments, information on, 46
Nightmares
   adolescents and, 305
   as late effects, 437
   from prednisone, 275
Nitrous oxide, 56
N-methylhydrazine, 236–237
NMRS scans, 145
NO CODE orders, 461
Noise and temporal lobe tumors, 18
Nolte, Dorothy, 325
Non-germinoma germ cell tumors, 40
Normalcy
   maintaining, 322–323
   returning to, 432–434
North American Brain Tumor Coalition, 386
North American Riding for the Handicapped Association (NARHA), 502
Notebooks for parents, 362
Notes on death of child, 468
Notice of Parents Rights, 412–413
Numbness of parents, 5–6
Numby Stuff, 54, 252
   for IVs, 73–74
Nurse practitioners, 4, 124
   surgery, preparation for, 152
Nurses
   hospital nurses, 124
   primary nurses, 130
   school class, talking to, 396
Nutrashake, 356–357
Nutrition, 254. *See also* Appetite changes
   advice from parents, 354–355
   balanced diet, 345–347
   calories, guidelines for boosting, 350–351
   commercial supplements, 356–357
   diarrhea, diet for, 271
   empty calories, 349
   enteral nutrition, 358–359
   food aversions, 280
   food obsessions, 343
   hospitalizations and, 84–85
   hospital nutritionist, consulting with, 352–353
   lactose intolerance, 344
   and nausea, 261

3D conformal radiation therapy, 192
Throat sores. *See* Mouth/throat sores
Thrombocytopenia, 286–287
Thumb sucking, 275
Thyroid function
    bone marrow transplants and, 299
    spinal radiation and, 209
    stem cell transplants and, 299
Thyroid hormone replacement, 436–437
Thyroid stimulating hormone (TSH), 209
Ticks, 269
Timberdoodle, 422
Time, sense of, 18
Tonic clonic seizures, 282
Tooth development
    bone marrow/stem cell transplants and, 299
    radiation therapy and, 210–211, 277
Toporek, Chuck, 148
Toposor, 43, 226–227, 449
Topotecan, 240–241
Torticollis
    as relapse symptom, 446
    as symptom, 2
Total parenteral nutrition (TPN), 357–358
TPN (total parenteral nutrition), 357–358
Tracheostomy, 157
Training hospitals, 131
Transplant centers, 288–290
    questions to ask, 289
Traumatic Brain Injury (TBI), defined, 416–417
Treatments, 41–46. *See also* End of treatment;
              Procedures; Stem; specific types
    advances in, 478
    for benign tumors, 35
    biologic modifiers, 46
    keeping track of, 132
    for malignant tumors, 35
    for medulloblastoma, 36
    new treatments, information on, 46
    observation, 45
    on relapse, 448–451
    standard treatment, defined, 151–162
    terminally ill children, 454–459
Trimethoprim, 77
Trimethoprim-sulfamethoxazole, 267
Trophies at end of treatment, 431
Trust
    in children, 313
    in family, 306–307
Tube feeding. *See* Nasogastric tubes
Tube feedings. *See* Gastronomy tubes, Intravenous
              nutrition
Tuberous sclerosis, 33

Tucker, Kathy, 12–14
Tumor board, 125
Tumor cells, 213–214
Tumor markers, 40
Tumor vaccine research, 46
Turcot syndrome, 33
Turkeys, 270
Turtles as pets, 269
Tympanic thermometers, 78

## U

Ulcer medications, 298
Ultrasonography, 147
United Way, 376
Urinary catheterization, 79
Urine
    chemotherapy, urinating after, 261
    collections, 79
    specimens, 79
Urokinase for external catheter clots, 176

## V

Valium, 54
Valsalva maneuver, 177
Vancomycin, 183
Varicella zoster, 267, 268
    from bone marrow transplants, 295
Varicella Zoster Immune Globulin (VZIG) injection,
            268, 401
Vascular access, 150
VCRs, 242–243
    in hospital rooms, 84
Velban, 241
Venoocclusive disease (VOD), 296
Venous catheters. *See* Central venous catheters
Ventilators, 151
Ventricular system, 26–28
Ventriculostomy for hydrocephalus, 147
VePesid, 43, 226–227, 449
Versed, 54, 55
    for MRIs, 68
Veterans of Foreign Wars, 376
Videos
    EEGs, videotaped, 65
    for siblings, 331
    for surgery preparation, 158
Vinblastine, 241
Vincristine, 43, 242–243, 449
    EMLA cream with, 74
Visceral nervous system, 30

# About the Authors

**Tania Shiminski-Maher** received her BSN and MS in pediatric primary care from Columbia University. She is certified as a pediatric nurse practitioner, clinical neuroscience registered nurse, and pediatric oncology nurse. She has worked as a pediatric nurse practitioner in pediatric neurosurgery and pediatric neuro-oncology for the past fifteen years. She has published extensively in the area of pediatric brain tumors, hydrocephalus, and multidisciplinary team communication. She has been a member of the nursing committee of the Children's Cancer Group for the past fifteen years and a member of the nursing steering committee for ten years. She holds academic appointments to the faculty of New York University School of Nursing and Hunter-Bellevue School of Nursing.

**Patsy Cullen** received her BSN in nursing from the University of California, her MS from the University of Kansas, and her pediatric nurse practitioner training from the University of Colorado. She has worked as a pediatric nurse practitioner in pediatric oncology for more than 20 years and is currently a member of the staff of Childhood Hematology-Oncology Associates and the Rocky Mountain Children's Cancer Center in Denver, Colorado. She has published extensively in the areas of general pediatric oncology, radiation oncology, and neuro-oncology. She has been a member of the Children's Cancer Group for twenty years, has served on the Nursing Discipline committee as Vice-Chair, and now chairs the clinical trials subcommittee. Additionally, Patsy is now a principal investigator in the Children's Oncology Group, administratively heading the program at Presbyterian–St. Luke's Medical Center, and was recently elected to serve on the group's nominating committee. She has held nursing appointments on many national pediatric CNS tumor trials and is currently on the CNS Tumor Steering Committee for the Children's Oncology Group.

**Maria Sansalone** has a Bachelor's in English from American International College and an Associate's in Science degree. She has worked in the past in hospital settings in the area of health information management, and for the last ten years as a Cross Reference editor for Merriam-Webster, Inc., the dictionary and reference publishers. Her position allows her access to information from almost every field. But nothing, she says, prepared her for her son's diagnosis of an optic glioma. "It was a completely shocking and shattering experience, and it's taken many years to find a balance. Listening to families relate their own experiences for this book was immensely influential. I think it helped to bring things back full circle."

# Colophon

Patient-Centered Guides are about the experience of illness. They contain personal stories as well as a combination of practical and medical information.

The cover of *Childhood Brain & Spinal Cord Tumors* was designed by Kristen Throop of Combustion Creative. The warm colors and quilt-like patterns are intended to convey a sense of comfort. The use of repetitive patterning was inspired by tile work seen by the designer on a trip to Turkey. The layout was created on a Macintosh using Quark 4.0. Fonts in the design are: Berkeley, Coronet, GillSans, Minion Ornaments, Throhand, and Univers Ultra Condensed. The design was built with tints of three PMS colors.

Rad Proctor designed the interior layout for the book based on a series design by Nancy Priest and Edie Freedman. The interior fonts are Berkeley and Franklin Gothic. The text was prepared using FrameMaker.

The book was copyedited by Paulette Miley and proofread by Marianne Rogoff. Tom Dorsaneo, Marianne Rogoff, and Katherine Stimson conducted quality assurance checks. Katherine Stimson wrote the index. The illustrations that appear in this book were produced by Rob Romano. Interior composition was done by Rad Proctor and Tom Dorsaneo.